CHILDREN AND YOUTH
ASSISTED BY MEDICAL TECHNOLOGY
IN EDUCATIONAL SETTINGS

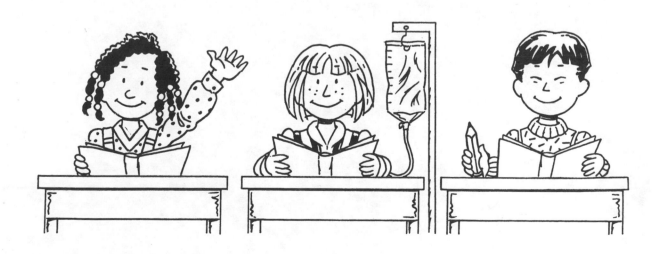

"This manual has been reviewed by representatives of the National Association of School Nurses, who have found these materials appropriate for use by school nurses in their practice."

National Association of School Nurses, Inc.

CHILDREN AND YOUTH ASSISTED BY MEDICAL TECHNOLOGY IN EDUCATIONAL SETTINGS

Guidelines for Care

Second Edition

edited by

Stephanie Porter, M.S.N., R.N.

Marilynn Haynie, M.D.

Timaree Bierle, B.S.N., R.N.

Terry Heintz Caldwell, Ed.D.

and

Judith S. Palfrey, M.D.

Project School Care
Children's Hospital
Boston

Illustrations by Marcia Williams

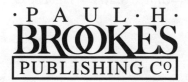

·P·A·U·L·H·
BROOKES
PUBLISHING C♀

Baltimore • London • Toronto • Sydney

Paul H. Brookes Publishing Co.
Post Office Box 10624
Baltimore, Maryland 21285-0624

www.brookespublishing.com

Typeset by Signature Typesetting & Design, Baltimore, Maryland.
Manufactured in the United States of America by
Versa Press, Inc., East Peoria, Illinois.

Second printing, January 1999.

Project School Care and the preparation of this volume were supported by grant nos. G0086C3511-88, G0086C3511-88A, MCJ259150, and MCH928 from the Bureau of Maternal and Child Health and Resources Development of the U.S. Department of Health and Human Services, the National Institute on Disability and Rehabilitation Research of the U.S. Department of Education, and the Dyson Foundation of New York. However, the contents of this publication do not necessarily represent the policy of these agencies and readers should not assume endorsement by the federal government.

The suggestions in this book are not intended as a substitute for professional medical consultation. The authors and publishers disclaim any liability arising directly or indirectly from the use of this book.

Permission to reprint the following materials is gratefully acknowledged:

Page 31: The Family's Role in Ensuring the Rights of Their Child excerpt from Anderson, B., & Vohs, J. (1992). Another look at Section 504. *Coalition Quarterly*, 10(1), 4; reprinted by permission.

Page 56: Excerpt from Ferrera, A. (1995). Sometimes I feel like I've always been there for her, and she's always been there for me. *The Inside Edition*, 3(2), 8; reprinted by permission.

The case studies in this book are true stories and are printed in this book by permission of the students and/or their families.

Users of this book are granted permission to photocopy the Individualized Health Care Plans forms provided in Chapter 6 and the Skills Checklists provided in Section II in the course of their service provision to students and their families.

Library of Congress Cataloging-in-Publication Data

Children and youth assisted by medical technology in educational settings : guidelines for care / edited by Stephanie Porter ... [et al.].—2nd ed.
   p. cm.
  Includes bibliographical references and index.
  ISBN 1-55766-236-3
  1. School health services—United States—Handbooks, manuals, etc. 2. Medical technology—United States—Handbooks, manuals, etc. 3. School children—Health and hygiene—United States—Handbooks, manuals, etc. I. Porter, Stephanie.
LB3409.U5C47   1997
371.7'12—dc20   96-46463
                                                      CIP

British Library Cataloguing in Publication data are available from the British Library.

CONTENTS

SECTION II   **Guidelines for Care**

Skills Checklists

CONTRIBUTORS

The Editors

Stephanie Porter, M.S.N., R.N.
Director of Nursing
Institute for Community Inclusion
University Affiliated Program
Program Coordinator
Project School Care
Children's Hospital
300 Longwood Avenue
Boston, Massachusetts 02115

Marilynn Haynie, M.D.
Director
Coordinated Care Service
Project School Care
Institute for Community Inclusion
University Affiliated Program
Children's Hospital
300 Longwood Avenue
Boston, Massachusetts 02115

Timaree Bierle, B.S.N., R.N.
Assistant Nurse Coordinator
Project School Care
Institute for Community Inclusion
University Affiliated Program
Children's Hospital
300 Longwood Avenue
Boston, Massachusetts 02115

Terry Heintz Caldwell, Ed.D.
Consultant
Project School Care
Inclusion Teacher
New Orleans Schools
120 Hesper Street
Metairie, Louisiana 70005

Judith S. Palfrey, M.D.
Director
Project School Care
T. Berry Brazelton Professor of Pediatrics
Harvard Medical School
Chief
Division of General Pediatrics
Children's Hospital
300 Longwood Avenue
Boston, Massachusetts 02115

The Contributors

Debra S. Alcouloumre, Ed.D.
Teacher of Children with Special Needs
New Orleans Schools
3411 Broadway
New Orleans, Louisiana 70125

Betsy Anderson
Federation for Children with Special Needs
95 Berkeley Street
Boston, Massachusetts 02116

Susanne Appel, M.D.
12 West 96th Street
Apartment 12A
New York, New York 10025

Jocelyn Bessette-Gorlin, R.N., P.N.P.
Hematology Nurse Consultant
51 Monument Avenue
Charlestown, Massachusetts 02129

Henry A. Beyer, J.D.
Director
N. Neal Pike Institute on Law and Disability
Boston University School of Law
765 Commonwealth Avenue
Boston, Massachusetts 02215

Ronald Blanchard
Southdown Care Center
1395 West Funnel Boulevard
Houma, Louisiana 70360

Denise P. Burns, R.N., B.S.N., C.E.T.N.
Staff Nurse II
Infant/Toddler Surgical Unit
Children's Hospital
300 Longwood Avenue
Boston Massachusetts 02115

Joan E. Daley, R.N., B.S.N.
Massachusetts Department of Public Health
Northeast Regional Health Office
Tewksbury Hospital
Tewksbury, Massachusetts 01887

Marguerite David, R.N.
Staff Nurse III
Infant/Toddler Surgical Unit
Children's Hospital
300 Longwood Avenue
Boston, Massachusetts 02115

Lois Doerr, R.N., B.A.
Allergy, Asthma Nurse
Department of Pediatrics
Allergy and Respiratory Division
Boston Medical Center
818 Harrison Avenue
Boston, Massachusetts 02118

Mary Jo Dunleavy, R.N., B.S.N.
Coordinator
Myelodysplasia Program
Children's Hospital
300 Longwood Avenue
Boston, Massachusetts 02115

Richard G. Giardina, R.N., B.S.N., C.I.C.
Infection Control Practitioner
Brigham and Women's Hospital–Channing Labs
181 Longwood Avenue
Boston, Massachusetts 02115

Rosemary H. Grant, R.N., B.S.N.
Nursing Coordinator
Division of Urology
Children's Hospital
300 Longwood Avenue
Boston, Massachusetts 02115

Andrea Rubin Hale, R.N., M.P.H.
Clinical Trials Nurse
AIDS Program
Children's Hospital
300 Longwood Avenue
Boston, Massachusetts 02115

Jacqueline Harrison, M.N., R.N.
Program Coordinator
National Maternal and Child Health Resource Center
   for Ensuring Adequate Preparation of Providers of
   Care
Children's Hospital
200 Henry Clay Avenue
New Orleans, Louisiana 70018

Elizabeth Hughson, M.S., R.N.
Program Coordinator
End Stage Renal Disease Program
Children's Hospital
300 Longwood Avenue
Boston, Massachusetts 02115

Laura Ibsen, M.D.
Division of Critical Care
Children's Hospital Medical Center of Akron
One Perkins Square
Akron, Ohio 44308

Janice Rutledge Janz, M.Ed.
Teacher of Children with Special Needs
New Orleans Schools
908 French Street
New Orleans, Louisiana 70124

Julie Jones, M.Ed.
Coordinator
Barnstable Special Education Preschools
2514 Main Street
West Barnstable, Massachusetts 02668

Susan Murray Larsen, B.S., R.P.T.
Physical Therapist
Kennedy Donovan Early Intervention Program
389 County Street
New Bedford, Massachusetts 02740

Arlene Swan Mahony, R.N., B.S.N.
Nurse Liaison
School Health Services
Boston Public Schools
515 Hyde Park Avenue
Roslindale, Massachusetts 02131

Ellen Meeropol, M.S., R.N.C.S., P.N.P.
Shriner's Hospital
516 Carew Street
Springfield, Massachusetts 01104

Cornelia Mercurio, B.S., R.R.T.
Respiratory Care Practitioner
133 Poplar Street
Roslindale, Massachusetts 02131

Dale O'Hayer, M.Ed.
Compass School
26 Sunnyside Street
Jamaica Plain, Massachusetts 02130

Lauren Perlman, R.R.T.
Respiratory Care Practitioner
Respiratory Care Department
Children's Hospital
300 Longwood Avenue
Boston, Massachusetts 02115

Christine E. Psota, B.S., M.T., C.I.C.
Epidemiologist
Children's Hospital
300 Longwood Avenue
Boston, Massachusetts 02115

Sandra Quigley, R.N., C.P.N.P., C.E.T.N.
Enterostomal Therapy Nurse
Children's Hospital
300 Longwood Avenue
Boston, Massachusetts 02115

Denise S. Richardson, R.N., B.S.N.
Gastroenterology and Nutrition Support Clinician
Children's Hospital
300 Longwood Avenue
Boston, Massachusetts 02115

Nadine Schwab, R.N., P.N.P., M.P.H.
Consultant for Health Services
Connecticut Department of Education
831 Oakwood Road
Middletown, Connecticut 06457

Thomas Silva, M.D.
Pediatrician
East Boston Neighborhood Health Center
10 Gove Street
East Boston, Massachusetts 02128

Barbara P. Sirvis, Ed.D.
Vice President for Academic Affairs
State University of New York College at Brockport
Brockport, New York 14420

Judy Still
26 Aurora Lane
South Yarmouth, Massachusetts 02664

Michael Still
26 Aurora Lane
South Yarmouth, Massachusetts 02664

Ann Tierney, M.S.N., P.N.P.
Pediatric Case Manager
Spaulding Rehabilitation Hospital
125 Nashua Street
Boston, Massachusetts 02114

FOREWORD

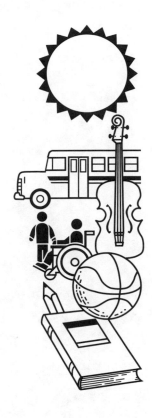

I salute the authors of this important and timely book. My mother and I can tell you how important this material will be to teachers and others as they plan for kids who need special technologies to join the classroom, receive an education, and stay happy and healthy.

As a person who has been living with a ventilator and who used to require treatments and gastrostomy feedings at school, I know that a tool like this book will make transition from home to school much easier for both students and family members. What many people don't realize is the effect, on the student who has special needs as well as on his or her peers, of active participation in the classroom.

This book provides an opportunity to challenge the perspective of both groups and to allow for a different, but equally important, kind of educational exchange to occur. It leads to mutual understanding and takes the fear out of health problems in general. It is such "mainstreaming" that will help students as they grow into adulthood to be prepared to work side by side and to support each other in the communities they build together. It is through such experience that *all* individuals recognize the importance of everyone's rights and responsibilities in society.

Katie Beckett
Freshman
Mount Mercy College
Cedar Rapids, Iowa
March 1997

PREFACE

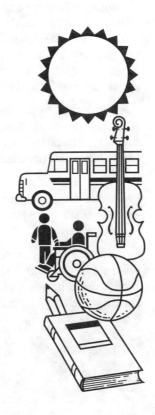

ifteen years ago, a small group of policy makers and professionals sat together in the Maternal and Child Health conference room on the third floor of the Harvard School of Public Health. Drawn together by common observations and concerns, the group included educators, nurses, and physicians. They were gathered because something new was happening. Children with increasingly complex medical conditions and nursing needs were appearing at the schoolhouse door. The children had chronic conditions but were not ill. They had disabilities but plenty of ability. They wanted to learn along with their neighbors and peers and didn't want their health needs standing in the way.

All over the United States, groups of professionals were seeing what our Massachusetts group saw. Medical technology was improving life chances and life functioning for children with a wide array of complex conditions. Parents were asking for new opportunities for their children; and, all over the country, groups were trying to respond.

Legislation and court precedent of the 1970s and 1980s had made it clear that children with disabilities and chronic illnesses had the right to a free, appropriate public education and to related services needed to ensure access to education. As a result, many schools were barreling headlong into the provision of a variety of health and nursing services with little or no guidance from nursing and medicine.

In Boston, our small task force concluded that there was a need for guidelines for the safe and appropriate provision of school health and nursing services. With funding from the National Institute on Disability and Rehabilitation Research and the Maternal and Child Health Bureau, we created Project School Care to develop guidelines for care and to provide technical assistance to school systems in Massachusetts and throughout the United States.

In some ways, Project School Care and this book have evolved as a series of concentric circles. The first circle was the public health and education policy makers who saw the new horizon and wanted to move toward it. The second circle was the large national group of professionals who joined together in 1988 at a consensus conference to ensure the accuracy and applicability of the guidelines. The consensus panel included nurses, physicians, educators, and parents; and it reflected our understanding that each widening circle must be composed of and informed by all groups involved in the education and care of children with complex medical conditions.

The original edition of this book was published in 1989 and distributed by the Maternal and Child Health Bureau and by Project School Care. Their dissemination led to ever-widening circles of colleagues and partners and to the realization that a second edition was needed to meet a new set of objectives. This new edition of our Guidelines for Care updates the original technical sections to reflect changes in medical practice, most notably the appearance of human immunodeficiency virus as a chronic childhood condition. Second, the book addresses a wider range of issues, including classroom educational considerations. Third, and most important, this new edition projects the voices of the widened circle of participants. Creating this volume has been a collaborative, interactive process involving parents, students, teachers, lawyers, nurses, and doctors. Each has brought a special perspective and a unique insight. Together, they have created a volume that reflects the reality in schools—the tension, the dilemmas, the weaknesses, and the strengths.

This second edition was written at a crossroads in time. The Individuals with Disabilities Education Act has been reauthorized and remains the legislative underpinning for educational and related service delivery. Nonetheless, mandates and federal standards are under substantial scrutiny, and responsibility for much programming has shifted to the community level, often without requisite resources.

For children with complex medical needs, any backward movement is indeed hazardous. In this book, we have held to the highest standards of care, underscored a central role for school nurses, and called on school systems that do not yet have adequate health services to develop responsible school nursing programs.

We are well aware that, for many school districts, the procedures outlined in this volume presuppose a system that either does not yet exist or is only marginally supported. The circles of people who have joined hands to create this book have shared their stories, their battles, and their solutions. Sustaining and expanding services depends completely on keeping those circles together and working in concert as partners.

Judith S. Palfrey, M.D.

ACKNOWLEDGMENTS

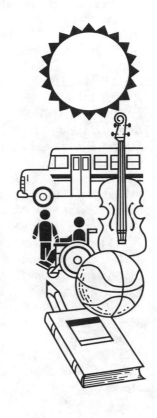

Development of this book has been generously supported by the National Institute on Disability and Rehabilitation Research, the Maternal and Child Health Bureau, and the Dyson Foundation. We are most grateful to Naomi Karp, Merle McPherson, and Anne Dyson for their commitment to children with complex medical problems and their families.

In addition, the contributions of many people made preparation of this manual possible. We thank Deidre Shaw and Catherine Carter, who provided their energy and expertise in manuscript preparation; Marcia Williams for her distinctive illustrations that enhance and enliven the text of the manual and Brenda Brooks for her illustration in the dedication; and Joan Lowcock for administrative support.

We also thank our families and friends for their patience and understanding during the countless hours involved in creating this manual. With their support and love, we were able to accomplish this task. The editors are indebted to many expert and knowledgeable people for their advice and assistance on Project School Care, as well as in the preparation and development of the guidelines in this volume.

Over the years, Project School Care has benefited enormously from the friendship and kind counsel of many wonderful, thoughtful people. This book has been enriched by the input of parents, educators, administrators, nurses, and physicians. We especially want to acknowledge the help of the following individuals:

Deborah Allen	Catherine Dunham	Judith McAuliffe
Carol Almeida	Stanley Eichner	Dorothy MacDonald
Anne Barrett-Dodwell	Beverly Farquahar	Trevor McGill
Anne Black	Louis Freedman	Joy McNeil
Patricia Blight	Jane Gardner	Nancy Miller
Ann Blood	Vince Hutchins	Anne Minichino
Richard Bourne	Judith B. Igoe	Mary Mitchell
Elaine Brainerd	Richard Incerto	Lois Moore
Jane Buckley	Lawrence C. Kaplan	Marie T. Mulkern
John Butler	Kay Keeney	LaRae Munk
Patricia Ciarleglio	Karl Kuban	David G. Nathan
Thomas Cohen	Russell Latham	Pearl O'Rourke
Molly Cole	Alan Leichtner	James Perrin
John Diggins	Merritt Low	Jo-Ellen Quinlan
Lori DiPrete	Barbara Marino	Julius B. Richmond
Mary Donar-Reale	Gerald Mazor	Michael J. Savage

Edith Siegel
Ann Smith
Lyle Stephens
Sally E. Tarbell

David Todres
Deborah Klein Walker
Michael Weitzman
Barbara Weston

Harland Winter
Lise Zeig

In addition, we extend our thanks to the following individuals who generously gave of their time to review portions of this book in the manuscript stage and whose suggestions are appreciated:

Betsy Anderson, Federation for Children with Special Needs, Boston, Massachusetts

Marilyn Ault, Ph.D., Department of Special Education, University of Kansas, Lawrence, Kansas

Lynwood Beekman, J.D., Beekman and La Pointe, P.C., Okemos, Michigan

Robert Bilenker, M.D., Metro Health Medical Center, Case Western Reserve, Cleveland, Ohio

Larraine Bossi, M.S., R.N., C.S., Children's Hospital, Boston, Massachusetts

Elaine Brainerd, R.N., M.A., C.S.N., Branford, Connecticut

Denise P. Burns, R.N., C.E.T.N., Infant/Toddler Surgical Unit, Children's Hospital, Boston, Massachusetts

Van Chauvin, M.S.N., M.H.S., R.N.C.S., F.N.P., C.S.N., Health Services, Dallas Independent School District, Dallas, Texas

Carol Costante, R.N., M.A., C.S.N., National Association of School Nurses, Office of Student and Employee Health Services, Baltimore County Public Schools, Baltimore, Maryland

Allen Crocker, M.D., Developmental Evaluation Center, Institute for Community Inclusion, University Affiliated Program, Children's Hospital, Boston, Massachusetts

Marguerite David, R.N., Infant/Toddler Surgical Unit, Children's Hospital, Boston, Massachusetts

Jean E. D'Amico, Oak Park, Illinois

Julia De Cicco, M.S., Fairview Elementary School, Milwaukee Public Schools, Milwaukee, Wisconsin

Mary E. Donar-Reale, R.N., M.S.N., Critical Care Service, Alfred I. duPont Institute, Wilmington, Delaware

Mary Jo Dunleavy, R.N., B.S.N., Myelodysplasia Program, Children's Hospital, Boston, Massachusetts

Arlene Evans, R.N., Placer City, Office of Education, Auburn, California

Steven Fishman, M.D., Department of Surgery, Children's Hospital, Harvard Medical School, Boston, Massachusetts

Robin Friedlander, M.S., Institute for Community Inclusion, Children's Hospital, Boston, Massachusetts

Nancy E. Goldberg, M.S.N., R.N., C.S., P.N.P., Division of Gastroenterology and Nutrition, Children's Hospital, Boston, Massachusetts

Rosemary H. Grant, R.N., B.S.N., Division of Urology, Children's Hospital, Boston, Massachusetts

Deb Hart, M.Ed., Institute for Community Inclusion, Children's Hospital, Boston, Massachusetts

Maura Heckmann, R.N.C., Children's Hospital, Boston, Massachusetts

Mary Horn, R.N., M.S., R.R.T., Nursing Staff Development, Children's Hospital, Boston, Massachusetts

Nancy Hurley, M.S., Institute for Community Inclusion, Children's Hospital, Boston, Massachusetts

Laura Ibsen, M.D., Division of Critical Care, Children's Hospital Medical Center, Akron, Ohio

Kathy Jabs, M.D., Dialysis and Renal Transplantation, Children's Hospital of Philadelphia, Philadelphia, Pennsylvania

Kim Kelley, Project School Care, Institute for Community Inclusion, Children's Hospital, Boston, Massachusetts

Virginia Kharasch, M.D., Division of Pulmonary Medicine, Children's Hospital, Boston, Massachusetts

Donna Lehr, Ed.D., School of Special Education, Boston University, Boston, Massachusetts

Ann Lowry, B.S., R.N., Lenox Public Schools, Lenox, Massachusetts

Helen Mahoney-West, M.S.N., P.N.P., Hemophilia Program, Children's Hospital, Boston, Massachusetts

Mary Ann Marchel, Ph.D., Department of Special Education, University of Wisconsin–Eau Claire, Eau Claire, Wisconsin

Ellen O'Donnell, R.N., B.S.N., School Age/Adolescent Surgical Unit, Children's Hospital, Boston, Massachusetts

Maryjane O'Malley, M.S.N., R.N.C.S., P.N.P., Medical Services, Italian Home for Children, Jamaica Plain, Massachusetts

Lori Parker-Hartigan, N.D., R.N., Division of Gastroenterology and Nutrition, Children's Hospital, Boston, Massachusetts

Sandra Quigley, R.N., B.S.N., C.E.T.N., Children's Hospital, Boston, Massachusetts

Alan Retik, M.D., Division of Urology, Children's Hospital, Boston, Massachusetts

Peggy Mann Rhinehart, Division of General Pediatrics and Adolescent Health, University of Minnesota, Minneapolis, Minnesota

Denise Richardson, B.S.N., R.N., Division of Gastroenterology and Nutrition, Children's Hospital, Boston, Massachusetts

Nadine Schwab, R.N., P.N.P., M.P.H., Connecticut Department of Education, Middletown, Connecticut

William Schwab, M.D., Department of Family Medicine, University of Wisconsin, Madison, Wisconsin

Margaret P. Smith, R.N., M.S., Kennedy Day School, Franciscan Children's Hospital, Brighton, Massachusetts

Tamara Stephensen, R.N., M.A., C.C.N., Phoenix Children's Hospital, Phoenix, Arizona

Aleece Stewart, R.N., C.S.N., Knox County Schools, Knoxville, Tennessee

Kathleen Sullivan, R.N., Department of Otolaryngology, Children's Hospital, Boston, Massachusetts

Arlene Swan Mahony, B.S.N., R.N., Boston Public Schools, Boston, Massachusetts

Judy Taylor, R.N., M.P.H., C.N.N., Pediatric Nephrology, Special Interest Group–American Nephrology Nurses Association, Tampa, Florida

Ann Tierney, M.S.N., P.N.P., Spaulding Rehabilitation Hospital, Boston, Massachusetts

Ann Todaro, M.N., R.N., Baylor College of Medicine, Texas Children's Hospital, Houston, Texas

Marilyn Z. West, R.N., M.S., Santa Clara County, Office of Education, San Jose, California

How to Use This Book

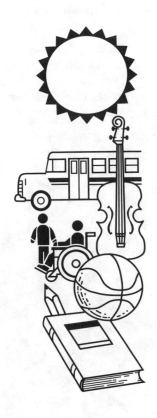

T his manual and its guidelines are intended for use by parents and professionals who care for children and youth who are assisted by medical technology. Parts of this manual are written for people with little or no medical background. Other parts detail the specific technical procedures that are needed by children with specific conditions on a daily basis. Many of the materials are intended for distribution and daily use. Forms to use to develop individualized health care plans (IHCPs), emergency plans, checklists, and an informational introductory letter about each procedure/ technology are included and may be photocopied.

The manual is divided into two sections. Section I, *Children and Youth Assisted by Medical Technology in Educational Settings,* comprises Chapters 1–6; and Section II, *Guidelines for Care,* comprises the various procedures, checklists, and guidelines themselves.

Chapters 1–3 outline important issues related to caring for children with special health care needs: Chapter 1 provides information about students' participation in school and includes an overview of medical technologies, educational needs of children, socioemotional considerations, and firsthand experiences of parents and professionals. Chapter 2 presents information about federal, state, and case laws, as well as regulations and professional standards, as they relate to children and their health providers. This chapter discusses PL 101-476, the Individuals with Disabilities Education Act of 1990; due process; Section 504 of PL 93-112, the Rehabilitation Act of 1973; fostering teamwork; and additional public laws and case laws. Policies and position statements related to do-not-resuscitate orders also are presented. Chapter 3 reviews the process of developing safe and educationally relevant school programs for students with special health care needs. Roles of various team members in a team approach are outlined; and specific steps are reviewed for meeting with the child and family after referral to assessment, planning, developing an IHCP, training, implementation, monitoring, and evaluation.

Chapter 4 provides overview information on planning and providing safe transportation for children with special health care needs. Several areas discussed include applicable laws and regulations, specialized seating and positioning, and personnel and training.

Chapter 5 reviews special health concerns including universal precautions, latex allergies, and human immunodeficiency virus (HIV) and acquired immunodeficiency syndrome. This chapter also addresses the recommended practices and supports for children who have HIV and are attending school.

Chapter 6 provides useful documents to assist families and school personnel in considering all elements of care for children. Tools to develop an IHCP are included, as are guidelines for cultural assessment, a checklist for considerations in developing an individualized education program, and a general classroom inclusion checklist. These documents are reprinted in this book by permission of the individuals who created them; they are provided here to be adapted by families and school staff to develop a specific plan of care for children in school.

Section II addresses procedural guidelines for enteral feeding, intravenous lines, dialysis, clean intermittent catheterization, ostomy care, and respiratory care. Each procedural section reviews physical anatomy and function, the purpose of the procedure and equipment, suggested settings and personnel, and issues for consideration in developing a child-specific plan for care. Each procedure highlights points to remember and possible problems that may require attention.

The procedural guidelines section is followed by skills checklists that can be used for teaching and training school staff. Each skills checklist assists the trainer in assessing the learner's knowledge of preparing for the procedure, identifying necessary supplies, and performing the procedure. Each skills checklist should be adapted to each specific student and his or her needs and concerns.

DISCLAIMER

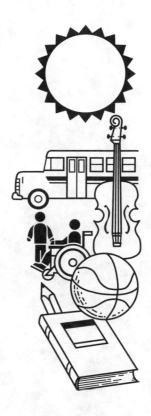

he recommendations contained in this volume reflect the best and most current medical, nursing, and educational advice that Project School Care could obtain.

Although it is expected that this book will play a part in establishing standards for the proper care of children assisted by medical technology in the school setting, there is no guarantee that the recommendations herein will be accepted by schools, courts, or others. Each school system must make its own determinations as to which recommendations to follow and which to reject.

This book was written to assist school systems in establishing a safe environment for students assisted by medical technology, conducive to receiving the public education to which they are entitled. The guidelines presented herein do not stand alone; they must be individually customized into a carefully developed health plan that takes into account the unique needs and circumstances of each student; establishes a comprehensive training program; and involves the student's primary health care provider, specialists who are knowledgeable about the student, the family, the school nurse, community health providers, and other medical and educational professionals. Together, this group can help establish a plan of care that best meets the student's schooling needs and possibilities.

This book is dedicated with love to the memory of Marilynn Haynie.

"Everything that limits us we have to put aside."
Jonathan Livingston Seagull
by Richard Bach

CHILDREN AND YOUTH ASSISTED BY MEDICAL TECHNOLOGY IN EDUCATIONAL SETTINGS

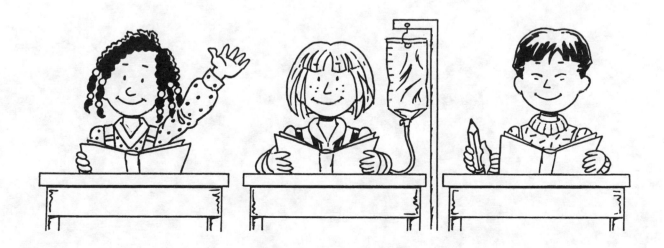

CHILDREN AND YOUTH
ASSISTED BY
MEDICAL TECHNOLOGY
IN EDUCATIONAL SETTINGS

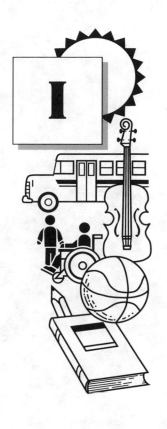

Students Who Require Medical Technology in School

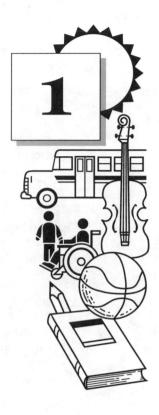

Terry Heintz Caldwell,
Barbara P. Sirvis, Judy Still, Michael Still,
Nadine Schwab, Julie Jones, Betsy Anderson,
Ronald Blanchard, and Susanne Appel

An increasing number of children and youth who are assisted by medical treatment and technology are living and attending schools in their home communities. Educators are challenged with developing school programs that prepare students academically and vocationally for adulthood and their future roles in society. This chapter provides information about students' school participation and includes an overview of the following:

- Medical technologies used by students
- Educational needs students may have in the school setting
- Social-emotional needs students may have in the school setting
- Experiences of some students and families
- Experiences of selected school personnel

This section includes case studies and relevant information and delineates the unresolved questions that continue to be voiced by families, school nurses, teachers, and administrators.

MEDICAL TECHNOLOGIES USED BY STUDENTS IN SCHOOL

Three student and family perspectives highlight school and community experiences:

Eddie is a 9-year-old who was diagnosed at birth with a lymphatic malformation in which parts of his lymph cells overgrew and replaced normal tissues in his face and neck. The lump was as big as a walnut at birth; 6 weeks later, it was the size of a cantaloupe and had to be removed surgically. Eddie required a tracheostomy to maintain an open airway so he could breathe and a gastrostomy tube so that he could receive feedings directly to his stomach. Eddie underwent frequent surgeries in early childhood and will continue to require surgery throughout his life when the lymph cells overgrow. He now is in fourth grade, does well in school, and has been invited to join the science club. He is an altar boy at his community church.

* * *

Robin is a 9-year-old who was born with a short intestine. Since birth, she has required a combination of intravenous and gastrostomy feedings. At home intravenous fluids go directly into her bloodstream through a central venous catheter, a permanent plastic tube in her upper chest that goes into a large blood vessel near her heart. Gastrostomy feedings go directly into her stomach through a gastrostomy tube. On occasion, Robin has used an automatic feeding pump that delivers continuous gastrostomy feedings while she is at school. Robin is now in fourth grade and in a program for gifted students; she rarely misses school. She wants to go to college and become a lawyer or an actor.

* * *

Brian is 18 years old and paralyzed from the neck down as a result of an accident that occurred when he was 11. Brian requires 24-hour ventilation through a tracheostomy tube, suctioning as needed, urinary catheterization (twice during the school day), body repositioning, and assistance with all activities of daily living, such as eating and grooming. In addition, he requires assistance with classroom activities, such as turning pages and taking notes. Brian is interested in technology, biology, and people.

Eddie, Robin, and Brian live in different parts of the United States; live in a rural, an urban, and a suburban community; and have a common need for medical technology and health care services in school. It is important to recognize that, although these children require special health care services or use medical devices, they are not sick children. They, like other students, are healthy most of the time.

Students who are assisted by medical technology are a small subset of the population of students who have special health care needs. One study found that approximately 1–2 of 1,000 (1–2:1,000) children require medical technology and treatment (Palfrey et al., 1994). The most common medical technologies include tube feedings; intravenous lines; clean intermittent catheterization; ostomy appliances; dialysis; and respiratory devices, such as tracheostomy tubes, oxygen tanks, and ventilators. Detailed information about these technologies is included in Chapters 4–6 and in Section II.

These guidelines focus on the services needed by students who require medical technology and health procedures. However, students who have a range of health care needs or those who do not require a procedure or medical technology, per se, may also require the special considerations that are discussed.

Throughout the first three chapters, special health conditions are considered in terms of *needs* rather than diagnoses. A student's actual needs influence the development of appropriate school programs. Does the student need care during the school day? What level of care is required? Are adaptations required in the school environment or in the curriculum? Eddie's mother discusses her son's needs:

Many people respond to my son Eddie in terms of his diagnosis rather than his humanness. First and foremost he is a child, not a diagnosis. He wants the same things as other children. The diagnosis distracts people from his total needs—an education and friends—because they think of everything in terms of his disease. In addition, they always assume he has mental retardation because he has a physical disability.

Students assisted by medical technologies have a range of health conditions that can affect a single organ system or multiple organ systems, as follows:

Congenital anomalies: central nervous system malformations (e.g., hydrocephalus, myelodysplasia, cerebral dysgenesis), gastrointestinal malformations (e.g., intestinal atresia), genitourinary malformations (e.g., cloacal exstrophy), and congenital heart conditions;

Chronic conditions: malignancies, cerebral palsy and other neuromuscular disorders, seizure disorders, immunodeficiency syndrome, asthma, chronic respiratory disorders (excluding bronchopulmonary dysplasia), congestive heart failure and other noncongenital heart conditions, renal disorders (e.g., chronic renal failure, glomerulonephritis), malabsorption, chronic malnutrition, and gastroesophageal reflux;

Perinatal factors: prematurity, bronchopulmonary dysplasia, meconium aspiration, perinatal asphyxia, necrotizing enterocolitis;

Hereditary/genetic: Cri-du-Chat, trisomy 18, trisomy 21, cystic fibrosis, Duchenne muscular dystrophy, mucopolysaccharidosis, other inborn errors of metabolism, Werdnig-Hoffman disease, Tay-Sachs disease, sickle-cell anemia, thalassemia, hemophilia, inherited immunodeficiencies;

Injuries: accidents, inflicted injuries, near-drowning, brain injury, spinal cord injuries, cardiopulmonary arrest, burns;

Infections: congenital viral infections, osteomyelitis, meningitis, viral encephalitis, acquired immunodeficiency syndrome;

Other nonspecific categories of primarily developmental and behavioral nature, such as severe developmental delay. (Palfrey et al., 1994, p. 231)

MEETING THE STUDENTS' EDUCATIONAL NEEDS

Eddie attends a general fourth-grade class and requires special assistance because of delays in motor and social skills. He spent a lot of time in bed during his first few years, so he didn't have the opportunity to practice motor skills. Eddie has trouble keeping up with his classmates at times. He has had multiple maxillofacial and tongue reduction surgeries, colds, and bouts of pneumonia, which have caused him to miss school. He missed 65 days in first grade, but several times the school provided a tutor. The chronic nature of his condition makes school progress difficult. In addition, he has trouble concentrating when he is anticipating surgery.

* * *

Robin is in a fourth-grade class for gifted students. She excels in her schoolwork and has not had any significant emergencies that would necessitate missing school or take her attention away from her schoolwork.

* * *

Brian is a senior in high school. At the time of his injury, he missed 7 months of school and, therefore, had to repeat sixth grade. Brian cannot write independently, manage school materials, or turn pages to read. Brian's concentration and stamina are not as good as they were before his injury. He takes more time than other students to complete all of his work, and, as a result, it takes him at least 12 months to complete what other students complete during a 9-month school year.

Special Health Care Needs Affect Development, Cognition, and Learning

Among students with chronic illness and disability, there is a wide variety of learning styles and abilities. Although many students who are assisted by medical technologies have conditions that have little or no impact on their cognition, other students, such as those with acquired brain injury, neurological conditions, or brain irradiation, may have substantial cognitive deficits that require special education intervention. Many of the following factors may impede a student's ability to learn:

- Lack of experience
- Frequent school absence
- Lack of concentration because of effects of the illness, including pain and fatigue
- Short- or long-term emotional/physical effects of undergoing medical treatments
- Anxiety, pain, and fatigue related to ongoing or periodic medical treatments
- Side effects of medication
- Less time for classes/studying as a result of time needed for health care procedures/therapies
- Personal concerns about health
- Acceptance and understanding of peers
- Poor self-image
- Lack of realistic expectations by program/service providers
- Specific learning disability/developmental delay/cognitive deficits

Many individual factors that affect learning are short-term problems (e.g., surgery, diabetic crisis). One factor or episode may not affect learning, but cumulative factors or repeated episodes need careful consideration. Many students with special health care needs can benefit from interventions that minimize the repeated effects of learning difficulties. These include the following:

- Logistical considerations, such as rest periods, shortened transportation, and an extra set of books at home
- Opportunities for experiences missed because of illness and hospitalizations
- Adaptation in the daily school schedules and time lines for academic requirements (e.g., 12-month program, summer services, after-school tutoring)
- Flexible, immediate home or hospital instruction services based on the student's condition
- Student education and counseling regarding the health condition, the effects of treatment, and self-management techniques
- Family education regarding health condition and effects on child's development and learning
- Special education services

People with Physical Disabilities or Health Conditions Sometimes Can Have Major Learning Problems

Families report that people often automatically connect obvious medical technologies and physical differences with cognitive delays. One mother, Betsy Anderson, relays her personal experiences:

Perhaps because my own child has a substantial physical disability and was mislabeled mentally retarded, I am more conscious of labels. I think the point is that labels can be very useful and important but they can also be very stigmatizing and sometimes...wrong. Our experiences clarified for me that even if my child had both a mental and a physical disability, I would still want the best for him and would still want him to achieve his fullest potential. I've always felt I wanted and needed to be his advocate. We don't want people just to make assumptions about physical/mental disabilities, but, because some of that seems inevitable, I think what we really need to do is work for appropriate quality care and services for everyone and emphasize that when planning programs and services, we must look at people as individuals with differing strengths and needs.

School Settings Adapted for Students Who Are Assisted by Medical Technology

School settings may need to be adapted to meet the educational, health care, and social needs of students assisted by medical technology. The following factors should be considered when determining a student's educational placement:

- Involvement of parents and students in planning and decision making
- Comprehensive knowledge of the student's health care and learning needs and the variety of ways these needs can be met
- Selection of the program on the basis of the student's educational needs, not program availability
- Comprehensive knowledge of the resources available in the school system and in the community
- Use of a more restrictive environment only when the student's educational needs cannot be met in the least restrictive classroom/setting (i.e., general education classroom) with appropriate aids and services

MEETING SOCIAL AND EMOTIONAL NEEDS IN THE SCHOOL SETTING

Because Eddie's tracheostomy needed constant attention, his mother or a nurse accompanied him everywhere he went when he was younger; as a result, he had very few school friends. At the insistence of his mother, he now completes his own health care. Eddie now has a larger circle of friends.

* * *

Robin has many friends, although she still struggles with issues regarding when and what they should know about her condition. She rarely requires health care in school. Robin does not complete her own health care but can direct it and is fully aware of the signs of problems.

* * *

Brian has few male friends but several female friends. He cannot participate in many of the activities his friends enjoy. For instance, he cannot participate in sports and is not interested in spectating. Specialized transportation is not available, so he cannot participate in activities in the community. Brian cannot complete any of his own health care and is not encouraged by his caregiver to direct his care.

Students with special health conditions have the same social, emotional, and educational needs as do other students. The social and emotional development of students can be enhanced by providing opportunities for

- Social interaction with peers
- Learning to provide or direct care
- Reaching the same expectations as peers regarding everyday functioning and learning
- Social interaction with adults with special health conditions

Social Interaction

Students with special health care needs may spend a large part of their time with caregivers and adults in medical settings and, as a result, may have little chance to interact with peers. Even when they are at home or school, they may have an adult with them constantly. The decision to foster independence and social interaction often depends on personal values, experiences, and culture. School staff should be encouraged to increase opportunities for social interaction. For these opportunities to occur, the following should be provided:

- Education of peers regarding specific health conditions and alternative forms of communication
- Attention of health caregivers to students' needs for privacy
- Sufficient time to spend with friends
- Special transportation for field trips and after-school activities
- Access to health care during field trips and after-school activities
- Architecturally accessible environments

Student Involvement in Health Care

Students frequently require health care procedures that are completed by adults. Students with special health care needs can participate in their care by completing it independently, directing care (e.g., letting the caregiver know when it is time for their treatment), assisting in care (e.g., handing caregiver the supplies), or cooperating with caregivers when verbal or physical participation is not possible (Caldwell, Todaro, & Gates, 1989). For example, Eddie's mother reports the following:

Autonomy [for Eddie] is important to me. I want him to learn how to provide his own care. The school put in a full-length mirror so he could learn to care for himself. He cleaned his tracheostomy with a cotton swab. He learned how to cough. He cleaned his inner-cannula as well as any 4-year-old could. If he has a tracheostomy in the future, I expect he will do his own care and he will need a private place for that. It is really hard to let him go, but if he never has the opportunity to do things on his own, he won't grow up. Even when he was little, I would pack his backpack and put it on him and send him to the grocery store with a coupon to match and pick out cereal or something else. Everyone in the store knew him. I did my homework and met everyone beforehand so I could trust they would come get me if something was wrong.

Relations with caregivers are important to his ability to socialize and learn to function autonomously. I know that his private duty nurse was trying to do too much for him. He didn't get to interact with other students. We finally scheduled time away from the nurse, and she used a walkie-talkie to keep in touch with him.

Not all students will have the physical capabilities necessary to provide their own care. These students can learn to direct their care, to arrange their schedule, and then direct the actual procedures. Brian, who is unable to provide self-care, described his independence this way:

> *I always did things by myself and made my own choices, which I still do. I'm stubborn just like my dad. He taught me to depend only on my family and on myself. I do have to depend on other people to do things for me, but I tell them what I want. When the technology gets better, I will be able to do more for myself. I make my own decisions. I learned that from my father. My sister and I were both independent when we were young. I always liked being independent.*

A student's participation in self-care efforts can be fostered by a number of factors. Self-care is encouraged when

- The family and student are involved in health care and education program development.
- Self-care goals are included in the student's individualized education and health care programs.
- The student's unique strengths, interests, and abilities are emphasized.
- Self-care is taught as early as possible and at a developmentally appropriate level.
- The student's self-care skills and changing health care needs are reviewed on a regular basis.
- A qualified caregiver is scheduled to teach and support the student in self-care.
- Family and other caregivers are counseled, if culturally acceptable, about the importance of maximizing student self-care skills.

Appropriate Expectations and Standards

The development of a student's social and emotional needs also depends on appropriate expectations of adults. Katie Beckett, a 16-year-old who has been supported by medical technology since infancy, reminded teachers that it was essential that they hold students with special health care needs to the same standards as other students for them to succeed educationally and vocationally (Beckett, 1994).

School personnel can create opportunities to achieve appropriate expectations by

- Working closely with the student's family and the student to determine what accommodations are necessary
- Allowing students to make mistakes and even fail, at appropriate times, so the student learns how to deal with mistakes
- Modifying the volume of the student's schoolwork while maintaining standards
- Providing extra time for the student to complete tasks (e.g., the high school student may require summer school or even 5 years to graduate, the elementary student may benefit from supplemental tutoring and extended school-year programs)
- Helping the student evaluate his or her own abilities, work pace, and progress
- Encouraging families and health care professionals to minimize the student's school absences that result from appointments
- Minimizing the effect of the student's time spent completing health care procedures by scheduling those procedures carefully
- Maximizing the student's academic participation by scheduling core subjects during periods when the student is least fatigued or affected by medication or undesirable side effects of medications
- Planning for school absences and initiating an alternative plan immediately when a student is absent
- Considering the use of communication technology to assist the student (e.g., personal computers, speaker telephones to listen to classes when absent, use of electronic mail to share assignments)

Parents, students, and teachers wonder whether to discuss a student's condition openly with peers and school staff. Does it make a difference whether the student's condition is obvious? Is there a "better" age at which to make the disclosure? This important issue rarely is discussed, but it can affect the student's social and emotional growth. Although no standard procedures regarding disclosure exist, the following guidelines are important:

1. Respect a student's and family's wishes if they do not want the student's condition discussed with anyone.

2. Offer to involve families and students in decisions regarding whether, when, and how to tell other students and staff about student's conditions.

3. Offer to involve families and students in decisions regarding who should provide education, what information should be disclosed, and which classmates or schoolmates should be included. Young students often will want their parents involved, but older students may prefer to invite one of their health care professionals or to conduct the session themselves. Younger students may want to include only their classmates; older students may want to include other schoolmates as well. Some students who are discussing a particular topic (e.g., catheterization) may want to include only students of the same gender (Caldwell et al., 1989).

4. Note that staff ideas and opinions regarding self-care and peer awareness may vary.

THE SCHOOL EXPERIENCE FOR STUDENTS WHO ARE ASSISTED BY MEDICAL TECHNOLOGY AND FOR THEIR CLASSMATES

Eddie's experience has been varied. He did not attend his neighborhood school in kindergarten and always has had adults with him, which impeded friendship development. He also has struggled to progress academically with his classmates. By second grade, he avoided talking about his tracheostomy or his illness. Recently, he found another student in his class who has a health condition, and they have developed a friendship. He no longer feels like he is the only one who has problems. Eddie and the other student have been educating their classmates together.

Eddie thinks the opinions of classmates vary. He stated, "Some kids don't care if you're different. They care about your insides. Other kids called me 'pipe neck.' I ignored it even though it hurt. I tell my friend who also has a trach and is scared, 'You will have friends.'"

* * *

Robin has not had many visible signs of her health condition and has not needed to have a caregiver with her all of the time. She always has succeeded in school and has developed close friendships.

During Robin's last year in nursery school, she required a nasogastric tube in her nose—a temporary, direct access to her stomach. Her teacher and the director of the school decided not to say anything to her classmates unless they brought up the subject. In retrospect, that probably was a mistake, because the other students stopped looking at Robin's face. When Robin was in kindergarten, a doll that had her equipment was used to orient her classmates. Some of the students were afraid of touching it, but they all wanted to put the clear dressing on the doll. One student talked about having stitches when he fell. In first grade, Robin's parents passed around a doll, and one girl said, "Ick, that is disgusting." Another student said, "I would say to the doll, 'I want to be your friend and it's not a big deal.'" Some students are afraid, but there always are students whose reactions help other students cope.

* * *

When Brian returned to school after his injury, the other students, especially the boys, avoided him because of the wheelchair and only one person remained his friend. Brian had two best friends in high school, both of whom were girls. As far as girls are concerned, Brian thinks he probably would be married someday were it not for his accident. Now, he plans just to have girlfriends, friends who are girls.

Brian doesn't think anything would have helped his friends to be more under-standing. They didn't associate with him because of his accident. Brian stated, "I don't think I would have been any different if it had been someone else [who had the accident]. I think that is the way they [boys] are."

Classmate Preparation

Students need encouragement to explore their attitudes and concerns regarding illness, disability, and death. Teachers and parents must be ready and willing to discuss these issues and to express their own concerns, discomfort, and understandings.

The decision to share information with classmates, teachers, and others in the school setting is a personal one that is based on culture, values, and experiences. A student's and family's specific needs and wishes concerning disclosure should be considered when planning peer awareness education. In the following excerpt, a teacher describes her efforts to provide orientation for a student assisted by medical technology:

It is important to prepare classmates and to model respect and expectation. I have used discussions, pictures, books, and dolls. It is important that the level of the presentation and answers to the students' questions be age appropriate. In my presentations to students, I emphasize that the individual is a student just like them and the student likes to do what they like to do but may not be able to do it in the same way.

I encourage students' help and participation to find ways things could be done differently to include the student, experience using adaptive equipment (e.g., wheelchairs, walkers), and learn alternative means of communication (e.g., sign language, communication boards).

The inclusion of students with health care needs offers opportunities for life experiences that few students have in school. We discovered that people learn in different ways and that everyone has strengths and weaknesses. Classmates also learned that people who look different can be their friends and playmates.

THE EXPERIENCE OF SCHOOL PERSONNEL

Teachers, administrators, and school nurses have different experiences and different reactions when a student who is assisted by medical technology is included in their school. One teacher stated

Several years ago I met with the family of a student who would be transferring into my classroom. The student had significant medical issues that required training of school staff and support of nursing personnel. After the support personnel (i.e., school nurse, speech-language therapist, occupational therapist, and physical therapist) gave their reports and recommendations for services, I turned to the parents and asked them to tell me their goals and dreams for their child. They told me that they had always expected him to "make it." They had this expectation despite what they had been told. They believed in him and gave him as many opportunities to develop his skills as they possibly could. After I heard their story, I was a little less overwhelmed by the special needs of this student. I thought, "I am only responsible for a school year! Parents are responsible for a lifetime. I can do this!"

The Teacher's Experience

It is important that teachers are involved in the decisions about, and process of, including a student with special health needs in the classroom.

Conversations with teachers who work with students who are supported by medical technology revealed some of the teachers' needs and wishes (Caldwell, 1995). Teachers want to interact physically with the student in a safe manner, to devote enough time and attention to all their students, to be supported adequately and trained to deal with health care and special education needs of students, to receive emergency backup they can depend on, and to receive accurate information about liability.

Teachers' Feelings

When a teacher first hears that a student assisted by technology will be entering his or her program, initial feelings may range from fear of the unknown to excitement about a challenge. Teachers will have many questions regarding

- The student's technological needs
- The type of assistance and support the teacher will receive
- The student's educational needs
- The impact of the student's special needs on his or her classmates
- Who will provide health care procedures in school

It is imperative that these questions be answered clearly and completely by a qualified person so that the teacher is comfortable with the student's entrance.

Teachers' Resource and Training Needs

Once the teacher's initial questions have been answered, it is valuable for the teacher to meet the student and the student's family and caregivers. Family members and caregivers can discuss the student's educational history and needs as well as the supports required by the student. This meeting gives family members the opportunity to express their goals and dreams for the student and to participate in planning for the student's transition into the classroom. It also gives the teacher the opportunity to meet the student in a situation outside of the classroom, to be comfortable with the student's equipment and health care needs, and to get a sense of the student's humanness beyond his or her documented medical needs. For example, one teacher stated the following:

I found that I needed information about the student's health and technological needs that was clear and easily understood by someone who does not have a medical background. I benefited from written materials, discussions with medical support staff and family/caregivers, and demonstration and practice of procedures I needed to know in the event of an emergency in the classroom. Meeting with colleagues who had worked with students who had similar medical or technological needs also was extremely valuable. Colleagues helped assure me that I could work comfortably with such students. They suggested materials or equipment that they had found useful, scheduling ideas, methods of including peers and the student in educational programming, and methods for working successfully with the family/caregivers. I also realized that I needed more than one training session to work with students. I required periodic review and updating of health information and equipment during the course of the school year.

In addition to specific information about the student, teachers need information about the roles of support staff who will be working with the student or who will be available as needed. In many cases, teachers may not have worked with specialists such as occupational or physical therapists. Teacher awareness of therapists' skills makes referrals and consultations more productive.

Teachers need experience collaborating with school nurses (and school nurses with teachers). Health procedures are only one of the issues in education. The school nurse can be a resource for teachers by monitoring the student's health status in school and interpreting health information. Together, the teacher and school nurse in collaboration with the family can ascertain the student's strengths and coping patterns and help to maximize the student's independence while ensuring that his or her health status is maintained at an optimal level.

The teacher's role in planning for the student's participation in school can be crucial to a smooth transition, yet teachers frequently are not notified about a prospective student's anticipated entry. To encourage the full participation of teachers, their involvement in all aspects of planning should be ensured.

The Administrator's Experience

Administrators' Responsibilities

School administrators set the tone for inclusion of students with special health care needs and have the overall responsibility for all aspects of their participation. The following questions are relevant to the school administrators' responsibility:

1. Are teachers, families, and students part of the educational and health teams that develop the philosophy, policies, and procedures for students with special health care needs? Do they participate in making placement decisions about individual students? Have the following been considered?

    *   The concerns and fears of parents, students, faculty, and staff
    *   Confidentiality and universal precautions issues
    *   Risk management, including preparation for natural disasters and emergencies
    *   Transitions

2. Do school personnel, families, and health care personnel communicate regularly and are the different branches coordinated? Have the following been considered?

    *   Gathering and sharing of relevant health information
    *   Time for planning
    *   Collaboration within the school community among general and special education, school health care personnel, related services personnel, and ancillary personnel, such as dietary and transportation staff
    *   Systematic access and updating of health information

3. Do school personnel have the training, technical assistance, orientation, and supervision they need? Have the following been considered?

    *   Universal precautions and infection control issues
    *   Preparation for emergencies and natural disasters
    *   Preparation for the provision of health care procedures
    *   Ongoing supervision for the provision of health care services

School administrators also must work closely with teachers, school nurses, families, and related services personnel to address these issues (Janz, Caldwell, & Harrison, 1995):

*   Risk management concerns
*   Securing of resources and funding
*   Arrangements for transportation
*   Need for adequate electricity, lighting, and heat, and sufficient electrical outlets and power
*   Storage space for supplies and back-up equipment
*   Building and playground accessibility

In addition, administrators, like other school personnel, must deal with their own personal responses (e.g., issues of their own comfort with chronic illness, medical technology, treatment). Has the administrator received training concerning the specialized administrative issues associated with these students? Does the administrator have the support of the school board and community? Does the administrator have assistance from qualified health care personnel and the family? Have collaborative roles been delineated? Administrators are in key positions to influence the placement and care that students will receive. Knowledge, support, and leadership regarding students with special health care needs are essential.

The School Nurse's Experience

School Nurses' Responsibilities

School nurses in the United States have varied roles and responsibilities. These variations depend on many factors:

- Traditions of public health and school/community characteristics and priorities
- Existence of legislation and labor agreements that mandate school health services and/or specific qualifications for school nurses, school medical directors, and school health supervisors
- Leadership in state and local agencies
- Geographical setting (i.e., rural, urban, suburban)
- Level of training

Hootman (1994) discussed the multiple roles of school nurses today, including the following:

- *Collaborator* with multiple state, school, and community agencies; health care providers; and families to resolve health concerns
- *Case manager* of students with special needs
- *Catalyst* for health education
- *Resource person* linking students and families with other health and community services
- *Interpreter* of health information to students, families, and school personnel
- *Clinician* for students presenting illness and injury concerns and for monitoring students with ongoing health care issues that may affect their learning ability and/or safety in school

According to the National Association of School Nurses, Inc. (NASN) (1989), the purpose of school nursing is to strengthen and facilitate the educational process by improving and protecting the health status of students. School nurses also provide assistance in the removal or modification of health-related barriers to the learning process. NASN Standards of School Nursing Practice (Proctor, Lordi, & Zaiger, 1993), based on the American Nurses Association Standards of Clinical Nursing Practice, are listed in Table 1.1. Examples of other nursing standards that apply to school nursing practice include the American Nurses Association's *Standards of Clinical Nursing Practice* (1991) and the National Association of State School Nurse Consultants' position paper, "Delegation of School Health Services to Unlicensed Assistive Personnel" (1995) (see Chapter 3).

With the varied roles, responsibilities, and caseloads of school nurses, meeting the special needs of students with more complex health problems is a challenge. Some school systems have a full-time school nurse with adequate administrative and clinical support in every school. In many districts, obstacles to providing safe and appropriate care for students with special health care needs are significant. Standards for safe care include the following:

- Adequate staffing and resources
- Availability of school nurse supervisors/directors to identify staffing needs; develop and evaluate health services programs; and provide support, consultation, and supervision for school nurses
- Opportunities for school nurses to update clinical knowledge and skills and consult with health professionals in the community
- Additional nursing coverage in schools when indicated (e.g., by nursing assessment) for the safe care of students
- Administrative support for nurse participation in evaluating and planning programs for students with special needs
- Adequate preparation of school nurses to contribute health-related educational goals and objectives to students' individualized education programs
- Knowledge of nursing licensure, delegation requirements, and nursing competencies at each level of preparation (e.g., licensed practical/vocational nurses; hospital-prepared registered nurses; associate-, bachelor-, and master-degreed registered nurses).

Many school systems throughout the United States recognize the need for increased nursing services to ensure the safe and appropriate education of students with special health care needs. These systems are using a number of creative mechanisms to provide

Table 1.1. NASN Standards of School Nursing Practice

1. The school nurse utilizes a distinct knowledge base for decision making in nursing practice.
2. The school nurse uses a systematic approach to problem solving in nursing practice.
3. The school nurse contributes to the education of the client with special health needs by assessing the client, planning and providing appropriate nursing care, and evaluating the identified outcomes of care.
4. The school nurse uses effective written, verbal, and nonverbal communication skills.
5. The school nurse establishes and maintains a comprehensive school health program.
6. The school nurse collaborates with other school professionals, parents, and caregivers to meet the health, developmental, and educational needs of clients.
7. The school nurse collaborates with members of the community in the delivery of health and social services and utilizes knowledge of community health systems and resources to function as a school–community liaison.
8. The school nurse assists students, families, and the school community to achieve optimal levels of wellness through appropriately designed and delivered health education.
9. The school nurse contributes to nursing and school health through innovations in practice and participation in research or research-related activities.
10. The school nurse identifies, delineates, and clarifies the nursing role, promotes quality of care, pursues continued professional enhancement, and demonstrates professional conduct.

From Proctor, S., Lordi, S., & Zaiger, D. (1993). *School nursing practice: Roles and standards,* pp. 226–233. Scarborough, ME: National Association of School Nurses, Inc.; reprinted by permission.

stable funding for school nurses. An article in the *American School Board Journal* (Essex, Schifari, & Bowman, 1994) recommended that a school nurse or other certified medical person be assigned to every school in the district to provide written instruction, technical assistance, and supervision to teachers as well as direct service to children with complex health care needs.

Relationships Between School Nurses and Families

The relationship between a school nurse (or home health nurse) and a family may be complex and takes time to develop. The only clear tool that the nurse and family have is open, honest communication. This means that the nurse, family, and school personnel will need to schedule time for regular meetings and be flexible about scheduling additional conferences on an as-needed basis. Open communication can help clarify roles and responsibilities and ensure that everyone has the information he or she needs to care adequately for the student's health, educational, and developmental needs.

In the following excerpts, Eddie's mother describes her relationships with nurses:

Initially, I was very clear that I did not trust nurses in the community or those at home or school. It is difficult because they are responsible for your child. You have to do it one relationship at a time and a day at a time. It is hard to let go once your child has had so many medical crises. Once we began to know each other better, the school nurse was able to help. For instance, she helps me balance what is normal childhood stuff and what is really related to Eddie's diagnosis. I have an excellent relationship with her now. I trust her, and we work things out together. For instance, when he needed an intravenous line at home, she was able to help me learn how to use it. For Eddie, the school nurse has the added role of counselor. Eddie knows he has a friend in her. I think this is true for many students with special health conditions. The nurse may be the only person in school who really understands what these students are going through.

I advocate that school nurses go to the primary hospital for updating skills. The relationship between the hospital personnel and the school nurse is an important one.

Relations with Eddie's private duty nurse were complex. Sometimes I felt she was trying to take him over. I bit my tongue many times and other times I said to her, "Well, that's how we do it." We had to write in the health plan that she would stop going everywhere with him.

SUMMARY

This chapter provides basic information about the population of students assisted by medical technology; the educational, social, and emotional implications of their participation in school; and the responsibilities of school personnel, including teachers, administrators, and nurses. Chapter 2 addresses aspects of school and advocacy law that affect the participation of students supported by medical technology and treatment in school. Chapter 3 addresses collaboration and teamwork; the process of developing safe, educationally relevant school programs; and the roles of teachers, administrators, nurses, and families in that process. Chapter 4 addresses transportation issues related to students with special health care needs; and Chapter 5 focuses on the special concerns related to universal precautions, latex allergies, and HIV and AIDS. Chapter 6 provides useful checklists and forms for people providing special health care needs, and Secion II addresses specific technologies and treatments.

Students who have special health care needs can participate successfully in school when they are given the appropriate supports. The three students and families who share their perspectives in this chapter have had good experiences. To make good experiences possible for other students, there is a need to continue to listen to students and their families, teachers, administrators, and health personnel to learn what to do to improve the education of these students. This chapter is only a beginning.

REFERENCES

American Nurses Association. (1991). *Standards of clinical nursing practice.* Kearneysville, WV: Author.

Beckett, K. (1994, April). *Students supported by medical technology: The student's experience.* Paper presented at the meeting of Project School Care, Boston, MA.

Caldwell, T.H. (1995). Students supported by ventilation in school: The experience of teachers and students (Doctoral dissertation, Teachers College, Columbia University, 1995). *Dissertation Abstracts International,* UMI9539814.

Caldwell, T.H., Todaro, A., & Gates, A.J. (1989). *Community provider's guide: An information outline for working with children with special health care needs in the community.* New Orleans, LA: Children's Hospital.

Essex, N., Schifari, J., & Bowman, S. (1994). Handle with care. *American School Board Journal, 181*(3), 50–53.

Hootman, J. (1994). Nursing our most valuable natural resource: School age children. *Nursing Forum, 29*(3), 5–17.

Janz, J., Caldwell, T.H., & Harrison, J. (1995). Children with special health conditions in school. In M.B. Goor (Ed.), *Case studies of leadership in special education* (pp. 200–228). San Diego, CA: Harcourt Brace Jovanovich.

National Association of School Nurses, Inc. (NASN). (1989). *Philosophy of school health services and school nursing.* Scarborough, ME: Author.

National Association of State School Nurse Consultants. (1995). Delegation of school health services to unlicensed assistive personnel: A position paper of the National Association of State School Nurse Consultants. *Journal of School Nursing, 11*(2), 16–18.

Palfrey, J.S., Haynie, M., Porter, S., Fenton, T., Cooperman-Vincent, P., Shaw, D., Johnson, B., Bierle, T., & Walker, D.K. (1994). Prevalence of medical technology assistance among children in Massachusetts in 1987 and 1990. *Public Health Reports, 109*(2), 226–233.

Proctor, S., Lordi, S., & Zaiger, D. (1993). *School nursing practice: Roles and standards.* Scarborough, ME: National Association of School Nurses, Inc.

SUGGESTED READINGS

Ahearn, E.I. (1993, September). *Medicaid as a resource for students with disabilities.* Alexandria, VA: National Association of State Directors of Special Education.

Ahmann, E., & Lipsi, K.A. (1991). Early intervention for technology-dependent infants and young children. *Infants and Young Children, 3*(4), 67–77.

Albrecht, D.G. (1995). *Raising a child who has a physical disability.* New York: John Wiley & Sons.

Anderson, P.P., & Fenichel, E.S. (1989). *Serving culturally diverse families of infants and toddlers with disabilities.* Washington, DC: National Center for Clinical Infant Programs.

Anderson, W., Chitwood, S., & Hayden, D. (1990). *Negotiating the special education maze: A guide for parents and teachers.* Rockville, MD: Woodbine House.

Ault, M.M., Graff, G.C., & Rues, J.P. (1993). Special health care procedures and teaching. In M. Snell (Ed.), *Systematic instruction of persons with severe disabilities* (4th ed., pp. 215–247). Columbus, OH: Charles E. Merrill.

Batshaw, M.L. (1991). *Your child has a disability: A complete source book of daily and medical care.* Boston: Little, Brown.

Bauer, D. (1994). School health services: Supporting students with special health needs. *Impact, 7*(2), 8–9.

Beckman, P.J., & Boyes, G.B. (1993). *Deciphering the system: A guide for families of young children with disabilities.* Cambridge, MA: Brookline Books.

Behrman, R.E. (1993). Update on children's health care. *American Journal of Disabled Children, 147*(5), 539.

Best, S., Carpignano, J., Sirvis, B., & Bigge, J. (1991). Psychosocial aspects of physical disability. In J. Bigge (Ed.), *Teaching individuals with physical and multiple disabilities* (3rd ed., pp. 102–131). Columbus, OH: Charles E. Merrill.

Bleck, E.E., & Nagel, D.A. (1982). *Physically handicapped children: A medical atlas for teachers.* New York: Grune & Stratton.

Blenk, K., & Landau-Fine, D. (1995). *Making school inclusion work: A guide to everyday practices.* Cambridge, MA: Brookline Books.

Budreau, G., & Chase, L. (1994). A family-centered approach to the development of a pediatric family satisfaction questionnaire. *Pediatric Nursing, 20*(6), 604–608.

Caldwell, T.H., & Kirkhart, K. (1991). Accessing the education system for students who require health technology and treatment. In N.J. Hochstadt & D.M. Yost (Eds.), *The medically complex child: The transition to home care* (pp. 122–138). New York: Harwood Academic.

Caldwell, T.H., & Sirvis, B.P. (1991). Students with special health conditions: An emerging population presents new challenges. *Preventing School Failure, 35*(3), 13–18.

Caldwell, T.H., Sirvis, B.P., Todaro, A., & Alcouloumre, D. (1991). *Special health care in the school.* Reston, VA: Council for Exceptional Children.

Caldwell, T.H., Todaro, A.W., & Gates, A.J. (1991). Special health care needs. In J. Bigge (Ed.), *Teaching individuals with physical and multiple disabilities* (3rd ed., pp. 50–74) Columbus, OH: Charles E. Merrill.

Caldwell, T.H., Todaro, A., Gates, A.J., Failla, S., & Kirkhart, K. (1991). *Community provider's guide: An information outline for working with children with special health care needs.* New Orleans, LA: Children's Hospital.

Commonwealth of Massachusetts Department of Education. (1994). *Fact sheet: Massachusetts municipal Medicaid program for special education services.* Malden, MA: Author.

Cutler, B.C. (1993). *You, your child, and "special" education: A guide to making the system work.* Baltimore: Paul H. Brookes Publishing Co.

Delaney, N., & Zolondick, K. (1991). Day care for technology-dependent infants and children: A new alternative. *Journal of Perinatal Neonatal Nursing, 5*(1), 80–85.

Diehl, S.F., Moffitt, K.A., & Wade, S.M. (1991). Focus group interview with parents of children with medically complex needs: An intimate look at their perceptions and feelings. *Children's Health Care, 20*(3), 170–178.

Eliades, D.C., & Suitor, C.W. (1994). *Celebrating diversity: Approaching families through their food.* Arlington, VA: National Center for Education in Maternal and Child Health.

Exceptional Parent. (1996, January). Resource guide: Directories of national organizations, associations, products & services [Special issue].

Fields, A.I., Coble, D.H., Pollack, M.M., & Kaufman, J. (1991). Outcome of home care for technology-dependent children: Success of an independent, community-based case management model. *Pediatric Pulmonology, 11*(4), 310–317.

Fuchs, D., & Fuchs, L. (1991). Framing the REI debate: Abolitionists versus conservationists. In J.W. Lloyd, N.N. Singh, & A.C. Repp (Ed.), *The regular education initiative: Alternative perspectives on concepts, issues, and models* (pp. 241–251). Sycamore, IL: Sycamore Publishing Co.

Gartner, A., & Lipsky, D.K. (1987). Beyond special education: Toward a quality system for all students. *Harvard Educational Review, 57*(4), 367–395.

Gaylord, C.L., & Leonard, A.M. (1988). *A guide to health care coverage for the child with a chronic illness or disability.* Madison, WI: Center for Public Representation.

Greey, M. (1994). *Honouring diversity: A cross-cultural approach to infant development for babies with special needs.* Toronto, Ontario, Canada: Centennial Infant and Child Centre.

Harry, B. (1992). *Cultural diversity, families, and the special education system.* New York: Teachers College Press.

Haupt, R., Fears, T.R., Robison, L.L., Mills, J.L., Nicholson, L.K., Zeltzer, A.T., Meadows, A.T., & Byrne, J. (1994). Educational attainment in long-term survivors of childhood acute lymphoblastic leukemia. *Journal of the American Medical Association, 272*(18), 1427–1432.

Hirsch, D. (1994, July). Questions about incontinence. *Exceptional Parent: Parenting Your Child With a Disability* [Special issue] p. 33.

Hixson, D.D., Stoff, E., & White, P. (1992). Parents of children with chronic health impairments: A new approach to advocacy training. *Children's Health Care, 21*(2), 111-115.

Hobbs, N., Perrin, J.M., & Ireys, H.Y. (1985). *Chronically ill children and their families.* San Francisco: Jossey-Bass.

Hochstadt, N.J., & Yost, D.M. (1991). The health care–child welfare partnership: The transition of medically complex children to the community. In N.J. Hochstadt & D.M. Yost (Eds.), *The medically complex child: The transition to home care.* New York: Harwood Academic.

Hostler, S.L. (1994). *Family-centered care: An approach to implementation.* Charlottesville: University of Virginia Press.

Igoe, J.B. (1994). School nursing. *Nursing Clinics of North America, 29*(3), 443–458.

Jackson, P.L., & Vessey, J.A. (1992). *Primary care of the child with a chronic condition.* St. Louis, MO: C.V. Mosby.

Joint Task Force for the Management of Children with Special Health Needs. (1990). *Guidelines for the delineation of roles and responsibilities for the safe delivery of specialized health care in the educational setting.* Reston, VA: Council for Exceptional Children.

Kaufman, J. (1991). An overview of public sector financing for pediatric home care: Part 1. *Pediatric Nursing, 17*(3), 280–281.

Kirk, J. (1993). They didn't tell teachers about students like Frankie. *The Special Edge, 7*(7), 16.

Kohrman, A.F. (1991). Medical technology: Implications for health and social service providers. In N.J. Hochstadt & D.M. Yost (Eds.), *The medically complex child: The transition to home care* (pp. 3–14). New York: Harwood Academic.

Krajicek, M.J., & Moore, C.A. (1993). Child care for infants and toddlers with disabilities and chronic illnesses. *Focus on Exceptional Children, 25*(8), 1–16.

Krementz, J. (1989). *How it feels to fight for your life.* Boston: Little, Brown.

Langer, J.C. (1995). What is the role of the pediatric surgeon in the care of children with motility disorders? *The Messenger: A Newsletter of the American Pseudo-Obstruction and Hirschsprung's Disease Society, Inc., 7*(2), 8–9.

Larson, G., & Kahn, J.A. (1990). *How to get quality care for a child with special needs: A guide to health services and how to pay for them.* St. Paul, MN: Lifeline Press.

Leff, P.T., & Walizer, E.H. (1992). *Building the healing partnership: Parents, professionals and children with chronic illnesses and disabilities.* Cambridge, MA: Brookline Books.

Lehr, D.H. (1990). Providing education to students with complex health care needs. *Focus on Exceptional Children, 22*(7), 9–12.

Lehr, D.H., & McDaid, P. (1993). Opening the door further: Integrating students with complex health care needs. *Focus on Exceptional Children, 25*(6), 1–7.

Lehr, D.H., & Noonan, M.J. (1989). Issues in the education of students with complex health care needs. In F. Brown & D.H. Lehr (Eds.), *Persons with profound disabilities: Issues and practices* (pp. 139–160). Baltimore: Paul H. Brookes Publishing Co.

Leibold, S. (1994, July). Achieving bowel continence. *Exceptional Parent, Parenting Your Child With a Disability* [Special Issue] p. 33.

Lieberman, G. (1995). Quality: It's everywhere. *Exceptional Parent, 25*(8), 34–35.

Lipsky, D., & Gartner, A. (1995). Common questions about inclusion. *Exceptional Parent, 25*(8), 36–39.

Lynch, E.W., Lewis, R.B., & Murphy, D.S. (1993). Educational services for children with chronic illness: Perspectives of educators and families. *Exceptional Children, 59*(3), 210–220.

Lynch, E.W., Lewis, R.B., & Murphy, D.S. (1993). Improving education for children with chronic illness. *Principal, 73*(2), 38–40.

Maternal and Child Health. (1990, May). *Improving state services for culturally diverse populations.* Work group session convened during the National Conference: "Cultural Perspectives in Service Delivery for Children and Families with Special Needs," Washington, DC.

McCarthy, M.M. (1993). Can costs be considered in special education placements? *Journal of Law and Education, 22*(3), 265–282.

McCormick, M.C., Gortmaker, S.L., & Sobol, A.M. (1990). Very low birthweight children: Behavior problems and school difficulty in a national sample. *Journal of Pediatrics, 117*(5), 687–693.

McManus, M.A. (1988). *Understanding your health insurance options: A guide for families who have children with special health care needs.* Washington, DC: Association for the Care of Children's Health.

Merkens, M.J. (1991). From intensive care unit to home: The role of pediatric transitional care. In N.J. Hochstadt & D.M. Yost (Eds.), *The medically complex child: The transition to home care* (pp. 61–78). New York: Harwood Academic.

Newacheck, P.W., Budetti, P.P., & McManus, M. (1984). Trends in childhood disability. *American Journal of Public Health, 74*(3), 232–236.

Newacheck, P.W., & Taylor, W.R. (1992). Childhood chronic illness: Prevalence, severity, and impact. *American Journal of Public Health, 82*(3), 364–371.

Palfrey, J.S., Haynie, M., McManus, M., Fenton, T., & Shaw, D. (1995, May). *A study of the financing of services for children with complex medical conditions.* Paper presented at the Annual Ambulatory Pediatric Association Meeting, San Diego, CA.

Palfrey, J.S., McGaughey, M.J., Cooperman, P.J., Fenton, T., & McManus, M.A. (1991). Financing health services in school-based clinics: Do nontraditional programs tap traditional funding sources? *Journal of Adolescent Health, 12*(3), 233–239.

Passarelli, C. (1993). *School nursing: Trends for the future.* Washington, DC: National Health Education Consortium.

Perrin, J.M., Shayne, M.W., & Bloom, S.R. (1993). *Home and community care for chronically ill children.* New York: Oxford University Press.

Pesata, V.L. (1994). Applying Benner's model to school nursing of multiple handicapped children. *Clinical Nurse Specialist, 8*(5), 230–233.

Peterson, N., Barber, P., & Ault, M.M. (1994). Children with special health care needs in early childhood special education. In B. Spodek & P. Stafford (Eds.), *Yearbook in early childhood education* (Vol. 5). New York: Teachers College Press.

Putnam, J.W. (Ed.). (1993). *Cooperative learning and strategies for inclusion: Celebrating diversity in the classroom.* Baltimore: Paul H. Brookes Publishing Co.

Rainforth, B., York, J., & Macdonald, C. (1992). *Collaborative teams for students with severe disabilities: Integrating therapy and educational services.* Baltimore: Paul H. Brookes Publishing Co.

Randall-David, E. (1989). *Strategies for working with culturally diverse communities and clients.* Bethesda, MD: Association for the Care of Children's Health.

Research and Training Center on Family Support and Children's Mental Health. (1994). Developing culturally competent organizations. *Focal Point, 8*(2), 1–29.

Rogers, J.J. (1991). Schools, insurance & your family's financial security. *Exceptional Parent, 21*(6), 76–78.

Rogers, J.J. (1993). *Third party billing for special education: Panacea or mirage?* Cambridge, MA: Brookline Books.

Rubovits, D.S., & Siegel, A.W. (1994). Developing conceptions of chronic disease: A comparison of disease experience. *Children's Health Care, 23*(4), 267–285.

Seligman, M., & Darling, R.B. (1989). *Ordinary families, special children.* New York: Guilford Press.

Shapiro, J.P. (1994). *No pity: People with disabilities forging a new civil rights movement.* Chicago: Times Books.

Shelton, T.L., Jeppson, E.S., & Johnson, B.H. (1992). *Family centered care for children with special health care needs.* Bethesda, MD: Association for the Care of Children's Health.

Sirvis, B. (1988). Students with special health care needs. *Teaching Exceptional Children, 20*(4), 40–44.

Sirvis, B.P., & Caldwell, T.H. (1995). Physical disabilities and chronic health impairments. In E.L. Meyer & T.M. Skrtic, *Special education and student disability: An introduction* (pp. 533–562). Denver, CO: Love.

Smokoski, F., & Paulmeno, C. (1991, January). A study of public school medical assistance pilot program. In Colorado Department of Education (Ed.), *Public school medical assistance pilot program* (Article 82, pp. 1–30). Denver, CO: Author.

Sobsey, D., & Cox, A.W. (1996). Integrating health care and educational programs. In F.P. Orelove & D. Sobsey, *Educating children with multiple disabilities: A transdisciplinary approach* (3rd ed., pp. 155–186). Baltimore: Paul H. Brookes Publishing Co.

Spector, R.E. (1991). *Cultural diversity in health and illness.* Norwalk, CT: Appleton and Lange.

Stainback, W., & Stainback, S. (Eds.). (1990). *Support networks for inclusive schooling: Interdependent integrated education.* Baltimore: Paul H. Brookes Publishing Co.

Stein, R.E. (1989). *Caring for children with chronic illness: Issues and strategies.* New York: Springer-Verlag.

Stutts, A.L. (1994). Selected outcomes of technology dependent children receiving home care and prescribed child care services. *Pediatric Nursing, 20*(5), 501–507.

Thousand, J.S., & Villa, R.A. (1990). Strategies for educating learners with severe disabilities within their local home, schools, and communities. *Focus on Exceptional Children, 23*(3), 1–24.

Tyler, J.S., & Colson, S. (1994). Common pediatric disabilities: Medical aspects and educational implications. *Focus on Exceptional Children, 27*(4), 1–16.

Walker, D.K. (1984). Care of chronically ill children in schools. *Pediatric Clinics of North America, 31*(1), 221–233.

Walker, D.K., Epstein, S.G., Taylor, A.B., Crocker, A.C., & Tuttle, G.A. (1989). Perceived needs of families with children who have chronic health conditions. *Children's Health Care, 18*(2), 196–201.

Wells, N., Anderson, B., & Popper, B. (1993). *Families in program and policy: Report of a 1992 survey of family participation in state Title V programs for children with special health care needs.* Boston: CAPP National Parent Resource Center, Federation for Children with Special Needs.

White, K.R., & Immel, N. (1990). *Medicaid and other third party payments: One piece of the early intervention financing puzzle.* Bethesda, MD: National Center for Family-Centered Care.

Legal Issues in the Education of Students with Special Health Care Needs

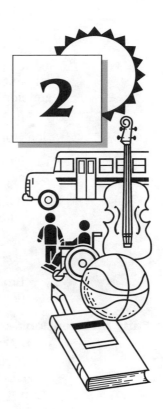

*Janice Rutledge Janz, Henry A. Beyer,
Nadine Schwab, Betsy Anderson,
Terry Heintz Caldwell, and Jacqueline Harrison*

A ll children in the United States have the right to a free appropriate public education. Since 1970, significant laws and legal precedents have established procedures for ensuring and protecting that right for children with disabilities. This chapter discusses federal, state, and case laws as well as a number of regulations and professional standards. Laws cannot, and do not attempt to, address every special health care need or every school situation. They leave room for interpretation that, at times, can frustrate and confuse educational personnel, families, and lawyers. That interpretation is dynamic, reflecting U.S. society's changing views and values regarding the rights of students with disabilities.

People who interact with students with special health care needs in school have diverse backgrounds and experiences. These people include parents, teachers, school nurses, secretaries, administrators, social workers, allied health professionals, community providers, volunteers, and paraprofessionals. An understanding of the services supported by the law is important for people working with students with special health care needs to facilitate quality educational programs.

THE INDIVIDUALS WITH DISABILITIES EDUCATION ACT (IDEA) OF 1990

The major legislation supporting children with disabilities is the Individuals with Disabilities Education Act (IDEA) of 1990 (PL 101-476), formerly the Education for All Handicapped Children Act of 1975 (PL 94-142). The purpose of IDEA is

> to assure that all children with disabilities have available to them, within the time periods specified in Sec. 1412(2)(B) of this title, a free appropriate public

Preparation of this chapter was supported in part by Project No. MCJ-225047 from the Maternal and Child Health Program (Title V, Social Security Act), Health Resources and Services Administration, U.S. Department of Health and Human Services.

education which emphasizes special education and related services designed to meet their unique needs. (20 U.S.C. § 1400[c])

This federal law entitles all children between the ages of 3 and 21 who have disabilities that interfere with their educational progress to a free appropriate public education. Some federal money helps states enact this law, but the amount from the federal government has never reached the levels originally targeted.

The language of the law is general, but detailed rules and regulations are contained in the Code of Federal Regulations (CFR). Each state also has a special education law and associated regulations. Local school system administrators also develop their own school policies and procedures, but these are not laws. Figure 2.1 illustrates IDEA's progression from the federal to the local level.

IDEA is divided into eight parts. The following four parts have significant implications for students with special health care needs:

1. Early intervention services provided for infants and toddlers (from birth to 3 years of age) (Part H)

2. IDEA's general purpose, applicability of IDEA, and definitions of children ages 3–21 who qualify (Part A)

3. State and local educational agency obligations in providing services for children ages 3–21 (Part B)

4. Process to be used in case of disagreement regarding special educational issues (Part E)

Early Intervention Services (Part H)

In 1986, Congress enacted the Education of the Handicapped Act Amendments (PL 99-457), which offered states financial assistance to implement early intervention services for children from birth through age 2 years, 11 months. In 1991 PL 99-457 was reauthorized as PL 102-119, the Individuals with Disabilities Education Act Amendments. The basic purpose of these services is to identify and evaluate children with disabilities and provide intervention services as early as possible. Families, service providers, and health care professionals can refer infants and toddlers who they suspect are at risk for or have developmental delays for early intervention services.

A multidisciplinary assessment is conducted to determine *eligibility* for early intervention services. Requirements for eligibility are met by children under the age of 3

with developmental delays or with a diagnosed physical or mental condition (e.g., cerebral palsy, Down syndrome) or who are at risk of having substantial developmental delays if early intervention services are not provided (e.g., low birth weight, mother addicted to cocaine). This particular criterion is at the discretion of each state. (20 U.S.C. § 1472[1])

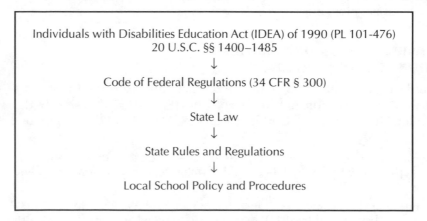

Figure 2.1. The progression of IDEA from the federal to the local level.

Early intervention services may include the following:

- Family training, counseling, and home visits
- Special instruction
- Speech therapy and audiology
- Occupational therapy
- Physical therapy
- Case management
- Diagnostic medical services
- Health services
- Social work
- Vision services
- Assistive technology
- Transportation
- Psychological services (Title 34, CFR § 1472[E])

An *individualized family service plan* (IFSP) refers to the actual meeting between parents and professionals in which the plan for early intervention services is discussed and to the written document that states the details of the plan. It is important that family members and professionals work as a team to develop the best IFSP for each child and family. Families know their children best and can give ideas for the best way to carry out the IFSPs.

The plan that is developed by the team is written down. The law explains that every IFSP document must include the following parts:

- The child's level of development
- The family's strengths and needs as they relate to the child's development
- Major outcomes expected for the child and accompanying time lines
- Early intervention services that are to be provided and the environments in which services will be delivered
- The dates on which services are expected to start and how long they will last
- The name of the case manager who will be responsible for implementing and coordinating the plan
- The steps to be taken to support the transition of the toddler to school programs (Part H) (20 U.S.C. § 1477[d])

Early intervention services can be offered at a variety of places, such as the home, clinic, center, or school.

General Purpose (Part A)

Part A of IDEA defines some of the key terms used in the laws. *Children with disabilities* are defined as children

> with mental retardation, hearing impairments including deafness, speech or language impairments, visual impairments including blindness, serious emotional disturbance, orthopedic impairments, autism, traumatic brain injury, other health impairments, or specific learning disabilities. (20 U.S.C. § 1401[a][1][A])

The Code of Federal Regulations further clarifies these terms. For example, *other health impairment* is defined as

> having limited strength, vitality or alertness, due to chronic or acute health problems such as a heart condition, tuberculosis, rheumatic fever, nephritis, asthma, sickle cell anemia, hemophilia, epilepsy, lead poisoning, leukemia, or diabetes that adversely affects a child's educational performance. (Title 34, CFR § 300.7[b][8])

The definition is phrased broadly; many students whose educational performance is delayed by frequent absences as a result of illness may qualify under this category. Students who have one of these conditions and are progressing in the general education program, however, may not need services under IDEA. Many state laws and regulations clarify the definition of *other health impairment* even further. Some states have added specific conditions such as Tourette syndrome (New York) and attention deficit disorder

(Arkansas and Louisiana) to the state definition. Furthermore, states may add additional categories of disability (e.g., Connecticut added neurologically impaired). *Note:* Many students not eligible under IDEA would receive services under Section 504 of the Rehabilitation Act of 1973 (PL 93-112) (see pp. 28–29).

Services for Children Ages 3–21 (Part B)

Part B of IDEA explains state and local educational responsibilities in providing services for children ages 3–21. This part of the law includes various components, such as identification, evaluation, confidentiality, and time lines, and addresses many important considerations for students with special health care needs. The following three considerations are addressed in this chapter: individualized education program (IEP), least restrictive environment (LRE), and related services. Also addressed in this chapter are transition services.

Individualized Education Program

An IEP is

> a written statement for each child with a disability developed in any meeting by a representative of the local educational agency or an intermediate educational unit who shall be qualified to provide, or supervise the provision of, specially designed instruction to meet the unique needs of children with disabilities, the teacher, the parents or guardian of such child, and, whenever appropriate, such child (20 U.S.C. § 1401[a][20])

The IEP serves as the agreement between the school district and the child and family. It is extremely important, therefore, that both education and health services required by the student for educational purposes are written in the IEP.

The IEP addresses the following:

- Present levels of educational performance
- Annual goals, including short-term instructional objectives
- Specific educational and related services to be provided
- When the child will participate in general educational programs
- A statement of transition services needed to prepare the student for life after leaving school
- When services will begin and how long they will last
- How to measure whether instructional objectives are being achieved (20 U.S.C. § 1401[a]20)

The IEP must be reviewed at least once each year, but it can be reviewed and modified more often if necessary. It is important for the IEP to contain goals that promote maximal independence in self-care (e.g., the student will assist in catheterization). The school nurse, families, and other health care professionals can provide important information about the scope and sequence of skills necessary for a particular child to achieve goals toward independence in self-care.

Least Restrictive Environment

The LRE principle stresses the importance of trying to include all students in the general classroom. IDEA clearly encourages the inclusion of students with disabilities and calls for each public school agency to ensure

> (1) that to the maximum extent appropriate, children with disabilities, including children in public or private institutions or other care facilities, are educated with children who are nondisabled; and (2) that special classes, separate schooling or other removal of children with disabilities from the regular educational environment occurs only when the nature or severity of the disability is such that education in regular classes with the use of supplementary aids and services cannot be achieved satisfactorily. (20 U.S.C. § 1412[5][B])

The regulations also state that each public agency shall offer a choice of placement options. Placement options include a general class, special instruction in addition to general class, a special class, a special school, home, and a hospital.

At times, students with health conditions have been placed in special programs or alternative settings on the basis of their health care needs alone. Although health and safety issues require careful consideration, they are not the only factors that should determine placement. The primary concern is the student's education. Issues such as availability of a school nurse, a room that can provide privacy during a health care procedure, or proximity to an emergency room should not be the primary reasons for deciding which school a child attends. The law requires that education in the general classroom always must be the first option; other classroom settings should not be considered unless it is clear that appropriate education with the use of supportive aids and services in the general classroom cannot be achieved satisfactorily.

The following is an example of one student's achievements in an LRE. The student, who was diagnosed with quadriplegia at age 11 as a result of a skateboard accident, depends on a ventilator. He recently graduated with his high school class after attending a general classroom in which a trained student-specific professional attended to his health care needs (e.g., suctioning, tracheostomy care, ventilator monitoring, catheterization, feeding), recorded class notes, and administered academic tests orally in the general classroom.

Related Services

The regulations define the term *related services* as

> transportation and such developmental, corrective, and other supportive services as are required to assist a child with a disability to benefit from special education, and includes speech pathology and audiology, psychological services, physical and occupational therapy, recreation, including therapeutic recreation, early identification and assessment of disabilities in children, counseling services, including rehabilitation counseling, and medical services for diagnostic or evaluation purposes. The term also includes school health services, social work services in schools, and parent counseling and training. (Title 34, CFR § 300.16 [a])

For a service to be considered a related service, the student must qualify for special education, and there must be some indication that a particular service is necessary for the student to benefit from special education. The menu of related services is extensive but not exhaustive. Families should be aware of the broad range of services that may be provided under the law. Families are encouraged to describe the student's needs to school personnel and to think with them about how best to address those needs, including which related services may apply. Goals and objectives for these related services should be written in the IEP to address how the related service is necessary to the student's ability to function in the school environment (e.g., occupational therapy goal: Student will demonstrate a purposeful grasp; Objective: Student will manipulate a computer mouse usefully).

The regulations distinguish between medical services and school health services. Medical services that are acceptable as related services are those provided by a licensed physician to determine a child's medically related disability that results in the child's need for special education and related services (Title 34, CFR § 300.16[b][4]) and those provided for diagnostic and evaluation purposes (20 U.S.C. § 1401[a][17]).

Additional health information may be needed to clarify the implications of the child's condition for his or her academic progress and learning environment (e.g., school absences, energy level, procedures during the day). The school system, therefore, may be required by IDEA to provide or pay for the diagnostic medical services to obtain this health information, because it influences student learning, but the school system is not required to provide the medical services or services of a licensed physician to treat the health condition. School health services are provided by a qualified school nurse or other qualified person (Title 34, CFR § 300.16 b[11]) and not limited to diagnosis or evaluation.

The school system may be required by IDEA to provide various other health services, such as nursing assessment, monitoring, catheterization, administration of medication, gastrostomy tube feeding, lifting and positioning, and teaching self-care in the school setting.

Transition Services (Part B)

IDEA includes provisions for planning the transition of children and youth from one service system to another (e.g., making a transition from school services [Part B] to adult living after school). *Adolescent/adult transition services* are defined by IDEA as a coordinated set of activities based on students' needs, preferences, and interests that promotes movement from school to postschool activities. Activities include the following:

- Postsecondary education
- Vocational training
- Integrated employment
- Continuing and adult education
- Adult services
- Independent living
- Community participation (20 U.S.C. § 1401[a][19])

Planning for transition should begin in early adolescence. Some of the important topics that must be considered in planning for adult living situations are the following:

- Independent living
- Financial arrangements
- Postsecondary training
- Job-related activities
- Recreation
- Medical services

Procedural Safeguards (Part E)

Part E of IDEA presents the process designed to ensure that families of children with disabilities are involved in education decisions affecting their children. Under these guidelines, parents have a number of options, including the right to

1. Request an administrative due process hearing to appeal an IEP.

2. File a complaint with the state's Department of Education to complain formally of a violation of IDEA and its regulations.

3. File a complaint with the U.S. Department of Education Office for Civil Rights (OCR).

4. Appeal a hearing officer's decision in court.

IDEA entitles families and students to an impartial hearing on any matter related to identification, evaluation, placement, and the provision of a free appropriate public education. Either school system staff or families can take a disagreement to a due process hearing. School systems have an obligation to inform parents of any free or low-cost legal services that the parents may wish to retain. Time lines for due process are as follows:

1. A final decision in the hearing is reached at the local level within 45 days after the receipt of such a request.

2. If a review is requested by the state agency, a decision is reached within 30 days after the receipt of such a request (Title 34, CFR § 300.504–300.512).

Some states offer a two-tier system of due process. The case is first heard at the local level, and, if dissatisfaction still exists, appeals can be made to the state education agency (Gerry, 1987). Other states conduct due process hearings only at the state level; in these states the decision can be appealed to a state or federal court.

For early intervention, the law requires states to set up a system to protect the basic rights of the children and families who are involved in the statewide early intervention program. The state's lead agency is responsible for establishing procedural safeguards and ensuring their effective implementation.

Table 2.1 lists a number of ways families and school personnel can work well together as teams to avoid disputes and formal complaint procedures. Collaboration with agencies outside the educational realm is essential. Individualized transition planning meetings should include the student, the family, and educational personnel, as well as representatives from agencies, such as vocational rehabilitation, independent living programs, and community resource programs. It is important for everyone on the transition team to foster an atmosphere in which the student and family can express their future goals honestly and be full and active participants at all stages of the plan's development. The team should identify people, such as rehabilitation counselors, health care providers, case managers (or service coordinators), and families, who will help with follow-through of the plan once the student leaves school.

Mediation

Mediation is one choice some states have implemented to settle differences between schools and families. The process is more informal than a due process hearing, which is the legal hearing held when mediation fails. Mediation involves a mediator, a trained neutral person, who hears the positions of both parties. The role of the mediator is to facilitate the process, create compromise between the parties, and assist in reaching an agreement. The mediator also may offer suggestions to school staff and families. Final decisions are made by families and school personnel, not the mediator. Mediation provides an opportunity for the school staff and families to settle their differences before a due process hearing starts. States, however, cannot mandate that mediation occur before holding a due process hearing.

Case Law Related to IDEA

Federal and state laws and regulations contain many terms that are subject to widely differing interpretations. One avenue for interpretation rests with the courts. The following section discusses litigation that has occurred as well as how these decisions may affect similar cases in different areas of the United States.

IDEA regulations state that any party who disagrees with a decision made in a due process hearing and who has exhausted his or her right of appeal in the state administrative process may file a civil action in federal district court (Title 34, CFR § 300.511). Both federal and state courts have the authority to order changes to the IEP of any student in a school system that receives federal financial assistance (e.g., *Oberti v. Board of Education*, 1992). Both federal and state courts also have the authority, in a lawsuit filed under federal special education law (which later became known as IDEA), to rule that a

Table 2.1. Fostering teamwork

- Communicate openly and frequently.
- Develop positive team relationships.
- Meet jointly with families, school personnel, insurance representatives, and community providers to discuss ways for financing services.
- Recognize the importance of establishing a personal rapport that fosters collaboration and respect.
- Discuss possible dilemmas in planning meetings.
- Collect and share reports, records, and summaries from health care providers that explain the need for health care services during the school day.
- Encourage physicians and other health care providers to communicate with school personnel.
- Stress that family members and professionals are equal partners on the team.
- Involve individuals who make financial decisions in the school system.
- Begin with points that people agree on and then discuss issues that need to be resolved.
- Ask what everyone wants for the student.
- Stress the student's best interests and actions that promote the student's educational interests.
- Consider all opinions and suggestions.
- Provide written recognition to supervisors of the significant role employees have played in meetings.
- Ask advocates to attend team meetings.

state's standard for the level of educational service be provided when the state standard is higher than the federal standard (e.g., *David D. v. School Committee*, 1985).

Rulings of the U.S. Supreme Court constitute the law of the land. Thus, the decision described next, which was reached in *Board of Education v. Rowley* (1982), although it directly involved only one student in New York State, established the definitive legal interpretation of the term *appropriate* education in PL 94-142, which must, thenceforth, be followed by all school systems and federal and state courts across the United States. To reverse a Supreme Court interpretation of the provisions of a federal law, Congress must amend the law or enact another law superseding it.

Although decisions by lower courts are binding precedents only within the boundaries of the particular court's jurisdiction (i.e., federal judicial circuit, state), they still carry persuasive value and often are relied on and cited by courts in other jurisdictions when deciding the same issue.

The following two legal cases address issues of educational benefit. The Supreme Court set the minimum federal standard for determining what constitutes appropriate education; this language was further interpreted to include students with the most severe disabilities.

Educational Benefit
Case 1

Issue:	What is the minimum federal standard for determining what constitutes appropriate education?
Case:	*Board of Education of the Hendrick Hudson Central School District v. Rowley*, 458 U.S. 116 (1982)
Description:	The parents of a child with a hearing impairment claimed she had a right under PL 94-142 to the services of a sign language interpreter as part of her free appropriate public education.
Outcome:	Supreme Court ruling:
	• PL 94-142 does not require schools to provide the best possible education, but only to provide students with disabilities "access" to an appropriate education.
	• Services provided must be sufficient to provide "some educational benefit" or a "basic floor of opportunity."

Educational Benefit
Case 2

Issue:	All students with disabilities are entitled to a free appropriate public education.
Case:	*Timothy W. v. Rochester N.H. School District*, 875 F. 2d 954 (1989)
Description:	Timothy W. had vision and hearing impairments, cerebral palsy, frequent seizures, mental retardation requiring pervasive care, and no discernable communication skills. He had made no observable educational progress in the school year, and the school district sought to exclude him from special education services by contending that he was "not capable of benefiting from special education."
Outcome:	First Circuit Court ruling:
	• "[N]ot only are severely handicapped children not excluded from the Act, but the most severely handicapped are actually given priority under the Act."
	• "'Zero-reject' policy is at the core of the Act, and . . . no child, regardless of the severity of his or her handicap is to ever again be subjected to the deplorable state of affairs which existed at the time of the Act's passage in which millions of handicapped children received inadequate education or none at all." (*Timothy W. v. Rochester N.H. School District*, 1989, pp. 960–961)

Several legal cases that distinguish school health services from medical services have been relied on in subsequent cases deciding the obligation of school systems to provide for the special health care needs of students in school. Several courts have been willing to strike down federal Medicaid regulations that limited a child's Medicaid-paid nursing services to home, hospital, or skilled nursing facility, thereby enabling the nurse to accompany the child to school (e.g., *Detsel v. Sullivan*, 1990; *Skubel v. Sullivan*, 1990).

School Health Services Rather than Medical Services
Case 1

Issue:	Is clean intermittent catheterization a school health service that must be provided by the school as a "related service"?
Case:	*Irving Independent School District v. Tatro*, 468 U.S. 883 (1984)
Description:	Amber Tatro had spina bifida and needed clean intermittent catheterization to empty her bladder during the school day. Was clean intermittent catheterization considered a related service (school health service) or a medical service?
Outcome:	Supreme Court ruling:

- Clean intermittent catheterization is a "related service" under the federal special education law; it must, therefore, be provided by the public school.
- To receive related services under federal special education law, a child must require special education.
- Only those services necessary to aid a child to benefit from special education must be provided.
- School health services must be provided only if they can be performed by a nurse or other qualified person, not if they must be performed by a physician, not if they can be provided other than during the school day, and only if the service will not prove unduly expensive for the school.

School Health Services Rather than Medical Services
Case 2

Issues:	1. Are catheterization; tracheostomy suctioning; manual resuscitation; emergency aid for autonomic hyperreflexia; monitoring for mechanical failures of the ventilator; and assistance with eating, drinking, and reclining "related services," which the school district is responsible for providing, or "medical services," which it is not responsible for providing?
	2. Must these services be provided by a registered nurse (R.N.) or a licensed practical nurse (L.P.N.), or will a "skilled and trained care provider" suffice?
	3. Is the school district required to provide "related services" even when the child does not need "special education" in the form of a special or modified program of instructions?
Case:	*GF v. Cedar Rapids Community School District*, 22 IDELR 278 (1994/1995)
Description:	GF, a 13-year-old, sixth-grade student, was paralyzed from the neck down, used a motorized wheelchair controlled by "a puff-and-suck straw," depended on a ventilator, and required someone to attend to some of his personal needs, including assisting with urinary bladder catheterization once a day; the suctioning of his tracheostomy tube "as needed, but at least once every 6 hours"; help with eating and drinking at lunch; assistance in assuming a reclining position for 5 minutes each hour; manual resuscitation (i.e., manual pumping of an airbag) when the ventilator is checked for proper functioning; monitoring of the ventilator for a malfunction or electrical problem; and the performance of emergency procedures if GF were to

experience autonomic hyperreflexia (i.e., an uncontrolled visceral reaction to anxiety or a full bladder), a condition that usually has been alleviated by catheterization and that he never has experienced at school.

In a written request in July 1993, GF's mother asked the school system to provide these services. The school district refused, arguing that GF needed "continuous care by an appropriate licensed practitioner" with supervision by a registered nurse. These, the school district explained, were "medical" rather than "health care" services, and this is "not the responsibility of the district to provide."

Outcome:

The administrative law judge concluded that several lower courts had misinterpreted the Supreme Court's *Tatro* opinion. He disagreed with the Federal District Court's statements in *Detsel* that the Supreme Court had held in *Tatro* that the expense and extent of the services required could be considered in determining whether a school system must provide them. The administrative law judge interprets *Tatro* to have "affirmed a bright line distinction between school health services (services provided by a qualified school nurse or other qualified person) and medical services provided by a physician that are not related to evaluation and assessment. If a nurse's services were needed, the school had to provide them as a related service" (22 IDELR 278, at 287). This is the test the administrative law judge applied. The Ohio Court of Appeals has reached a very similar conclusion (*Tanya v. Cincinnati Board of Education,* 1995).

The administrative judge ruled

- The health care services required by GF are "related services" that must be provided by the school district. The district must reimburse GF's mother for the cost of health care he has received at school since her 1993 written request.

- The question of whether an R.N., an L.P.N., or a nonlicensed person is required to provide that care "should be better resolved by the Board of Nursing" (22 IDELR 278, at 289).

- The school district must provide the required "related services," although GF does not need a special or modified program or instruction. As in *Tatro*, "related services can stand alone for those students who need only those services to succeed" (22 IDELR 278, at 289) in general education.

THE REHABILITATION ACT OF 1973 (PL 93-112), SECTION 504

Section 504 of PL 93-112 is a civil rights law that prohibits discrimination on the basis of a disability. Individuals with disabilities have a right to obtain the same programs and services available to their peers without disabilities. Section 504 does not provide federal monies to help agencies provide services; however, child care, preschool, and public and private elementary and secondary education programs that receive federal funds have an obligation to provide the necessary accommodations.

Eligibility

An individual with a disability, according to Section 504, is anyone who "(i) has a physical or mental impairment which substantially limits one or more of the person's major life activities, (ii) has a record of such an impairment, or (iii) is regarded as having such an impairment" (29 U.S.C. § 706[8][B]). The regulations define major life activity as "functions such as caring for one's self, performing manual tasks, walking, seeing, hearing, speaking, breathing, learning, and working" (Title 34, CFR § 104.3 [j][2][ii]). This definition of an individual with an eligible disability is considerably broader than is the definition under IDEA and **should include virtually any child with a special health care need**. Section 504, unlike IDEA, does not require that the child's disability adversely affect educational performance or that the desired accommodation is necessary for the child to benefit from special education.

School Services Supported by Section 504

Section 504 regulations require that schools receiving federal aid offer the following:

- Free appropriate public education
- Related services
- A process for implementing an IEP or its equivalent
- Transportation
- Preplacement evaluation, evaluation procedures, and reevaluation
- Appropriate placement
- Procedures to guarantee the rights of students (Title 34, CFR §§ 104.33–104.36)

The regulations that implement Section 504 mirror those that implement IDEA. Many states acknowledge these similarities and have established specific state regulations reflecting these requirements. Students with ongoing health care needs (e.g., diabetes, seizure disorders, cystic fibrosis), who may not qualify for services under IDEA, qualify for services necessary to attend and benefit from school programs under Section 504.

Section 504 and Decisions of the Office for Civil Rights (OCR)

A parent can file a grievance under a school district's Section 504 policy, seek a due process hearing, or seek a court ruling regarding an alleged violation of Section 504. OCR cases regarding the rights of students with health care needs have involved such issues as the right to an evaluation to determine eligibility for accommodations during the school day and the right to related services, including medication administration. Complaints regarding violations in the area of education may be filed with the U.S. Department of Education OCR and the regional office of the OCR. Section 504 complaints are investigated and ruled on by regional offices of the OCR. The decision on a specific complaint is called a *Letter of Findings.*

THE AMERICANS WITH DISABILITIES ACT (ADA) OF 1990 (PL 101-336)

The Americans with Disabilities Act (ADA) of 1990 (PL 101-336) gives civil rights protection to individuals with disabilities in employment, all public services, public accommodations, transportation, and telecommunications. Compliance with the ADA is mandatory. The law states that

> no qualified individual with a disability shall, by reason of such disability, be excluded from participation in or be denied the benefits of the services, programs, or activities of a public entity, or be subjected to discrimination by any such entity. (42 U.S.C. § 12132)

The ADA strengthens and expands the rights guaranteed to individuals with disabilities under IDEA and Section 504 and their state counterparts.

Eligibility

The ADA and Section 504 use the same definition of an individual with a disability (42 U.S.C. § 12102; 29 U.S.C. § 706[8][B]).

School Services Supported by the Americans with Disabilities Act

The ADA extends the educational rights of students with disabilities to include private schools. Also included are private child care programs, preschool settings, and post-secondary institutions, although these receive no federal funds. In addition, the ADA expands the opportunities for daily living activities for people with disabilities (e.g., accessibility of stores, restaurants, hotels, entertainment and recreational facilities, employment). The ADA provides greater access for students with disabilities to both schools and the larger society they encounter outside of the classroom and after exiting school.

Americans with Disabilities Act Enforcement

Federal agencies have begun to apply the accessibility provisions of the ADA to public and private school systems. The U.S. Department of Justice, for instance, has determined an ADA Title II requirement that public school programs, "when viewed as a whole, be accessible to and usable by persons with disabilities," to mean that a public school's field trip to a local museum must be made accessible to students with disabilities (Department of Justice, 1995). After a complaint investigation by the U.S. Department of Education OCR, a Massachusetts university has agreed to take corrective actions to remove the architectural barrier posed by three steps leading into a cafeteria (U.S. Department of Education, Office for Civil Rights, 1994). The courts also have begun to consider ADA education issues. A federal district court in Pennsylvania has refused to dismiss a lawsuit filed by a boy with spina bifida against a public school district seeking to have high school facilities, and in particular its stadium, made accessible to his wheelchair (*Bechtel v. School District*, 1994). In addition, the father of a 6-year-old has filed a complaint against the Philadelphia School District, claiming that he is unable to attend parent–teacher conferences because of the steps at every entrance to his daughter's school (*Kates v. School District of Philadelphia*, 1995). Because many cases are settled before they reach the administrative or judicial decision stage (many, in fact, before a formal complaint is even filed), the ADA's actual effects on school systems have been much more widespread than is indicated by reported decisions.

Complaints against public schools thought to be violating the ADA may be filed with the U.S. Department of Education OCR and are handled exactly like Section 504 complaints. ADA complaints against private child care centers, nursery schools, schools, and other "public accommodations" may be filed with the U.S. Department of Justice, Office on the ADA, Civil Rights Division.

Americans with Disabilities Act and Decisions by the Office for Civil Rights (OCR)

Some courts have found the ADA to be "redundant" of IDEA, Section 504, or both in the school context and have granted no additional rights under the ADA. Others have found ADA claims to validly supplement those rights guaranteed under IDEA and Section 504.

The OCR regional offices investigate and issue decisions on complaints concerning the ADA. OCR's interpretations of ADA are not binding in court, but they may be influential.

The following are decisions of two cases in violation of the ADA:

Americans with Disabilities Act
Case 1

Issue:	Is a school system in violation of ADA if it does not allow students with severe to profound hearing loss the right to choose the type of signing used by interpreters provided by the school?
Case:	*Petersen v. Hastings Public Schools*, 831 F. Supp. 742 (1993)
Description:	Several parents of students with severe to profound hearing loss requested that the school system allow them to choose the type of signing interpreters used with the students.
U.S. District Court Ruling:	• "If only an 'effective' auxiliary aid is needed when a requested aid is vastly superior to the school district, the principal purpose of the Act may be circumvented. (831 F. Supp at 752 [D. Neb.], 1993)"
	• Students were not able to prove the superiority of the system they devised and thus failed to demonstrate any discrimination on the part of the school.

Americans with Disabilities Act
Case 2

Issue:	Is a university in violation of ADA if a student with disabilities, requiring a personal care attendant, does not have a roommate randomly assigned as is the case for other students attending that university?
Case:	*Coleman v. Zatechka,* 824 F. Supp. 1360 (1993)
Description:	A college student, who required a personal care assistant, applied for student housing and requested a roommate who did not smoke. The university assigned the student a room but not a roommate. The student repeated her request that the university randomly assign her a roommate.
U.S. District Court Ruling:	• The university's blanket policy of excluding students who use attendant care from the roommate assignment program violated both the ADA and Section 504 of PL 93-112.

THE FAMILY'S ROLE IN ENSURING THE RIGHTS OF THEIR CHILD

In discussing laws and regulations regarding school services for students with health care needs, one must first think of the students' best interests.

Anderson and Vohs (1992) offer four strategies for families to use in securing an IEP and services for their child:

1. Families should believe absolutely that their children have a right to attend school and to do so in a safe environment. Many of the accommodations needed by children, such as medication administration, should be offered in the context of the support services available to all students. For many families, the first approach, after discussion with the child's health professionals, simply is to meet with school officials, describe the child's needs, and problem-solve with the officials about the best way to address those needs.

2. Families should review information about eligibility and the process for obtaining services under Section 504 and IDEA.

3. Families may choose to request services under Section 504 without considering IDEA first. School systems have not paid much attention to Section 504 and few typically give families information about it. All public, and some private, schools, however, must sign assurances that they are in compliance with Section 504 as a prerequisite to receiving federal funds.

4. If the child is found not to have a disability as defined by IDEA or Section 504, the family may appeal the decision. If, however, the child is found to have a disability, but the family is dissatisfied with the child's IEP or plan under Section 504 or believes that the child is being discriminated against because of his or her disability, the family also may file an appeal. Filing a complaint under either of these provisions sets into motion the mechanisms for an impartial due process hearing. Hearing officers and courts can order a school system to take any number of actions to correct violations of both IDEA and Section 504. Under both laws, compensatory education, reimbursement for special education and related services that have been paid for by families, and reimbursement of attorneys' fees may be available remedies.

Along with the major considerations of *what* will be provided, *how* services will be provided often is extremely important to students and families.

OTHER LAWS, REGULATIONS, AND STANDARDS

In addition to federal and state laws related to the education and civil rights of students with disabilities, state laws and regulations related to health care may influence the education of students who have special health care needs. For example, state licensure laws and regulations define and control the practice of physicians, nurses, and other health care professionals. Other state laws may address issues such as the responsibilities of health and education professionals to maintain confidentiality of client health information or the administration of medications. In addition, professional standards of practice and state guidelines that set standards for the quality of health care services affect the services students receive in school.

Legal Aspects Related to the Practice of Nursing

State legislatures pass licensure laws for nursing to protect the health, safety, and welfare of their citizens. Although these laws vary from one state to another, in general, state legislatures delegate the function of regulating the practice of nursing to a state board of nursing or board of nurse examiners. These boards are given the power and authority within their state to regulate nursing practice; monitor nursing activities; determine the scope of practice of the professional registered nurse (R.N.), advanced practice nurse (A.P.N.), licensed vocational nurse (L.V.N.), or licensed practical nurse (L.P.N.); and set disciplinary standards. The scope of nursing practice in a state is the same no matter where a nurse works (e.g., hospital, school, home), unless specific state laws specify otherwise, and legal standards set forth in a nurse practice act take priority over school district policies. According to the American Nurses Association (1994), "institutional policies cannot contradict state law."

Nurse practice acts generally prohibit unlicensed individuals from practicing nursing for compensation and may define the limits of a penalty, such as monetary fines, jail terms, or both, for those found guilty of violating the law (e.g., *Connecticut General Statutes* §§ 20-102). School employees who are not licensed nurses, therefore, can be held civilly and even criminally liable if they provide services within the scope of nursing practice that have not been properly delegated and supervised by a nurse. Medical practice acts address the physician's scope of practice.

In general, school district administrators need to understand the jurisdiction and specifics of their state's medical and nursing practice acts. Variations in nursing practices regarding delegation to and supervision of unlicensed assistive personnel primarily are based on differences in each state's nursing practice act and associated rules or regulations (Schwab & Haas, 1995). Other practice differences are influenced by leadership of a state's board of nursing, availability of nurses within the region, and opinions of attorneys general or other state agency administrators.

National Standards and Guidelines

Many national organizations have produced publications, position statements, and/or guidelines that are relevant to the provision of health care services in schools. Such organizations include the American Federation of Teachers, the American Nurses Association, the National Association of School Nurses, Inc., the National Association of State School Nurse Consultants, the American Academy of Pediatrics, and the National Education Association. It is important to review documents created by such organizations when planning and evaluating school health service programs for students with special needs. As with state guidelines, they are not the law, per se, but they offer standards for high-quality practice and services.

Several state departments of health or education have produced guidelines that affect the education of, and services provided for, students with special health care needs. These guidelines, although generally not adopted into law or regulation, are used as a standard against which a school district might be measured in a due process hearing or court of law. State agency guidelines that address school services for students with special health care needs may include such issues as staffing requirements, infection control, universal precautions, medication administration, guidelines for nursing procedures, classroom modification, transportation, and school policy recommendations. In a state that has a school nurse consultant in either the department of health or department of education, the school nurse consultant may be a resource for school administrators, school nurses, families, and staff in other state agencies, such as departments of protection and advocacy. Parent education advocacy and training centers also may have staff who are knowledgeable about these issues.

Local School Policies

Policies and procedures of local school districts, including job descriptions, personnel qualifications, and staffing patterns of school nurses and assistive personnel, also influence the standards and quality of services available to students with special health care needs. Despite state and national standards, local districts may or may not adopt standards that are not specifically mandated by law. In some school districts, a school nurse may be available in every building. In other districts, a school nurse may be available to a school for only one-half day per week or perhaps not at all. In the first instance, it is not difficult for the school to make available a school nurse to monitor and provide treatments for a student with severe asthma. In the latter instance, the district may not even consider the assignment of a full-time school nurse to the student's neighborhood school an option. To what extent school districts are required to provide school health care services as a related service under IDEA, the ADA, or Section 504, regardless of their usual staffing pattern, is not yet fully clear; therefore, a wide variation in practice exists.

There have been few court cases to date specifically related to issues of scope of practice, supervision, and delegation in school settings. The following are two examples:

Scope of Nursing Practice, Delegation, and Supervision Issues
Case 1

Issue:	Can a school principal assign a school health assistant the responsibility for performing clean intermittent catheterization for a middle school student with spina bifida?
Case:	*Mitts v. Hillsboro Union High School,* C.A. No. 87-11420 (1988/1989)
Description:	A school health assistant was directed by the school principal to perform clean intermittent catheterization for a student. She was trained by the student's parent but observed by the school nurse. The health assistant maintained she was not qualified or competent to perform the procedure.
Declarative ruling:	• The court asked the State Board of Nursing for a declarative ruling. The Board concluded that the principal was unlawfully practicing nursing without a license.
	• The state Board of Nursing also disciplined the school nurse who had acted contrary to nursing standards by passively accepting the decisions of the principal rather than actively pursuing appropriate responsibility for delegating and training the health assistant.

Scope of Nursing Practice, Delegation, and Supervision Issues
Case 2

Issue:	Does the school district need to provide a private duty nurse or a trained paraprofessional to meet the needs of a 5-year-old child with paraplegia and ventilator dependence?
Case:	*Caledonia Public Schools,* 19 IDELR 1125 (1993)
Description:	The parents of a 5-year-old child with paraplegia and ventilator assistance requested that the school district provide a private duty nurse or trained paraprofessional to meet the health needs of their child during the school day and during transportation.
Due process ruling:	• The district must provide the child with the school health services necessary to meet her health care needs during school and transportation.
	• Appropriate delegation should be made in accordance with Michigan's Public Health Code allowing delegation by physicians and nurses (i.e., to unlicensed individuals who function under the supervision of the delegating professional).

Related School Health Issue—Do Not Resuscitate (DNR) Orders

Because some children and youth in the latter stages of terminal illness are attending school, their parents may ask school districts to be informed of and respect DNR orders. Such orders are issued by a student's physician in collaboration with the parents or guardians who have concluded that they want their child who is terminally ill to be allowed to die with maximum comfort and minimum suffering. They do not want cardiopulmonary resuscitation (CPR) to be performed for life-extending or lifesaving purposes. DNR orders, always extremely complex, originally were developed for medical teams in hospitals and other clinical settings. In school, they become even more complicated. Questions such as "What are the actions that are in the best interest of the student?" and "Who can accept a DNR order from a physician?" must be explored and answered.

Because the clinical, legal, administrative, and ethical issues are so complex, it is essential that the school health care and education personnel, representatives of the emergency transportation system, families, physicians, other health care providers, and local hospital staff work together to educate each other, explore all of the relevant issues, and develop a collaborative plan that ensures high-quality care for each student with a DNR order.

It is essential for the team to know whether its state has produced guidelines, laws, court decisions, an attorney general's opinion, and/or ruling of the state's board of nursing or board of medicine on DNR orders in schools. Such guidelines or standards, when they exist, should be used as a basis of planning for individual students. In states in which such guidelines do not exist, state or local communities should collaborate to address the many complex issues involved and to develop general guidelines for school policies and procedures. Members may include representatives from education and health professions, educational and health law, families, the emergency medical system, the board of nursing, state agencies, and the field of medical ethics.

In addition to the material in Figure 2.3 (on p. 35), which is adopted by the National Education Association, the National Association of School Nurses, Inc., has published a position paper on DNR orders in schools (see Figure 2.2 below).

POSITION STATEMENT "DO NOT RESUSCITATE"

(Adopted by the National Association of School Nurses, Inc., September 1994)

History: Increased numbers of medically fragile, chronically ill students are in school.

Description: In some instances, parents of chronically ill students do not wish CPR to be initiated in the case of respiratory or cardiac arrest. The school district may be petitioned to honor a DO NOT RESUSCITATE order.

Rationale: DO NOT RESUSCITATE orders are a sensitive issue. School health nurses will often need assistance in developing a plan of care for medically fragile students and learning when it is possible to honor a DNR order.

Conclusion: It is the position of the National Association of School Nurses that DO NOT RESUSCITATE orders for medically fragile students must be evaluated on an individual basis at the local level, according to state and local laws. The local Board of Education should refer this matter to school district legal counsel for guidance. Each student involved should have an Individualized Health Care Plan developed by the professional school health nurse with involvement from the parents, administrator, physician, teacher, and student, when appropriate. It needs to include a written DNR request from the parent(s) as well as the physician's written DNR order. The plan should be reviewed at least annually. The health plan also should state the steps to be taken in case of respiratory or cardiac arrest.

Figure 2.2. National Association of School Nurses, Inc., position statement: "do not resuscitate." (From National Association of School Nurses, Inc. [1994, September]. *Position statement on "do not resuscitate."* Scarborough, ME: Author; reprinted by permission.)

"DO NOT RESUSCITATE ORDERS"

(Adopted by the NEA Executive Committee June, 1994)

Advances in medical technology now make it possible for some severely ill students to attend school and participate in the learning environment. However, there exists an ever-present threat that such students may go into cardiac/respiratory arrest while in school. In some instances, parents of such students, in conjunction with their physicians, have determined that certain emergency procedures, such as cardiac pulmonary resuscitation, would be too invasive and painful, might cause severe brain damage, or might otherwise result in worsening the student's physical problems. In such a case, the physician will issue a "do not resuscitate" ("DNR") order, directing that no life-saving procedures be utilized.

While DNR orders have been common phenomena in hospitals and nursing homes, they have only recently surfaced in several school districts around the country. This has prompted a number of inquiries and requests for guidance from NEA members and affiliates.

Of particular concern is the question whether a classroom teacher or other school employee must obey a directive from the school employer to comply with a DNR order. As a general rule, a school employee always should obey a specific directive from the employer. Since this is a developing area of the law, however, NEA members should consult with counsel at the state level to determine whether any special state laws or policies address this situation.

While many districts honor requests to follow DNR orders, others have refused, and still others require parents to obtain a court order before honoring DNR orders. The Maryland Attorney General, for example, has taken the position that school officials in Maryland must comply with DNR orders, while the Iowa Attorney General has said that a school "has no duty to comply with a decision by parents and the physician to withhold life-sustaining procedures" because a school is not a licensed health care provider under state law.

The proposed policy does not take a position on whether school districts *should,* as a matter of public policy, honor DNR orders; that is an issue that should be resolved at the state and/or local level. However, in considering a request to honor a DNR order, the school district should consult with counsel to determine what legal rights and responsibilities it has, including the applicability of a collective bargaining agreement.

While requests to honor DNR orders must be handled on a case-by-case basis, NEA recommends that no request be granted unless the following minimum conditions are met:

1. The parents' or guardians' request is submitted in writing and accompanied by a written DNR order signed by the student's primary licensed physician.

2. The school district establishes a "team" consisting of the parents/guardians, student's physician, school nurse, student's teacher(s), appropriate support staff, and school superintendent or designee to consider the request. The team first considers all available alternatives. If no other option is acceptable to the parents/guardians, then the team develops a "medical emergency plan," which includes the following essential elements:

    a. The plan specifies what actions the student's teacher or other school employee should take in the event that the student suffers a cardiac arrest or other life-threatening emergency, e.g., telephone the local emergency medical service, apply emergency procedures as determined by the team, contact the parents/guardians, evacuate other students from the classroom, etc.

    b. All school employees who have supervision of the student during the school day are fully briefed on the procedures to follow in the event of a medical emergency involving the student.

    c. The student wears an ID bracelet while at school indicating that he/she is subject to a DNR order and a medical emergency plan.

    d. The parents execute a contract with the local emergency medical service providing that the service will honor the DNR order, a copy of the contract is made available to the school superintendent/designee.

Figure 2.3. National Education Association policy on do not resuscitate orders. (From National Education Association. [1994, June]. *National Education Association policy on "do not resuscitate" orders.* Washington, DC: Author; reprinted by permission.)

SUMMARY

This chapter briefly outlined laws that support services for students with special health care needs in school. The discussion covered IDEA, Section 504, and the ADA and provided information on how other laws, such as licensure, affect services for students with special health care needs. These laws have differing purposes but many overlapping provisions. Sometimes, the provision of one law rather than another may be useful to achieve particular outcomes. A resource list is provided at the end of the chapter to assist the reader in exploring these issues.

Much has been accomplished since the 1980s in expanding and ensuring the rights of students with special health care needs. However, there continue to be unresolved challenges that promise future discussion and resolution that will affect children with special health care needs at school.

REFERENCES

American Nurses Association. (1994). *Registered professional nurses and unlicensed assistive personnel*. Washington, DC: Author.

Americans with Disabilities Act (ADA) of 1990, PL 101-336, 42 U.S.C. § 12101 *et seq.*

Anderson, B., & Vohs, J. (1992). Another look at Section 504. *Coalition Quarterly, 10*(1), 1–4.

Bechtel v. School District, 1994 U.S. Dist. LEXIS 1327 (E.D. Pa 1994).

Board of Education of the Hendrick Hudson Central School District v. Rowley, 458 U.S. 116 (1982).

Caledonia Public Schools, 19 IDELR 1125 (SEA MI 1993).

Coleman v. Zatechka, 824 F. Supp. 1360 (D. Neb. 1993).

Connecticut General Statutes, § 20–102, 44.

David D. v. School Committee, 775 F.2d 411 (1st Cir. 1985).

Department of Justice. (1995). Policy letter. *National Disability Law Reporter, 6*(81).

Detsel v. Sullivan, 895 F.2d 58 (2d Cir. 1990).

Education for All Handicapped Children Act of 1975, PL 94-142, 20 U.S.C. § 1401 *et seq.*

Education of the Handicapped Act Amendments of 1986, PL 99-457, 20 U.S.C. § 1400 *et seq.*

Gerry, M. (1987). Procedural safeguards insuring that handicapped children receive a free appropriate public education. *NICHCY News Digest, 7,* 1–8.

GF v. Cedar Rapids Community School District, 22 IDELR 278 (No. SE-98, Iowa Dept. of Ed., decided 12/16/94, reported 1995).

Individuals with Disabilities Education Act (IDEA) of 1990, PL 101-476, 20 U.S.C. § 1401 *et seq.*

Individuals with Disabilities Education Act Amendments of 1991, PL 102-119, 20 U.S.C. §§ 1400 *et seq.*

Kates v. School District of Philadelphia, 6:12. *National Disability Law Reporter (Highlights)*5 (reported 7/20/95).

Mitts v. Hillsboro Union High School, C.A. No. 87-11420 (D. Ore., 1989).

National Association of School Nurses, Inc. (1994, September). *Position statement on "Do not resuscitate."* Scarborough, ME: Author.

National Education Association. (1994, June). *National Education Association policy on "do not resuscitate" orders.* Washington, DC: Author.

Oberti v. Board of Education, 789 F. Supp. 1322 (D.N.J. 1992).

Petersen v. Hastings Public Schools, 831 F. Supp. 742 (D. Neb., 1993).

Rehabilitation Act of 1973, PL 93-112, 29 U.S.C. § 794 *et seq.*

Irving Independent School District v. Tatro, 468 U.S. 883 (1984).

Skubel v. Sullivan, C.A. No. 90-279 (EBB) (U.S.D.C., D. Conn., Prelim. Inj., 7/6/90).

Schwab, N., & Haas, M. (1995). Delegation and supervision in school settings: Standards, issues and guidelines for practice (Part I). *Journal of School Nursing, 11*(1), 26–35.

Tanya v. Cincinnati Board of Education, 100 Ohio App. 3d52 (1995).

Timothy W. v. Rochester, N.H. School District, 875 F.2d 954 (1st Cir. 1989).

U.S. Department of Education, Office for Civil Rights. (1994). Letter of findings: University of Massachusetts at Amherst. *National Disability Law Reporter 4*(431).

SUGGESTED READINGS

American Nurses Association. (1985). *Code for nurses with interpretive statements*. Kansas City, MO: Author.

Anderson, B. (1989). Why should your child receive instruction when not in school. In L. Wetherbee & A. Neil (Eds.), *Educational rights for children with arthritis* (pp. 5-1–5-12). Atlanta, GA: Arthritis Foundation.

Anderson, N. (1991). Section 504: A tool for obtaining services for children with special health needs. *Exceptional Parent, 21*(1), 6.

Baltimore County Public Schools. (1994). *The child with a DNR order: Sample nursing care plan.* Baltimore: Author.

Beekman, L. (1994). DNR orders: What should a school district do? *EDLAW Briefing Papers, 4*(6), 1–12.

Birenbaum, A., Guyot, D., & Cohen, H.J. (1990). *Health care financing for severe developmental disabilities.* Washington, DC: American Association on Mental Retardation.

Brown, S.E. (1995). Do not resuscitate orders in early intervention settings: Who should make the decision. *Infants & Young Children, 7*(3), 13–27.

Cohen, R., Hart, D., Hunt, A., & Komissar, C. (1995). Moving on...Planning for the future. *The Institute Brief.* Available from Institute for Community Inclusion, Children's Hospital, Boston.

Connecticut State Department of Education. (1992). *Serving students with special health care needs.* Hartford, CT: Author.

Copenhaver, J. (1995). *Section 504: An educator's primer.* Logan, UT: Mountains Plains Regional Resource Center.

Council of Administrators on Special Education, Inc. (1992). *Student access: A resource guide for educators.* Albuquerque, NM: Author.

Crowley, T. (1994). *Settle it out of court: How to resolve business and personal disputes using mediation, arbitration, and negotiation.* New York: John Wiley & Sons.

Disability Law Center of Massachusetts. (1992). *Discrimination on the basis of disability: Federal and Massachusetts laws.* Boston: Pike Institute on Law and Disability, Boston University School of Law.

Essex, N., Schifani, J., & Bowman, S. (1994). Handle with care: Your school's tough new challenge—educating medically fragile children. *American School Board Journal, 181*(3), 50–52.

First, P.F., & Curcio, J.L. (1993). *Individuals with disabilities: Implementing the newest laws.* San Francisco: Corwin Press.

Graff, J.C., Ault, M.M., Guess, D., Taylor, M., & Thompson, B. (1990). *Health care for students with disabilities: An illustrated medical guide for the classroom.* Baltimore: Paul H. Brookes Publishing Co.

Herlan, E.R. (1994). *The legal framework for responding to DNR orders on school grounds. Individuals with Disabilities Education Law Report, Special Report #11.* Horsham, PA: LRP Publications.

Honoroff, B., Matz, D., & O'Connor, D. (1990). Putting mediation skills to the test. *Negotiation Journal, 6*(1), 37–46.

Koenig, K.L., & Tamkin, G.W. (1993). "Do not resuscitate" orders: Where are they in the prehospital setting? *Prehospital and Disaster Medicine, 8*(1), 51–55.

Krajicek, M., & Steinke, G. (Eds.). (1994, August). *A summary of the proceedings on the national conference on developing policy and practice to implement IDEA related to invasive procedures for children with special health care needs.* Paper prepared from National Conference on Developing Policy and Practice to Implement IDEA Related to Invasive Procedures for Children with Special Health Care Needs, Denver, CO.

Marcus, L.J. (1995). Negotiation, arbitration, and mediation. In L.J. Marcus (Ed.), *Renegotiating health care: Resolving conflict to mild collaboration* (pp. 317–363). San Francisco: Jossey-Bass.

Martin, R. (1991). *Extraordinary children, ordinary lives: Stories behind special education case law.* Champaign, IL: Research Press.

Martin, R. (1991). *Medically fragile/technology dependent students: Drawing the line between education and medicine.* Unpublished manuscript, Carle Center for Health, Law and Ethics, Urbana, IL.

McGonigel, M.J., & Johnson, B.H. (1991). An overview. In M.J. McGonigel, R.K. Kaufman, & B.H. Johnson (Eds.), *Guidelines and recommended practices for the individualized family service plan* (2nd ed., pp. 1–5). Bethesda, MD: Association for the Care of Children's Health.

McWilliam, P.J., & Bailey, D.B., Jr. (Eds.). (1993). *Working together with children and families: Case studies in early intervention.* Baltimore: Paul H. Brookes Publishing Co.

Morse, M.T. (1990). PL 94-142 and PL 99-457: Considerations for coordination between the health care and the education systems. *Children's Health Care, 19*(4), 213–218.

National Association of State Directors of Special Education. (1993, November). *Leading and Managing for Performance: An Examination of Challenges Confronting Special Education.* Alexandria, VA: Author.

National Council of State Boards of Nursing, Inc. (1990). *Concept paper on delegation.* Chicago: Author.

Ordover, E.L., & Boundy, K.B. (1991). *Education rights of children with disabilities: A primer for advocates.* Cambridge, MA: Center for Law and Education.

Proctor, S. (1993). *School nursing practice: Roles and standards.* Scarborough, ME: National Association of School Nurses, Inc.

Rushton, C., Will, J., & Murray, M. (1994). To honor and obey—DNR orders and the school. *Pediatric Nursing, 20*(6), 581–585.

Schrag, J. (1993). Response to inquiry: Medical v. school health services distinguished. *Individuals with Disabilities Education Law Report, 19*(6), 348–350.

Schwab, N. (1991). *Guidelines for documentation in school nursing practice.* Scarborough, ME: National Association of School Nurses, Inc.

Singer, L. (1994). *Settling disputes: Conflict resolution in business, families, and the legal system* (2nd ed.). Boulder, CO: Westview.

Turnbull, H.R. (1993). *Free appropriate public education: The law and the children with disabilities* (3rd ed.). Denver: Love Publishing Co.

U.S. Dept. of Education, Office of Civil Rights, and Adaptive Environment Center, Inc. (1995). *Compliance with the Americans with Disabilities Act: A self-evaluation guide for public elementary and secondary schools.* Washington, DC: U.S. Government Printing Office.

Vitello, S.J. (1987). School health services after *Tatro. Journal of School Health, 57*(2), 77–80.

Whitted, B.R. (1991). Educational benefits after *Timothy W.*: Where do we go from here? *West's Education Law Reporter, 68*(3), 549–555.

Advocacy, Inc.
7800 Shoal Creek Boulevard, 171-E
Austin, TX 78757
(This organization publishes *SPECIAL EDition* quarterly.)

Center for Law and Education
955 Massachusetts Avenue, Suite 3A
Cambridge, MA 02139

Collaboration Among Parents and Professionals (CAPP) Centers
National Parent Resource Center (NPRC)
Federation for Children with Special Needs
95 Berkeley Street, Suite 104
Boston, MA 02116

EDLAW, Inc.
Post Office Box 59105
Potomac, MD 20859-9105

Exceptional Parent
209 Harvard Street, Suite 303
Brookline, MA 02146

National Association of School Nurses, Inc.
Post Office Box 1300
Scarborough, ME 04074

National Association of State Directors of Special Education
1800 Diagonal Drive, Suite 320
Alexandria, VA 22314

National Association of State School Nurse Consultants, Inc.
Post Office Box 708
Kent, OH 44240-0708

National Center for Community Based System of Services for Children with Special Health Care Needs and Their Families
University of Iowa
Boyd Law Building
Iowa City, IA 52242

National Council of State Boards of Nursing, Inc.
676 North St. Clair Street, Suite 550
Chicago, IL 60611-2921

National Information Center for Children and Youth with Disabilities (NICHCY)
Post Office Box 1492
Washington, DC 20013-1492

New England Disability and Business Technical Assistance Center
145 Newburg Street
Portland, ME 04101

Parent Training Information Centers
Protection and Advocacy Agency
Each state has a Parent Training Information Center as well as an advocacy agency. For specific information for the contact in your state, call NICHCY.

Pike Institute on Law and Disability
Boston University School of Law
765 Commonwealth Avenue
Boston, MA 02215

State Board of Registration in Nursing
For specific information needed to contact the board in your state, refer to State Government listing in the telephone directory.

State Department of Education
For specific information needed to contact the department in your state, contact NICHCY.

Transition Research Institute
University of Illinois
61 Children's Research Center
51 Gerty Drive
Champaign, IL 61820

U.S. Department of Education
Office of Civil Rights
600 Independence Avenue, SW
Washington, DC 20202

Entrance and Planning Process for Students with Special Health Care Needs

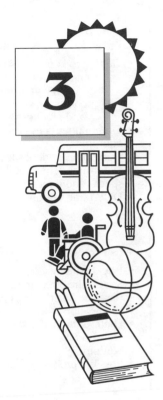

Terry Heintz Caldwell, Janice Rutledge Janz,
Debra S. Alcouloumre, Stephanie Porter,
Marilynn Haynie, Judith S. Palfrey, Timaree Bierle,
Thomas Silva, Judy Still, Barbara P. Sirvis,
Nadine Schwab, and Arlene Swan Mahony

This chapter examines the process for inclusion of students with special health care needs, particularly those who are assisted by medical technology. School systems share a common goal to provide safe and educationally sound programs for all students. This goal can be accomplished best by using a team approach. This chapter outlines the process of school entry and the roles of team members in creating an environment that fosters students' academic success and social competence while meeting their unique health needs. Figure 3.1 provides an outline of the steps in the entrance process.

Eddie requires suctioning and tracheostomy care on an as-needed basis, as well as gastrostomy feedings twice during the school day. His care originally was provided by a private duty nurse who stayed with him throughout the school day. The nurse eventually moved out of the room but was in constant contact.

* * *

Robin requires scheduled assistance with parenteral and enteral feedings in school. Care is provided in the nursing office. From the beginning, the school nurse also worked with Robin's schoolmates, although she was hired specifically to care for Robin. The nurse is available for immediate intervention if Robin has problems.

* * *

Brian's care is provided by a trained assistant who stays with him throughout the day. The assistant, who is supervised by the school nurse, was selected by a team that included his family, teacher, and school nurse. Brian requires continuous ventilation, suctioning as needed, periodic checks of his ventilator, gastrostomy feedings to supplement his oral intake, intermittent catheterization twice a day, periodic emptying of his leg bag (attached to a

ENTRANCE PROCESS FOR STUDENTS WITH SPECIAL HEALTH CARE NEEDS

EARLY IDENTIFICATION AND NOTIFICATION

IDENTIFY THE STUDENT'S TEAM

ASSESSMENT

- Getting to know the student and family
    - Obtain health history records from parents and health care providers
    - Incorporate knowledge of diverse cultural beliefs and practices
- Obtain physician's orders for health procedures and equipment
- Determine student's level of care required
- Determine school building accessibility and student space requirements
- Determine student's ability to participate in care

PLANNING

- Determine and delegate roles and responsibilities to team members
- Review transition into school
- Determine safe, appropriate class placement
- Discuss and determine necessary services and personnel
- Plan for student participation in health care
- Plan for training
- Plan for scheduling modifications
- Plan for follow-up team meetings

DEVELOPMENT OF AN INDIVIDUALIZED HEALTH CARE PLAN

- Brief health history
- Special health care needs
- Baseline health status
- Medication
- Diet/nutrition
- Transportation
- Equipment
- Possible problems and interventions

- Emergency plans for school and transportation
- Notification of Fire Department/EMT/local emergency room of possible student emergency needs
- Plan reviewed by physician, and signed by parent, educational administrator, and school nurse
- Incorporate Individualized Health Care Plan into pertinent student records

TRAINING

General

For persons who have contact with a student but are not responsible for providing necessary direct health service).

Review of Individualized Health Care Plan and Emergency Plan Awareness Training
- School personnel
- Community providers
- Peers

Student-Specific

Training in health procedures and emergency interventions for direct health care providers, teacher(s), and community providers

Student Training

Improved tolerance
Learn to direct care
Increased independence in learning and providing own care

STUDENT ATTENDS SCHOOL
IMPLEMENTATION, MONITORING, AND EVALUATION

- Provide direct care as appropriate and supervise student care providers
- Update the assessment of the student's health status
- Update and evaluate student's individualized health care plan
- Document, review, and update skills and provide annual training

Figure 3.1. An outline of the school entrance process for students with special health care needs. (From Palfrey, J.S., Haynie, M., Porter, S., Bierle, T., Cooperman, P., & Lowcock, J. [1992]. Project school care: Integrating children assisted by medical technology into educational settings. *Journal of School Health, 62*(2), 51; adapted by permission of American School Health Association, Kent, Ohio. This is not a transfer of copyright; the American School Health Association maintains copyright ownership and authorship of the use of said material, and the American School Health Association or others authorized by the American School Health Association are in no way restricted from republication.)

condom catheter and used to keep him dry between intermittent catheterization), pres-sure relief or repositioning every 30 minutes to restore circulation to his buttocks and back, and assistance with all activities of daily living and education.

The entrance process for students with special health care needs requires several key steps:

1. Identify the child early and notify the education system.

2. Designate the student-specific team responsible for assessment and planning.

3. Develop an individualized health care plan (IHCP).

4. Provide general and student-specific training.

5. Implement and provide ongoing follow-up and evaluation.

EARLY IDENTIFICATION AND NOTIFICATION

Notification about a student's health care needs should provide enough information for the school system to prepare for the student's needs and identify key family members and health personnel to assist in the assessment and planning process.

Who Should Be Referred to the School System for Evaluation?

Students Who Need Health Care During the School Day

Early notification of school personnel is important for students who have special health care needs that must be met during the school day. When possible, notification should be made 3–5 months before the child begins school to allow sufficient time for the child to make a smooth transition into school. Students who have conditions that affect learning (e.g., traumatic brain injury, Down syndrome) should be referred as soon as they are identified. Early notification allows time for team identification, assessment, and planning and time to 1) determine the level of health care required by the child in the school setting; 2) determine who will provide direct health care services, whether care can be delegated to unlicensed personnel, and what kind of training and supervision will be needed; 3) determine what special education or modifications and adaptations under Section 504 of PL 93-112, the Rehabilitation Act of 1973, are appropriate for the student's education program; and 4) orient and teach staff.

It is sometimes difficult to determine whether students with special health care needs will have learning problems or require special education services. For instance, students who have seizure disorders, diabetes, or heart or liver conditions may miss school because of illness and treatments. At times, their energy level and ability to concentrate may be reduced. Therefore, students may be identified because of increased absenteeism, which interferes with educational progress.

Children Identified Between Birth and 3 Years Old

All states have early intervention programs identified for children between birth and 3 years of age (see Chapter 2), but the types of early intervention services offered differ by state. Early intervention services are administered by different agencies, including state health departments, state departments of education, state social services agencies, and interagency coordinating committees. School departments will know to which agency referrals for early intervention should be made.

Students Identified with Health Care Needs During Hospitalization

Students who have had traumas or illnesses that have resulted in the potential for learning problems or a need for medical technology or health care in school should be referred to the school system during hospitalization. Early referral allows education and health care personnel to begin planning, so that school services will begin when the student is discharged from the hospital. Referral during hospitalization allows school health care personnel the opportunity to learn student-specific health procedures.

Who Should Make the Referral?

Referrals for education services can be made by the family, education personnel, and community or health care providers. Assistance with a referral may come from case managers or service coordinators, the primary pediatrician, visiting nurses, home care providers, and staff of any public or private developmental or education program in which the student is currently enrolled. If individuals other than family members make the referral, parental consent must first be obtained. The family will be asked to indicate the names and addresses of health care providers who have health information about the child and sign a "release of information" statement that authorizes sharing of appropriate information.

Who Should Be Notified?

Referral should be made directly to the school principal, guidance counselor, or school nurse. It also is appropriate to notify the director of special education for the school district. When determining whom to notify, consider the following:

- Is this the student's first school experience?
- Is the student already in a school placement?
- Does the student require accommodations and/or related services?

What Will Happen After the Referral Is Made?

The education staff will use referral information to contact the family and obtain consent, select an appropriate assessment and planning team, and coordinate meetings with the family and health care personnel. It is important for a family representative and the education and health teams to communicate frequently. Frequent communication will facilitate the timeliness of the process.

IDENTIFICATION OF THE STUDENT'S TEAM FOR ASSESSMENT AND PLANNING

Members of the student-specific team include the following people:

- Family, including the student when appropriate
- Health care and education personnel
- Community personnel who will provide resources or emergency care (i.e., fire department, emergency medical response system, home care agency)
- Team coordinator, selected by the school system, who will be responsible for coordinating meetings and collecting and disseminating information
- Related services personnel
- Other team members suggested by the family and/or education staff

Role of the Family

The family's and student's unique understanding of the student's health care needs is integral to assessment, planning, implementation, and continuation of the student's educational program. The family and student are an expert source of information and resources. Their role may include the following activities:

- Advocacy
- Providing information about student-specific health care needs
- Providing information about health care providers and equipment vendors
- Participating in planning and training meetings
- Assisting in developing and approving the individualized education program (IEP), IHCP, and emergency plan
- Coordinating the exchange of information regarding changes in the student's condition or health care requirements
- Maximizing the student's educational and social opportunities
- Identifying team participants (e.g., community providers, physicians, clinical nurse specialists)
- Planning transitions

Role of the Teacher

The teacher's primary role is to provide the best educational program for the student by using his or her knowledge of student learning styles and curricula. As the primary educator on the student's educational team, the teacher is responsible for evaluating student strengths and areas for improvement, identifying specific educational goals, implementing the IEP, and monitoring student progress.

When a student has learning problems, the teacher's role will include collaborating with special education staff to

- Identify specific or potential learning problems that should be evaluated by support staff in such areas as fine motor development, language processing, and expressive language development.
- Refer the student to, or work with, specialists in designing, implementing, and evaluating instructional programs, aids, and services that will maximize the student's learning.
- Work with support personnel who can help modify and adapt equipment, suggest alternative equipment for classroom use, and adapt an activity so that the student is included in the classroom program.

Additional teacher roles in the community may be to

- Educate other students, teachers, administrators, school committee, and community members by modeling interactions.
- Speak publicly to parent advisory groups and the school committee/board of education.
- Attend conferences with peers or parent groups.
- Share personal and professional experiences in working with students assisted by medical technology.

Another important teacher role is to communicate with the student's family. Students who are assisted by medical technology often require frequent communication with family members (i.e., telephone calls, meetings, and keeping records to coordinate services and educational planning). The focus of communication should be on health and education. With the family's permission, teachers can offer information to the student's physicians and therapists. Teachers have information about their students that can be critical to care planning and evaluation.

Role of the School Nurse

The school nurse is a member of the education team. The school nurse serves as a liaison among family, community health providers, and educators to ensure that the special health care needs of the student are addressed in school. In most cases, the school nurse is the appropriate person for this role. Figure 3.2 outlines the major responsibilities of the school nurse. **When a school does not employ a school nurse, the student's health care coordination should be supervised by one of the following:**

- **School district/community physician with child health or adolescent expertise**
- **Pediatric home care nurse**
- **Public health nurse with child/adolescent health expertise**
- **Hospital- or community-based pediatric nurse practitioner or specialist**

In summary, the school nurse must take a leadership role within the school in planning and providing services for students with special health care needs. To do so, the nurse must be

- An integral member of the school's multidisciplinary team
- Competent to provide necessary clinical services
- Sensitive to the individual needs and cultural differences of students and families
- Able to identify and communicate health issues relevant to the student's educational program

KEY HEALTH ASSESSMENT COMPONENTS

Student assessment

- Health history
- Current health status
- Medical diagnoses
- Current development status
- View of health condition
- Level of self-help skills
- Personal strengths
- Sense of differentness
- Home care routine
- Health needs in school

Student's health care system

- Health care providers, primary and specialists
- Communications required
- Physician orders
- Procedural guidelines
- Necessary emergency planning and communications

Family assessment

- Parents' vision for the child
- Family priorities
- Family strengths and resources
- Family support/liaison needs
- Sibling considerations
- Cultural variables

School environment

- Access to buildings, classrooms, and other spaces
- Safety for the student and others
- Availability and preparation of personnel to provide service
- Special supplies, equipment, and back-up equipment
- Maintenance of, storage of, and access to equipment
- Special electrical and climate considerations
- Privacy considerations
- Preparation of peers

KEY MANAGEMENT RESPONSIBILITIES

Participate in planning before/at school entry

- Obtain consultations and updating in special techniques or procedures.
- Obtain written parental permission to share health information with the student's health care providers.
- Initiate an IHCP based on nursing diagnoses and collaborative medical and education problems.
- Recommended program modifications and adaptations.
- Finalize the IHCP in collaboration with family and, as appropriate, with other members of the school team.
- Include the IHCP in the IEP for special education students.
- Provide personnel in-service education/training as needed.
- Ensure availability of equipment/supplies/other resources.
- Develop back-up plans.

Participate in interventions after school entry

- Promote normal development and student independence in health maintenance.
- Provide expert health services—direct nursing care.
- Supervise and monitor care provided by others.
- Consult with school personnel regarding student's health status, needs, and education programs.
- Promote integration of health services into the student's education program.
- Collaborate, communicate, and coordinate with the student's family and health care providers; refer as appropriate.
- Advocate for the child and family.

KEY EVALUATION RESPONSIBILITIES

Conduct ongoing evaluation

- Continue to assess the student's health status.
- Assess IHCP outcomes with the student, family, and team.

- Evaluate delegations and supervision plans.
- Recommend further assessment by others.
- Revise the IHCP accordingly.

Figure 3.2. The major responsibilities of the school nurse. (From Schwab, N. [1995]. Role of the school nurse. In Schwab, N. [Ed.], *Guidelines for the management of students with genetic disorders: A manual for school nurses* [3rd ed.]. Mt. Desert, ME: New England Regional Genetics Group; adapted by permission.)

- Prepared to educate, train, and supervise other members of the school team when appropriate
- In regular communication with the student's parent or guardian and health care providers (Schwab, 1995)

Role of the Pediatrician/Primary Care Provider

Primary care physicians and nurse practitioners can make several important contributions to the planning process for students with special health care needs. Pediatricians often are the first professional involved with families and may be the first to make a referral to an early intervention program. As the child moves into school, the primary care provider may be called on to help outline the needed services and to prescribe services, therapies, and equipment for use in home and school. Pediatricians also provide continuity from year to year through the transitions from an early intervention program into school and at the various junctions in school. It is especially critical that the child's primary care provider monitor the child's health and well-being and that the physician communicate with the school if the child's condition prohibits school attendance.

For the education process to run smoothly, the student's physician should be an equal member of the planning team. Through his or her knowledge of the student's health status, the physician collaborates with other team members by

- Referring the student and family to appropriate community agencies
- Providing an up-to-date, relevant health history
- Establishing a student's return to, and attendance at, school
- Reviewing and writing orders for procedures, medications, equipment, therapies, and services
- Making recommendations for personnel/staff in collaboration with the team
- Assisting in the training of staff
- Providing consultation regarding the health care and emergency plans
- Coordinating information from medical specialists
- Attending or remaining informed about team meetings when possible

Other Members on the Student-Specific Team

Important participants on the team may include representatives from the student's health specialty team (e.g., pediatric subspecialist; subspecialty nurse clinician; registered nurse; respiratory therapist; social worker; nutritionist; occupational, speech-language, and physical therapists) and community personnel (e.g., visiting nurses, home care or emergency response personnel, transportation personnel, and other team members suggested by the family and/or education staff).

Roles of Additional Team Members

Representatives from the student's health care team, in conjunction with the family, can

- Provide a description of the student's condition, including special health care requirements
- Provide information about precautions, warning signs and symptoms, and emergencies related to the student's condition
- Recommend the specific skills needed to provide the health care required by the student in the academic setting
- Assist education personnel in assessing the effect of the student's condition on his or her ability to learn and participate in school activities

Roles of Other Community Participants

Each community will have different individuals who are available to participate in the team process or serve as resource people for the family during the school entrance process. In some communities, federal Title V programs, frequently called Children with Special Health Care Needs (CSHCN) programs, provide case management and other services for students with complex health care needs. Private companies, including home health care agencies, also may provide case management, direct care, therapy, and training. Vendors of equipment and supplies also can be good resources for training and technical assistance, but they may not need to be part of regularly scheduled student team meetings.

Representatives from parents' groups may have experience with the transition-to-school process and can suggest ways to help plan the student's participation in school. They also can link the family with other families in the community for information and support.

Members of community emergency medical services, Red Cross branches, and fire departments can assist education personnel in planning for all types of potential emergencies. Emergencies can arise as a result of physiological or technological problems or natural disasters, such as fire, tornado, hurricane, earthquake, and ice or snow storm. The school principal and the school nurse will work with emergency personnel or school medical advisers to ensure that adequate plans are made for any type of emergency that may occur.

THE TASKS INVOLVED IN ASSESSMENT AND PLANNING

Making assessments and planning for a student's education require many steps.

Assessment

Family and education and health personnel should participate in assessments. Assessments should be timely, complete, nonjudgmental, and confidential, and they should reflect an awareness and knowledge of diverse cultural beliefs and practices. Health care and education information must be presented in understandable language and in the family's primary language. The information from the family, school, and health personnel needs to be synthesized to ensure a full picture of the student's need and strengths.

The following are steps in the assessment process:

1. ***Get to know the child and family***   The assessment process involves collecting the necessary health and education information needed to plan the best possible school program for the child. This information may consist of written documents, interactions with the child, and conversations with individuals associated with the child. It is essential to be knowledgeable about health beliefs and practices across cultures. Awareness of and respect for this diversity will enhance the ongoing relationships among the family, school staff, and community providers. Meeting with the child and family provides the opportunity to

    *   Establish a working relationship
    *   Obtain parental and student permission for the release of information
    *   Interact with the child and identify his or her strengths and needs
    *   Obtain existing documents from the family
    *   Obtain and clarify health and education information
    *   List the names of health care, education, and resource providers who can provide information and assistance

2. ***Obtain physician's orders for health procedures and equipment***   School systems require specific orders from the child's physician outlining the procedures, medications, and equipment the child will need during the school day. Some school systems will have specific forms that must be completed by the physician. To expedite the process, school personnel should provide families with the required forms. Physician's orders should include the student's name, date of birth, diagnosis, treatment or medication required, and specific procedures to be followed in administering treatment or medication (e.g., time of day; amounts; signature, address, telephone number of person completing the order).

3. ***Determine student's need for care and level of care required***   The school nurse, in collaboration with the student's physician and family, will determine the student's health needs and levels of care required during school. The school nurse should base recommendations on information gathered from the family, student, and health care providers, as well as from a nursing assessment of the student.

4. ***Determine student space requirements***   The school site should be assessed to determine the following (Ventilator Assisted Care Program, 1989):

    *   Safety and environmental concerns (e.g., allergens)
    *   Accessibility to all school programs and activities (i.e., to and from the cafeteria, assembly centers, library, elective programs, classrooms, upper floors of school, bus-loading area, playground, emergency exits, elevators, ramps)

- Availability and location of electrical outlets necessary for equipment and need for back-up generator
- Location of a room or space with running water, privacy for the child, and an area for storage of necessary equipment
- Location for disposal of used equipment/supplies
- Information regarding the heating and cooling system in the school (e.g., some seizure disorders may be triggered by extremes in temperature)
- In-school communication systems that may be needed in case of emergency (e.g., intercom, mobile telephone)

5. ***Determine student's ability to participate in his or her own care***   The student's ability to participate in self-care can be assessed using information from the following sources:
- Reports from family members regarding the student's current level of self-care and goals for the future
- Nursing assessment of and discussion with the student
- Reports from and discussions with the health care team
- Reports from and discussions with allied health professionals, such as occupational therapists and physical therapists

Planning

Family and education and health personnel participate in the planning process. The following are steps in the planning process:

1. ***Review the transition process***   Considerations in aiding the student's transition into the education setting may include the following (Caldwell, Todaro, & Gates, 1989b):
- Need to make a gradual transition to school
- Need for tutoring program
- Assessment of student's energy level
- Family observation of school program
- Need for time to make architectural changes or to hire and train personnel

The following is an example of a family's review of the transition process for their daughter:

Working together took work on everyone's part. The move from elementary school to middle school was scary for Tamika and me. My husband or I always help her with her bladder catheterization because her hands still shake when she tries to do it. She still needs reminders to wash her hands and not let the catheter touch the sides of the toilet. If she gets an infection it could mean terrible things because she has only one kidney, has a brain shunt, and needs heart surgery to replace her aorta.

We called a team meeting in June to plan for middle school and tried to work on her IEP then. All the elementary school staff attended—physical therapist, teacher, guidance counselor, school nurse, speech therapist, and occupational therapist—and so did some of the middle school people. That summer I toured the school with Tamika, the middle school nurse, and one of her teachers. Tamika wasn't too glad to visit the school—she dragged her feet and was very quiet. All she could think about was the upcoming heart surgery, but we had to work together to have her start middle school in September. In the building, we planned how much help she'd need to get from class to class because she's a bit unsteady walking in crowded hallways. We went over her class schedule and agreed on times for her to do the catheterization. "Cool" was what she said when we got to the social studies classroom, because she just loves geography, flags, and maps. We found a private bathroom where she'd do the procedure; the place needed a lot of cleaning, but the assistant principal and the school nurse said they'd work with the custodian to get it ready. We talked over who would help her change clothes in the locker room.

Finally, on our way out the door, she said, "I'm glad we came today, Mom." We set up a team meeting for the week before school started to iron out all the details. I hope people follow through with things they say they'll do, but so far everyone's tried to work together.

2. ***Determine roles and responsibilities of team members*** It is important for members of the team to know the specific steps that are required for entry/reentry to school. Specific assignments and clear role definition will alleviate greatly the reservations and questions of the family, student, and school personnel.

3. ***Determine safe, appropriate class placement*** Appropriate class placement is a decision that should be based on the child's educational needs. Health needs, although not a placement factor, are important when considering the child's safety in school.

    The following steps outlined by Caldwell, Todaro, Gates, Failla, and Kirkhart (1991) can be used to promote safety in the school setting:

    a. Obtain individualized prescriptions and protocols for the specialized care and procedures to be performed.

    b. Review physician-approved protocols with parents, and have them sign a form indicating their agreement with the procedures as outlined in the protocol.

    c. Determine care needs of student and the need for additional personnel and other resources.

    d. Document that appropriate training, based on protocols, has occurred. Include parents and community health professionals in conducting the training. List names of individuals trained, specific procedures demonstrated, and dates for scheduled supervision and follow-up.

    e. Train all staff involved in the student's care (i.e., bus driver, playground monitors). The level of training may vary.

    f. Establish back-up plans. Train other personnel to substitute when primary care providers are unavailable. Train those who will assist in an emergency situation.

    g. Establish emergency procedures.

    h. Develop and document plans, with input from physician and parents, for transport and provision of services in the local emergency room.

    i. Establish priority utility service reinstatement with agencies (e.g., electric and telephone companies).

    j. Acquaint emergency agencies (e.g., fire department, Red Cross) with the particular needs of the child.

    k. Document effectively the educational and health care needs of the student and the process of how they will be met in the IHCP and IEP when indicated. Include a list of the necessary services and personnel.

4. ***Discuss and determine necessary services, personnel, and funding*** The student's team will meet to discuss and decide which services the student needs and how those services will be delivered. At this time, school program scheduling modifications and adaptations should be reviewed. **The school nurse, in collaboration with the family and primary health care providers, will assess the skill level required of the child-specific health care provider at school, be aware of laws and nursing standards that govern the delegation of health procedures, and determine the appropriate individuals to provide health care procedures.** Finally, the school nurse is responsible for managing all of the health care services that the student receives, including those delegated to others (see Figure 3.3). The team also considers and identifies back-up personnel to provide child-specific health care procedures. Depending on the skill level required, back-up personnel may include school nurses, pediatric home care nurses, staff from visiting nurse associations/public health nurses, parents/relatives, health care aides, and teachers, teaching assistants, integration specialists, and other related services personnel.

NASN POSITION PAPER:
DELEGATION OF SCHOOL SERVICES TO UNLICENSED ASSISTIVE PERSONNEL

There are two critical questions involved in delegating and supervising a nursing activity:

1. **Is the activity a nursing task under the state's definition of nursing?**

    Nursing activities are defined by state statute and interpreted by the state board of nursing. A state's attorney general's opinion, court decision, or other mandate may modify the state's definition of nursing or interpretation of its scope of practice. On the basis of these definitions and interpretations, the nurse decides whether the activity or procedure is one that can be performed only by a registered nurse (RN).

2. **Can the activity be performed by unlicensed assistive personnel (UAP) under the supervision of a registered nurse?**

    The delegation of nursing activities to UAPs may be appropriate when

    *   It is not otherwise prohibited by state statute or regulations, legal interpretations, or agency policies.
    *   It does not require exercising nursing judgment.
    *   It is delegated and supervised by an RN.

Determinations Required in Each Case

According to the National Association of School Nurse Consultants (1995), the delegating and supervising RN makes the following determinations, on a case-by-case basis, for *each student with health care needs and each required nursing care activity:*

a. The RN validates the necessary physical orders, including emergency orders, parent/ guardian authorization, and any other legal documentation necessary to implement the nursing care.
b. The RN conducts an initial nursing assessment.
c. Consistent with the state's nursing practice act and the RN's assessment of the student, the RN determines what level of care is required—care by RNs, licensed practical or vocational nurses, other professionals, or UAP.
d. Consistent with the state board of nursing regulations, the RN determines the amount of training required for the UAP. If the individual to whom the nurse will delegate care has not completed standardized training, the RN must ensure that the UAP obtains such training in addition to receiving child-specific training.
e. Prior to delegation, the nurse evaluates the competence of the individual to perform the task safely.
f. The RN provides a written care plan to be followed by the unlicensed staff member.
g. The RN indicates, within the written plan, when RN notification, reassessment, and intervention are warranted as a result of a change in the student's condition, the performance of the procedure, or other circumstance.
h. The RN determines the amount and type of RN supervision necessary.
i. The RN determines the frequency and type of student health reassessment necessary for ongoing safety and efficacy.
j. The RN teaches the UAP to document the delegated care according to the standards and requirements of the state's board of nursing and agency procedures.
k. The RN documents activities appropriate to each of the nursing actions listed above.

Figure 3.3. The position paper of the National Association of State School Nurse Consultants addresses questions about delegating care and outlines determinations to be made on a case-by-case basis. (From National Association of State School Nurse Consultants. [1995]. Delegation of school health services to unlicensed assistive personnel: A position paper of the National Association of State School Nurse Consultants. *Journal of School Nursing, 11*(2), pp. 17–19; reprinted by permission of American School Health Association, Kent, Ohio. This is not a transfer of copyright; the American School Health Association maintains copyright ownership and authorship of the use of said material, and the American School Health Association or others authorized by the American School Health Association are in no way restricted from republication.)

Funding for necessary school health care services continues to be a concern. Some school districts finance personnel to provide care through their special education budgets. Others consider it the responsibility of general education. The following resources have been helpful in funding or supplementing school health care services:

- Medicaid reimbursement for school-based health services when such reimbursement does not adversely affect the availability of home-based services
- Nursing services from town/city public health departments
- Family's health insurance policy, with family consent, when there is no additional cost to the family (e.g., lifetime cap, premiums, home care services)
- Local funding
- Special state-designated funds
- State-funded grants (e.g., school reform, educational enhancement, systems change, specialized taxes)
- Local philanthropic organizations or foundations
- Several funding sources sharing the cost

5. ***Plan for the student's participation in his or her own health care*** Collaboration among families, health care providers, and school personnel is important for establishing consistent student expectations in terms of participation in self-care. Collaboration will help delineate the sequence of tasks required in self-care and identify methods that have been or may be useful in promoting maximum student involvement.

   An assessment of the student's current level of participation in self-care forms the basis for establishing realistic goals and assessing improvement. Student involvement in self-care on three levels is possible (Caldwell et al., 1989b):

   a. Tolerance for the position or procedure
   b. Ability to assist with or direct the care required
   c. Ability to perform self-care independently with or without supervision

   Developing appropriate goals in the three levels of involvement is discussed later in the Training section.

6. ***Plan for training*** The school nurse must review the state's public health code and/or Nurse Practice Act to determine whether health care can be delegated (see Chapter 2). The school nurse will determine the skill level required for individuals who will serve as health care providers during the school day. Frequently, in schools, one or more individuals are appointed as the student's health care providers. Other school personnel will serve as back-up and will need the skills to identify and respond to changes in a child's health status. School personnel who frequently serve as health care providers are the school nurse, health aides, teacher(s), assistants, or home health care personnel. The following considerations or questions are important when planning for training:

   a. Is the confidentiality of the student and family respected?
   b. What is the skill level necessary for the student's health care provider?
   c. Which individuals and groups require training?
   d. What amount of detailed information is appropriate for various training needs?
   e. Who will conduct the training?
   f. Which health professionals in the community are available to the school system to provide consultation and training?
   g. How will the family and student be involved in training?
   h. Is there a cost involved?
   i. Where will the training be conducted?
   j. How much time will be required?
   k. Are substitutes/back-up personnel needed to perform the existing responsibilities of the individuals being trained?
   l. Who will provide supervision, follow-up, and support?
   m. How often will training updates be needed?

DEVELOPMENT OF AN INDIVIDUALIZED HEALTH CARE PLAN

Several IHCP formats are available, and one format is included in Chapter 6. Other formats can be found in manuals listed in Suggested Readings at the end of this chapter. Key points about IHCPs include the following:

- IHCPs are based on health assessments of the students by the school nurse. Consideration should be given to varied cultural beliefs and health practices (see Chapter 6).
- IHCPs outline the goals and strategies needed to maintain and/or improve student health and increase student participation in self-care activities.
- IHCPs are important documentation for health and education staff.
- IHCPs foster consistency for health care across all environments for students (i.e., in transit to and from school, in school, on field trips, in after-school programs).

Components of the Individualized Health Care Plan

The following is a list of the components of the IHCP:

1. *Brief health history*   A description of the course and severity of the child's condition is useful. The history may indicate how the child's condition may affect educational functioning.

2. *Special health care needs of the child*   Special health care needs may include procedures and medications that the child requires at home and school, socioemotional concerns, child's communication method and ability to communicate needs, modifications or alternative methods needed in caring for the child (e.g., bathroom modifications for children needing catheterization), infection control procedures, restrictions and/or precautions, and possible problems and symptoms of impending emergencies.

3. *Basic health status*   Knowledge of the student's baseline status provides comparative information about stability or improvement in the child's overall health. The student's physical endurance, baseline weight, and level of involvement in self-care are points to consider.

4. *Medications (refer to individual state regulations regarding medication administration)*   The IHCP should
   - Designate the individual responsible for dispensing medication
   - List medications administered at home
   - List medications needed at school
   - Indicate dose and time of medication administration
   - List medication side effects and interaction effects that may affect school functioning or child's safety
   - List any adverse reactions to the medication the child may have experienced and appropriate responses
   - Identify medications that are administered on an as-needed basis and the circumstances that indicate the medication is needed
   - Indicate known allergies
   - Delineate protocols for administering experimental medications

5. *Diet/nutrition*   IHCPs should address the individual nutrition needs of the students. Nutritional considerations may include
   - Need for special or modified diet
   - Known allergies and reactions
   - Special fluid requirements/restrictions
   - Route of feeding (e.g., oral, tube, both)
   - Feeding problems and management techniques
   - Oral/dental concerns
   - Need to schedule snacks and meals around administration of medication or a health procedure (e.g., chest physiotherapy, exercise routine)

6. *Transportation (see Chapter 4)*   The transportation section of a health care plan should include information about the following:
   - Accessible vehicle
   - Need for safety-tested car seats
   - Appropriate equipment to secure the wheelchair to guarantee student safety

- Appropriate method for securing the equipment
- Temperature-controlled vehicle when indicated
- Listing of trained personnel who are ready to provide routine and emergency care
- Written emergency care plan in the vehicle
- Communication device in vehicle

The following is an example of a plan for safe transportation to and from school that was incorporated into a student's IHCP.

At first I was nervous about my new assignment as Maria's bus monitor. Maria is a little girl who will be coming to school in a wheelchair and will need assistance with all of her daily activities. She is unable to speak, but her mother said that she communicates with her eyes and by laughing and crying. When she is happy, her eyes light up, she laughs and her whole body tenses up as if she could jump out of her wheelchair. I was taught how to secure her wheelchair into the van safely with a four-point restraint system. Because Maria could not move her extremities voluntarily, I had to ensure that her arms and legs were always resting properly on her wheelchair and that her head was positioned on her head rest. Sometimes at the end of a busy school day, Maria would be tired and her head would drop down to her chest.

Maria also has a gastrostomy tube and needs to receive formula continuously by a feeding pump, even on the bus. Maria's mother and the school nurse briefly reviewed with me the purpose of the gastrostomy tube, how the pump works, and when I might need to shut off the pump. For example, if Maria has a sad cry and her body becomes rigid, I have been instructed to shut off her pump. We have the emergency plan posted in the school bus, and Maria's mother feels more secure knowing that the bus driver can notify her by his cellular phone if a problem arises.

I'm not nervous traveling with Maria anymore. She loves to see the yellow bus pull up to her house and always greets me with her big smile and cries of delight.

7. ***Equipment***   Considerations for equipment include the following:
   - Type and size of equipment required by the child
   - Who provides the equipment
   - Who provides other materials (e.g., clean wipes, cotton balls, gloves)
   - Who maintains the equipment
   - Contingency plans when the equipment is not working (e.g., back-up battery for a ventilator)
   - Need for back-up or emergency supplies and equipment (e.g., extra catheters)
   - Convenient storage area for equipment and supplies in school
   - Resources for learning how to use equipment

8. ***Possible problems and interventions***   The student's team is responsible for anticipating possible child-specific problems that may occur at school and in transit. Anticipation of possible problems and concerns allows the team to plan and provide child-specific training and interventions. Each of the procedures in the Guidelines for Care section includes a list of possible problems.

9. ***Emergency plan for school and transit***   Planning for emergencies is vital to coordinate efforts and reduce or improve response time. Plans must be developed for both student-specific emergencies and natural disasters (see the Individualized Health Care Plan in Chapter 6).
   a. *Child-specific emergencies*   Students with special health care needs require individualized emergency plans. The emergency plan should be discussed and reviewed with families and should address warning signs and symptoms of problems/distress, interventions, time frame necessary to respond to an emergency, and emergency contact names and telephone numbers (alternate telephone numbers). The emergency plan also should include the following information:

- Closest agreed-upon emergency room that is equipped to meet the child's emergency needs
- Roles and responsibilities of transportation personnel during student emergency
- Communication system that enables the driver to obtain emergency assistance
- How a student will be transported to an emergency care facility (e.g., driver transports student, driver calls for emergency vehicle).

b. *Natural disasters and fire* It is important to plan for natural disasters, such as hurricanes, floods, tornadoes, and ice and snow storms. Team members must consider back-up equipment, supplies, and emergency evacuation plans in the event that the student is required to stay for an extended time at the school during the disaster.

Individuals developing the plan for school evacuation in the event of fire may need to consider the special assistance that some students require. Adults outside of those in the student's classroom may need to be assigned to help a particular child evacuate the building. It is critical to check the accessibility of each emergency exit. Fire department personnel can assist in developing a student-specific fire evacuation plan.

c. *Agencies to contact regarding emergencies* Notify the Red Cross, fire department, telephone company, electric company, emergency room, and emergency medical services concerning the diagnosis and special health care needs of identified students. These organizations will utilize the information when planning for prioritizing the people and places to evacuate, reinstating services, and securing necessary equipment that emergency medical services or emergency rooms need for pediatric emergencies.

10. ***IHCP, reviewed by physician and signed by parent, educational administrator, and school nurse*** Agreement on the IHCP is documented by the signatures of the above-listed parties.

11. ***Incorporation of the IHCP into pertinent student records*** Many students with special health care needs may qualify for special education under IDEA and will need IEPs. Information from the IHCP (developed by the school nurse) should be incorporated into the IEP and it should be noted in the IEP or the individual student accommodation plan (mandated by Section 504) that school health care services are required. The IHCP should then be attached. Inclusion of school health care services in these plans ensures the delivery of those services. Goals and objectives for increasing student involvement in self-care should be part of the child's IEP or individual student accommodation plan.

Each student should have a cumulative permanent record that follows him or her throughout his or her school career. For students not receiving special education services, the cumulative record should include the IHCP. Documentation may assist with continuity and consistency of services in school.

TRAINING

Training includes *general training, child-specific training,* and *training for student involvement in self-care.* Training promotes safe and effective care for the student, competence and confidence on the part of the care providers at school, and family confidence in the service provided and provides a forum, if necessary, to discuss chronic illness, coping, grief, and bereavement. Training also respects and includes knowledge of diverse cultural beliefs and practices.

Steps in General Training

General training or orientation is designed for people who have contact with a student with a special health care need but who are not responsible for providing the necessary health care (e.g., peers, school staff, parents, administrators). General training is designed to create positive attitudes among teachers, administrators, and classmates toward including students with a range of diverse needs in the school community; creates an opportunity for education staff to discuss concerns; addresses the concerns parents, teachers, and students may have about the social, emotional, and educational impact of attending school with a peer who has a disability or a chronic illness; and provides an overview of the child's health care needs and emergency plan.

1. ***Include the health care plan in general training*** The team should review the health care plan to determine appropriate information to include in a general training. Any general training should include a brief description of the health condition and appropriate associated health care needs the student may have. If a child is assisted by medical technology, it may be useful to display the equipment and describe how it works.

2. ***Explain the emergency plan*** A brief explanation of the child's emergency plan should be presented during general training. It is important to include

   - A review of the emergency plan and universal precautions
   - Assurances that a procedure is in place
   - Known location of copies of the plan
   - Recognition of emergency situations and appropriate responses
   - A clear designation of people who will perform emergency services and how to reach them
   - Times and places for practice/emergency drills

3. ***Develop awareness training*** The following is an excerpt from *The Inside Edition* (Ferrera, 1995) of a child discussing awareness of her sister's disability:

   > *I was four years old when my sister Elia was born. She had cloacal exstrophy and a lot of problems because of it. . . . One time we had learning about handicapped in my classroom. I asked my teacher and my mom if I could go in my class and tell them about what happened with Elia. They said ok, and I got to tell them about Elia and answer their questions. I knew a lot of the answers. They wanted to know what her prosthesis looked like, so I took her to the bathroom to take off her tights, and we showed them. It went great. Everybody understood and didn't make fun of her. She showed them her wheelchair and did wheelies, and everybody laughed. Elia loved it. She felt good because they could understand.*
   >
   > *Some people don't understand. Like in the grocery store or at the beach. They stare because of her prosthesis and they don't leave her alone. That doesn't make me feel very good, even though I try to ignore it.*
   >
   > *I think it's going to be hard for Elia as she grows up. She might need my help. But one thing that's important is that no matter what, I would always love her.* (p. 8)

   Some school districts and community programs have age-based disability/diversity awareness programs. Topics covered as part of such programs include, but are not limited to, noticing and understanding similarities and differences in people; learning about types of disabilities and health care conditions; feeling included and experiencing barriers; and showing cooperation, curiosity, and respect. Awareness programs provide a beginning for students, school staff, and families to work together and answer questions.

   Students assisted by medical technology and their families may want to share specific information with school personnel, classmates, and community providers. Awareness training often includes questions and answers about a child's condition and equipment. The family and student should understand that they can refuse to answer any questions. The following list includes questions frequently asked:

   - What is that tube for? Does it hurt?
   - How do you eat, drink, go to the bathroom, and get dressed?

- Why is that grown-up with you in school?
- What games and television shows do you like?
- How fast does your wheelchair go?
- Do people make fun of you? What do you say or do?
- What is it like in the hospital?
- What is the best way to help you with everyday simple things?
- Would you rather spend your life like this or would you rather have not lived?
- Do people treat you differently now?
- Do you go on dates?
- How do you drive your car? Can we see you drive?
- What are your plans for the future?

Steps in Student-Specific Training

Student-specific training is always necessary, even if school personnel have provided similar care to other students. Although published protocols describing general procedures may exist, individual students may require or prefer variations that school staff must become familiar with to ensure each student's comfort and to maintain consistency with home regimens. Individualized student-specific training is divided into three components: 1) an overview of the student's health condition, 2) health care procedures, and 3) an emergency plan. People who are directly responsible for providing health care services to the student need comprehensive training.

1. *Provide an overview of the training*   The following is a brief list of the topics to discuss in student-specific training:
   a. Description of the health issues or condition and required procedures
   b. Universal precautions
   c. Psychosocial implications, including privacy, confidentiality, and dignity; maximum involvement of student in self-care; and attitudes and preferences of the student and family
   d. Pertinent information from the IHCP
   e. Communication network within school and among school, home, and health care providers

2. *Discuss health care procedures*   The following are topics on health care procedures to discuss:
   a. Basic anatomy and body mechanics
   b. Name and purpose of the procedure
   c. Time(s) to be performed and length of time involved
   d. Teaching methods, such as trainer demonstration of the procedure (e.g., using a mannequin, viewing videotapes or slides); trainee demonstration of the procedure on a mannequin; trainee observation of the parent or trainer performing the procedure on the student; and documentation using skills checklists.
   e. Site where student's care will take place
   f. Hygienic practices, including universal precautions
   g. Equipment and supplies required
   h. Lifting and positioning of the student
   i. Level of student involvement in self-care
   j. Precautions
   k. Signs and symptoms requiring attention
   l. Documentation of the procedure
   m. Scheduled supervision and follow-up

3. *Review emergency plan*   It is important to review the following steps and responsibilities in an emergency plan:
   a. Signs of possible problems
   b. Recognition of and response to problems and emergency situations
   c. Individual responsibilities in an emergency situation

d. Location of the emergency plan
e. List of people to contact in case of an emergency
f. Mock emergency plan drill

Steps in Student Training

The ability of students to provide their own health care can provide them greater freedom in school and in the community. It will promote the goal of independent living in their adult years. Students can improve their self-care skills by improving their tolerance, direction, and/or independent completion of health care (Caldwell, Todaro, & Gates, 1989a).

1. *Increase tolerance for care*   Students achieve independence in and tolerance of self-care at varying levels depending on cognitive, physical, emotional, social, and cultural factors. Appropriate goals should be developed to increase their tolerance of care. For instance, a student who has difficulty tolerating gastrostomy tube feedings may allow the procedure if it is paired with listening to a favorite piece of music.

2. *Direct the care provider*   Many students with physical disabilities learn to direct the care provider and assist during aspects of the procedure. For example, a student who has hemiplegia and has limited use of his or her extremities may inform the care provider when it is time for his or her gastrostomy feeding and may assume the correct position for the feeding.

3. *Achieve independence*   Other students will be able to learn to perform procedures independently. The degree of supervision needed may vary depending on the complexity of the care and the developmental level of the child. Depending on the preference of the child and family, procedures can be performed to facilitate inclusion with peers.

IMPLEMENTATION, MONITORING, AND EVALUATION

The following list provides steps for families and health care and school personnel to assist in the implementation, monitoring, and evaluation of a student with special health care needs in school:

1. ***Provide direct care as appropriate or supervise student's health care provider(s).***
   In some cases, the school nurse or another competent licensed nurse will provide the health care services delineated in the student's IHCP. When care is delegated to unlicensed personnel, the school nurse supervises the student's health care provider(s) (see Figure 2.2).

2. ***Update assessment of the student's health status annually.***
   Doctor's orders and prescriptions for health care services in the school should be reviewed at least annually; some may need review every 3 months. For many students with special health care needs, periodic visits to the physician are common. Any change in the health status of a child and/or health care procedures should be reported to the school nurse and will require new physician's orders. Reporting procedures will need to be established in the initial stages of school entry/reentry.

3. ***Update and evaluate student's IHCP.***
   The student's IHCP should be reviewed at least yearly. Based on changes in the student's condition, reassessment and revision of the health care plan may need to be done more frequently.

4. ***Document, review, and update skills training.***
   There are many reasons to *document* health care services. Documentation provides a clear understanding of required health care needs, indicates the time and date that health care has been provided, indicates any problems observed, assists in answering questions or concerns of parents or health care providers, provides evidence of risk management, and provides information to school administrators as to number of students needing health care procedures in school.

The team *reviews* and *updates* the child's IHCP and IEP at specified intervals and as necessary. This process helps prevent and manage problems and helps identify the need to modify an existing program. Team review provides the opportunity to assess whether the services are being delivered as planned and whether the plan is effective.

People responsible for the school-based health care of students with special health care needs benefit from continuing education opportunities to improve and maintain their knowledge and skills. In addition, care providers need to learn new approaches and techniques, which are developed and updated every year.

SUMMARY

Can children who have special health needs safely attend school? Eddie's mom expresses the fears of families, health providers, and educators:

Eddie needed his inner cannula cleaned every 2 hours, suctioning as needed about twice a day, and gastrostomy feedings. Could they really do that in a school building? What about dust, air quality, and access to water? He didn't need an intensive care unit anymore; he needed a school. I had to let go.

We now know that children with special health care needs can safely attend school. We also know that their attendance requires team processes involving families, school staff, and medical personnel, and we know that those team processes must include careful planning and thorough training in the school district and on the school site.

This chapter has addressed basic information about the processes necessary for the development of safe and appropriate education programs for children with special health care needs. The remaining chapters are related to special health care procedures. They provide specific information that can be used to provide training and education about special health care needs and daily and emergency procedures.

REFERENCES

Caldwell, T.H., Todaro, A.W., & Gates, A.J. (1989a). *Community provider's guide: An information outline for working with children with special health care needs.* New Orleans, LA: Children's Hospital.

Caldwell, T.H., Todaro, A.W., & Gates, A.J. (1989b). Special health care needs. In J. Bigge (Ed.), *Teaching individuals with physical and multiple disabilities* (3rd ed., pp. 50–75). New York: Macmillan.

Caldwell, T.H., Todaro, A.W., Gates, A.J., Failla, S., & Kirkhart, K. (1991). *Community provider's guide: An information outline for working with children with special health care needs* (1991 addendum). New Orleans, LA: Children's Hospital.

Ferrera, A. (1995). Sometimes I feel like I've always been there for her, and she's always been there for me. *The Inside Edition, 3*(2), 8.

National Association of State School Nurse Consultants. (1995). Delegation of school health services to unlicensed assistive personnel: A position paper of the National Association of State School Nurse Consultants. *Journal of School Nursing, 11*(2), 17–19.

Palfrey, J.S., Haynie, M., Porter, S., Bierle, T., Cooperman, P., & Lowcock, J. (1992). Project school care: Integrating children assisted by medical technology into educational settings. *Journal of School Health, 62*(2), 50–54.

Rehabilitation Act of 1973, PL 93-112, 29 U.S.C. § 701 *et seq.*

Schwab, N. (Ed.). (1995). *Managing students with genetic disorders: A manual for school nurses* (3rd ed.). Mt. Desert, ME: New England Regional Genetics Group.

Ventilator Assisted Care Program. (1989). *School facility assessment for students who are ventilator assisted.* New Orleans, LA: Children's Hospital.

SUGGESTED READINGS

Ahmann, E., & Lipsi, K. (1992). Developmental assessment of the technology-dependent infant and young child. *Pediatric Nursing, 18*(3), 299–305.

American Federation of Teachers. (1992). *The medically fragile child in the school setting.* Washington, DC: Author.

American Nurses Association. (1995). *The ANA basic guide to safe delegation.* Washington, DC: Author.

Anderson, W., Chitwood, S., & Hayden, D. (1990). *Negotiating the special education maze: A guide for parents and teachers.* Rockville, MD: Woodbine House.

The Annenberg Washington Program in Communications Policy Studies of Northwestern University. (1994). *Communications technology for everyone: Implications for the classroom and beyond.* Washington, DC: Author.

Ault, M.M., Guess, D., Struth, L., & Thompson, B. (1988). The implementation of health related procedures in classrooms for students with severe multiple impairments. *Journal of The Association for Persons with Severe Handicaps, 13*(2), 100–109.

Batshaw, M.L., & Perret, Y.M. (1992). *Children with disabilities: A medical primer* (3rd ed.). Baltimore: Paul H. Brookes Publishing Co.

Bishop, S.G. (1991). Creating partnerships: A hospital-based newsletter for teachers. *Journal of School Health, 61*(8), 361–362.

Blenk, K., & Fine, D.L. (1995). *Making school inclusion work: A guide to everyday practices.* Cambridge, MA: Brookline Books.

Bristow, D., & Pickering, G. (1993). A primer on assistive technology. *The Special Edge, 7*(7), 8–9.

Chauvin, V.G. (Ed.). (1994). *Students with special health care needs: A manual for school nurses* (Vol. 1). Scarborough, ME: National Association of School Nurses, Inc.

Cox, J., & Jonson, E. (1994). Self-care in the classroom for children with chronic illness: A case study of a student with cystic fibrosis. *Elementary School Guidance & Counseling, 29*(2), 121–128.

Dychkowski, L.B. (1990). Caring for the terminally ill child in the school setting. *School Nurse, 6*(2), 8–12.

Ellerton, M., & Turner, C. (1992). Back to school: An evaluation of a reentry program for school-aged children with cancer. *Canadian Oncology Nursing Journal, 2*, 8–11.

Freedman, R., & Fesko, S. (1995, August). Consumer and family perspectives on the meaning of work. *Research Practice.* Boston: Institute for Community Inclusion, Children's Hospital.

Graff, J.C., Ault, M.M., Guess, D., Taylor, M., & Thompson, B. (1990). *Health care for students with disabilities: An illustrated medical guide for the classroom.* Baltimore: Paul H. Brookes Publishing Co.

Harbeck, D. (1990). Individual health care plans. *School Nurse, 6*(1), 19–21.

Hass, M.B., Villars Gerber, M.J., Kalb, K.M., Luehr, R.E., Miller, W.R., Silkworth, C.K., & Will, S.I.S. (1993). *The school nurse's sourcebook of individualized healthcare plans.* North Branch, MN: Sunrise River Press.

Hootman, J. (1990). *Procedure manual for quality nursing intervention in the school* (Rev. ed.). (Available from Multnomah Education Service District, School Health Services, 11611 NE Ainsworth Circle, Portland, OR 97220)

Igoe, J.B. (1994). Project ASSIST: Preparation for paraprofessionals working with school nurses serving children and youth with special health needs. *Issues: A Newsletter of the National Council of the State Boards of Nursing, 15*(2), 4–8.

Illinois State Board of Education, Illinois Association of School Nurses, & Illinois Department of Public Health. (1992). *Management of students with health impairments in the school setting.* Springfield: Illinois State Board of Education.

Jackson, P., & Vessey, J. (1996). *Primary care of the child with a chronic health condition.* St. Louis, MO: Mosby Yearbook.

Jarrow, J., Baker, B., Hartman, R., Harris, R., Lesh, K., Redden, M., & Smithson, J. (1993). *How to choose a college: Guide for the student with a disability.* Columbus, OH: Association on Higher Education and Disability and The HEATH Resource Center.

Johnson, M.P., & Asay, M. (1993). Who meets the special health care needs of North Carolina schoolchildren? *Journal of School Health, 63*(10), 417–420.

Kozloff, M.A. (1994). *Improving educational outcomes for children with disabilities: Guidelines and protocols for practice.* Baltimore: Paul H. Brookes Publishing Co.

Krajicek, M.J., & Moore, C.A. (1993). Child care for infants and toddlers with disabilities and chronic illnesses. *Focus on Exceptional Children, 25*(8), 1–16.

Krajicek, M.J., & Steinke, G.D. (1994, August). *Summary of proceedings: The national conference of developing policy and practice to implement I.D.E.A. related to invasive procedures for children with special health care needs.* Denver, CO: ED383162.

Krier, J. (1993). Involvement of educational staff in the health care of medically fragile children. *Pediatric Nursing, 19*(3), 251–254.

Larson, G. (1988). *Managing the school age child with a chronic health condition.* Wayzata, MN: Division of Chronimed, Inc. Publishing.

Larson, G.L. (1990). *Managing the student with a chronic condition: A practical guide for school personnel* (Rev. ed.). Wayzata, MN: DCI Publishing.

Lash, M. (1992). *When your child goes to school after an injury.* Medford, MA: Tufts University.

Liptak, G.S., & Weitzman, M. (1995). Children with chronic conditions need your help at school. *Contemporary Pediatrics, 12*(9), 64–80.

Michael, M.G., Arnold, K.D., Magliocca, L.A., & Miller, S. (1992). Influences on teachers' attitudes of the parents' role as collaborator. *Remedial and Special Education, 13*(2), 24–30, 39.

Moffitt, K., Reiss, J., & Nackashi, J. (1992). *Special children, special care.* (Available from South Florida Bookstores [813] 974-2631)

Moore, C. (1992, July). *Maximizing family participation in the team process.* Paper prepared for the Second National Symposium on Effective Communication for Children with Severe Disabilities, McLean, VA.

National health and safety performance standards: Guidelines for out-of-home child care programs. (1992). Arlington, VA: National Center for Education in Maternal and Child Health.

Parette, H.P., Jr., Bartlett, C.R., & Holder-Brown, L. (1994). The nurse's role in planning for inclusion of medically fragile and technology-dependent children in public school settings. *Issues in Comprehensive Pediatric Nursing, 17*(2), 61–72.

Parette, H.P., Jr., & Holder-Brown, L. (1992). The role of the school counselor in providing services to medically fragile children. *Elementary School Guidance & Counseling, 27*(1), 47–55.

Parette, H.P., Jr., & Parette, P.C. (1992). Young children with disabilities and assistive technology: The nurse's role on multidisciplinary technology teams. *Journal of Pediatric Nursing, 7*(4), 237–245.

Porter, S., Burkley, J., Bierle, T., Lowcock, J., Haynie, M., & Palfrey, J.S. (1992). *Working toward a balance in our lives: A booklet for families of children with disabilities and special health care needs.* Boston: Project School Care, Children's Hospital.

Rabin, N.B. (1994). School reentry and the child with a chronic illness: The role of the pediatric nurse practitioner. *Journal of Pediatric Health Care, 8*(5), 227–232.

Santilli, N., Dodson, W.E., & Walton, A.V. (1991). *Students with seizures: A manual for school nurses.* Cedar Grove, NJ: HealthScan, Inc.

Schwab, N. (1995). *Guidelines for the management of students with genetics disorders: A manual for school nurses* (3rd ed.). Mount Desert, ME: New England Regional Genetics Group.

Schwab, N., & Haas, M. (1995). Delegation and supervision in school settings: Standards, issues, and guidelines for practice (Part 1). *Journal of School Nursing, 11*(1), 26–35.

Seager, D. (1993). *Guidelines for the care of children assisted by medical technology in the educational setting.* Sarnia, Ontario, Canada: Lambton County Board of Education.

Sexson, S.B., & Madan-Swain, A. (1993). School reentry for the child with chronic illness. *Journal of Learning Disabilities, 26*(2), 137.

Silkworth, C.S., Haas, M., Villars, M., & Luehr, R.E. (1988). *Responding with support: An individualized health plan for a student with AIDS virus infection.* Minneapolis: School Nurse Organization of Minnesota and Minnesota Department of Education, Division of Development and Partnerships Learner Support Services.

Special education school nurse procedure manual. (1988). (Available from Michigan Education Association, 1216 E. Kendall Blvd., East Lansing, MI 48823).

Special health care: Recommended practices for the early childhood educator. (1993). Vancouver, British Columbia, Canada: Early Childhood Educators of British Colombia.

Stainback, S., & Stainback, W. (Eds.). (1992). *Curriculum considerations in inclusive classrooms: Facilitating learning for all students.* Baltimore: Paul H. Brookes Publishing Co.

Steele, N.F., & Morgan, J. (1989). Emergency planning for technology-assisted children. *Journal of Pediatric Nursing, 4*(2), 81–87.

Supervisor's guide for transporting children with special health needs. (1991). Baltimore: Maryland State Department of Education and Maryland State Department of Health and Mental Hygiene.

Thompson, B., Wickham, D., Wegner, J., Ault, M.M., Shanks, P., & Reinertson, B. (1993). *Handbook for the inclusion of young children with severe disabilities: Strategies for implementing exemplary full inclusion programs.* Lawrence, KS: Learner Managed Designs, Inc.

Todaro, A.W., Failla, S., & Caldwell, T.H. (1993). A model for training community-based providers for children with special health care needs. *Journal of School Health, 63*(6), 262–265.

Torres, I., & Corn, A.L. (1990). *When you have a visually handicapped child in your classroom: Suggestions for teachers.* New York: American Foundation for the Blind.

Turner-Hanson, A., Holaday, B., Corser, N., Ogletree, G., & Swan, J.H. (1994). The experiences of discrimination: Challenges for chronically ill children. *Pediatric Nursing, 20*(6), 571–575.

Valluzzi, J.L. (1995). Safety issues in community-based settings for children who are medically fragile: Program planning for natural disasters. *Infants and Young Children, 7*(4), 62–67.

Wadsworth, D.E., Knight, D., & Balser, V. (1993). Children who are medically fragile or technology dependent: Guidelines. *Intervention in School and Clinic, 29*(2), 102–104.

Waterman, B.B. (1994). Assessing children for the presence of a disability. *NICHCY News Digest, 4*(1), 1–27.

Wold, S. (1981). *School nursing: A framework for practice.* North Branch, MN: Sunrise River Press.

Ylvisaker, M., Hartwick, P., & Stevens, M. (1991). School reentry following head injury: Managing the transition from hospital to school. *Journal of Head Trauma Rehabilitation, 6*, 10–22.

MANUALS

Bradley, B. (1994). *Occupational exposure to bloodborne pathogens: Implementing OSHA standards in school settings*. Scarborough, ME: National Association of School Nurses, Inc.

California State Department of Education. (1990). *Guidelines and procedures for meeting the specialized physical health care needs of pupils*. Sacramento, CA: Author.

Chauvin, V.G. (1994). *Students with special health care needs: A manual for school nurses* (Vol. 1). Scarborough, ME: National Association of School Nurses, Inc.

Connecticut State Department of Education. (1992). *Serving students with special health care needs*. Hartford, CT: Author.

Crimlisk, J.T., Murray, S.V., Judas, M.L., Jorgensen, K.M., & Thompson, J.A. (1990). *Your child has a tracheostomy: A guide for home care*. Boston: Department of Health and Hospitals.

Early Childhood Educators of British Columbia. (1993). *Special health care: Recommended practices for the early childhood educator*. Vancouver, British Columbia, Canada: Author.

Goodman, I.F., & Sheetz, A.H. (1995). *The comprehensive school health manual*. Boston: Massachusetts Department of Public Health.

Haas, M.B. (Ed.). (1993). *The school nurse's source book of individualized healthcare plans* (Vol. 1). North Branch, MN: Sunrise River Press.

Hootman, J. (1990). *Procedure manual for quality nursing intervention in the school* (Rev. ed.). Portland, OR: Multnomah Education Service District, School Health Services.

Illinois State Board of Education, Illinois Association of School Nurses, & Illinois Department of Public Health. (1992). *Management of students with health impairments in the school setting*. Springfield: Illinois State Board of Education.

Larson, G.L. (1990). *Managing the student with a chronic condition: A practical guide for school personnel* (Rev. ed.). Wayzata, MN: DCI Publishing.

Maryland State Department of Education & Maryland State Department of Health and Mental Hygiene. (1991). *Supervisor's guide for transporting children with special health needs*. Baltimore: Author.

Michigan Education Association. (1988). *Special education school nurse procedure manual*. East Lansing, MI: Author.

Moffitt, K., Reiss, J., & Nackashi, J. (1992). *Special children, special care*. Tampa: University of South Florida.

National Center for Education in Maternal and Child Health. (1992). *National health and safety performance standards: Guidelines for out-of-home child care programs*. Arlington, VA: Author.

Santilli, N., Dodson, W.E., & Walton, A.V. (1991). *Students with seizures: A manual for school nurses*. Cedar Grove, NJ: HealthScan, Inc.

Schwab, N. (1994). *Guidelines for the management of students with genetics disorders: A manual for school nurses* (2nd ed.). Mt. Desert, ME: New England Regional Genetics Group.

Scott, J., & Brandstaetter, P. (1995). *Students with other health impairments: Guidelines for educational assessment and services*. Virginia, MN: State Physically and Other Health Impaired Network, Northeast Service Cooperative.

Seager, D. (1993). *Guidelines for the care of children assisted by medical technology in the educational setting*. Sarnia, Ontario, Canada: Lambton County Board of Education.

Silkworth, C.S., Haas, M., Villars, M., & Luehr, R.E. (1988). *Responding with support: An individualized health plan for a student with AIDS virus infection*. Minneapolis: School Nurse Organization of Minnesota and Minnesota Department of Education, Division of Development and Partnerships Learner Support Services.

Special Education Program Services Unit, Rhode Island Department of Education. (1991). *Children with special health care needs in the school setting in Rhode Island: Guidelines for care*. Providence: Rhode Island Department of Education.

Urbano, M.T. (1992). *Preschool children with special health care needs*. San Diego, CA: Singular Publishing Group.

Utah State Office of Education. (1992). *Guidelines for serving students with special health care needs*. Salt Lake City, UT: Author.

Ventilator Assisted Care Program and Respiratory Care Department. (1987). *Getting it started and keeping it going: A guide for respiratory home care of the ventilator assisted individual* (manual and accompanying videotape). New Orleans, LA: Children's Hospital.

Viele, E. (1988). *Procedure guidelines for health care of special needs students in the school setting*. Denver: Colorado Department of Education and Colorado Department of Health.

Wetherbee, L.L., & Neil, A.J. (1989). *Educational rights for children with arthritis: A manual for parents*. Atlanta, GA: Arthritis Foundation and Ronald McDonald Children's Charities.

Transportation of Students with Special Health Care Needs

Joan E. Daley and Susan Murray Larsen

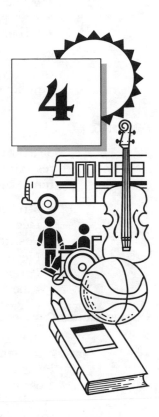

P lanning for and providing safe transportation for children with special health care needs are important components of the health care planning process. A student-specific transportation plan should be developed as part of the health care plan and accompany the student in transit. The transportation provider and a specialist who is familiar with the transportation safety issues and the student's special health care and positioning needs should be added to the planning team.

These areas must be taken into consideration:

- Applicable laws and regulations
- Type of car seat or specialized seating required for the child to be well positioned and safe
- Personnel and training
- Special considerations

APPLICABLE LAWS AND REGULATIONS

PL 101-476, the Individuals with Disabilities Education Act (IDEA) of 1990, lists transportation as a related service available to children who receive special education (who need specialized transportation services). Section 504 of PL 93-112, the Rehabilitation Act of 1973, requires that services and programs provided to students who have disabilities must be equal to those provided to students without disabilities. This includes transportation for nonacademic and extracurricular activities if transportation is provided to students without disabilities. Both laws speak to the right to transportation services but provide little guidance for specific issues.

Federal regulations set standards for vehicle specifications and safety seats for children. Federal Motor Vehicle Safety Standard 213 (FMVSS 213) applies to child-restraint systems designed for children who weigh less than 50 pounds. Conventional and specialized devices for children under 50 pounds that are marketed for use in motor vehicles must meet the criteria of crashworthiness, adequate labeling with instructions for use, and adequate materials used in construction. Although not directly covered by FMVSS 213, some restraint systems and positioning devices for bigger children are constructed using suggested materials and crash-testing guidelines specified in the federal standard.

An amendment to Federal Motor Vehicle Safety Standard 222 (FMVSS 222) establishing some requirements for the transportation of wheelchairs and their occupants became effective in January 1994. This amendment requires that, for newly purchased or outfitted vehicles, the following criteria must be met:

- Wheelchairs transported in a forward-facing position
- Four point tie-downs used
- Occupants secured by separate three-point belts

Some states' laws provide for additional specific standards, including vehicle specifications, types of occupant restraints, types of wheelchairs that may be transported, and number of staff.

SEATING

Seating choices vary. These may include conventional car seats and/or the vehicle's own restraint system, specialized seats and restraints, or a wheelchair with a tie-down system. Seating decisions should address the following:

- Student's height and weight
- Degree of support needed for head or trunk
- Positioning
- Need for supervision (health/behavior)
- Potential for interference with devices (e.g., tracheostomy site and tubes, gastrostomy tubes, central venous lines, casts, braces, eyeglasses)

Conventional Car Seats

Students who are smaller than 40 pounds and 40 inches should, whenever possible, use a conventional child safety seat. The student should be evaluated in the seat to see that he or she can tolerate the position and that the seat belts do not create pressure on gastrostomy tubes, catheters, and so forth. Students with tracheostomy tubes should use seats with 5-point harnesses and avoid seats with front crossbars to prevent the possibility of blocking the tracheostomy tube if the student's head falls forward. Seating devices always should be used exactly according to manufacturers' specifications, including those for adding additional straps and tethering for students over a certain size. Harnesses always should be comfortable, snug, and adjusted properly for the student's height.

Specialized Car Seats

A broad range of specialized car seats and convertible seats (i.e., seats that serve as both car seats and mobility devices) is available. As stated previously, a number of these products have been tested for compliance with the standards set by FMVSS 213. The seat chosen should be determined by the student's positioning and activity needs. Most of these seats will be placed in the transportation vehicle with the mobile base collapsed or removed. The seats' manufacturers will provide instructions for securing the seating device to the car seat with seat belt and possible tethers.

Regular Bus Seat with Restraint System

Many students with special health care needs who weigh more than 40 pounds and are more than 40 inches tall do not need specialized devices for transport; for these students, a general restraint system is sufficient. Seat belts should fit snugly. Lap belts should be placed across the hip bones and should never be placed on the abdomen. Shoulder straps must go across the collarbone and should not cross the front of the neck. Care should be taken to ensure that the seat belts do not press on items such as gastrostomy tubes and central venous lines. There are crash-tested safety vests available for students who cannot use conventional seat belts but do not require the positioning assistance of an assistive device.

Some students who use specialized mobility devices may be able to be transferred to the bus seat and use the regular restraint system or a vest. The team will need to consider the following factors in making a decision:

- Student's weight, health condition, and trunk and head control
- Number of staff needed to transfer the student safely
- Adequate training of staff involved in the transfer

An approved specialized seating device should be obtained if the student's condition or the mechanics of the transfer make using the bus seat infeasible, and if the student is transferred mainly because his or her current device is not appropriate for use on a vehicle.

Transportation in a Wheelchair

Children in wheelchairs, travel chairs, and strollers with crash-tested bases can be transported in their seating system when necessary. Students in wheelchairs and other seating systems should be transported facing forward with a four-point restraint system in place to hold the chair secure in the vehicle. A separate three-point system to secure the student in the chair should be used. In cases in which students are using motorized chairs or chairs that have respirators or other equipment attached, make certain weight does not exceed that recommended for the tie-down system. If equipment weight does exceed limits, some equipment (e.g., spare batteries) may need to be removed and stowed separately. Many wheelchair models currently are not tested for crashworthiness.

Other Areas of Consideration for All Seating Devices

The following are some factors to consider when using seating devices:

- Crashworthiness of seating system should be checked.
- The restraint system that holds the child in the seat must be separate from the system that holds the seat in the car.
- Soft does not equal safe. Care should be taken in adding cushions and padding. Padding that can shift or that is easily compressed should be avoided. Padding to enhance positioning may be added along the sides or between the legs outside the restraint system.
- Velcro does not protect and should *not* be used for belts that secure the child in the device (e.g., seat belts, shoulder harnesses).
- The need for head support (i.e., high seats, head rests) should be assessed. Neck supports designed to improve head control are just beginning to be tested for transport. Care should be taken to follow manufacturers' directions for these devices.
- Students who have protective helmets usually should wear these during transport unless specified by the physician and family.
- Trays *always* should be removed during transport and stored safely. If the tray is a permanent part of wheelchair, ensure there are no loose pieces of equipment on tray.
- All drivers and others responsible for assisting children in and out of vehicles must be trained carefully in the proper use of each child's seating device.
- All seating devices and tie-downs should be clean, in good working order, and installed according to manufacturers' directions. Someone should be designated responsible for checking seating devices, especially those provided by school districts or transportation providers.

PERSONNEL AND TRAINING

The school nurse, in consultation with the student's parents and health care providers, should use information from a thorough health assessment of the student to determine the following:

- Level of care needed
- Equipment needed
- Personnel qualified to provide the student's health care in transit

Designation of personnel in transit may vary according to state laws and regulations governing health care delivery.

Vehicle drivers and any other adults accompanying the student(s) in transit should be trained. Training should be coordinated by the school nurse and can be provided by home health care staff, equipment vendors, clinic or school nurses, and parents. Consider involving any substitute transportation staff in training sessions. This is an ideal time for transportation staff and parents to be introduced. Topics for training include the following:

- Confidentiality of information covered in training
- Overview of the student's health condition
- Signs of possible health problems/emergencies and action to be taken
- Student-specific health care procedures needed in transit
- Roles and responsibilities of the vehicle driver
- Roles and responsibilities of any other adults accompanying the student(s)
- Cardiopulmonary resuscitation
- First aid
- Universal precautions
- Equipment and supplies used in transit
- Securement/storage of equipment and supplies during transit
- How to obtain community emergency assistance (e.g., fire department, ambulance, emergency department)

Training should be provided and updated on an annual basis or when the student's health condition, equipment, and/or seating device change.

SPECIAL CONSIDERATIONS

The following vehicle accommodations may be necessary to ensure safe transit:

- Communication system (i.e., cellular phone, two-way radio)
- Climate control for students with temperature instability
- Scheduled route modifications to decrease amount of transport time
- Back-up power source for electrical equipment used in transit
- Lead acid batteries on electrically powered wheelchairs and respiratory systems converted whenever possible to gel-cell or dry-cell batteries
- An external battery box to house and protect batteries used in transit
- Precautions for when oxygen is transported

Additional regulations and safety standards for transportation of children with special health care needs are being developed both on national and state levels across the United States. Teams are urged to contact their states' transportation experts for updated information especially in the area of wheelchair transport.

REFERENCES

Individuals with Disabilities Education Act (IDEA) of 1990, PL 101-476, 20 U.S.C. § 1400 *et seq.*
Rehabilitation Act of 1973, PL 93-112, 29 U.S.C. § 701 *et seq.*

SUGGESTED READINGS

A report from the National School Bus Standards conference. (1995). *Exceptional Parent, 25*(8), 66.
American Academy of Pediatrics. (1989, Spring). The challenge of transporting children with special needs. *Safe Ride News.*[1]

---

[1]For more information regarding topics addressed by *Safe Ride News*, contact Safe Ride News Publications, 5223 N.E. 187th, Lake Forest, WA 98155, (202) 364-5696.

American Academy of Pediatrics. (1993, Winter). Policy statement: Transporting children with special needs. *Safe Ride News* insert.

American Academy of Pediatrics. (1994, Spring). Progress made at special needs transport meeting. *Safe Ride News.*

Automobile transportation: Car seats, wheelchair carriers, and van lifts. (1989). *Exceptional Parent, 19*(4), 28–33.

Barbera, M.C. (1992). Unsung heroes: Special ed. bus drivers. *Exceptional Parent, 22*(6), 24–26.

Bluth, L.F. (1993, April). Transporting infants, toddlers, and preschool children with disabilities. *School Business Affairs, 59*(4), 13–16.

Bluth L.F., & Hochberg, S.N. (1994, April). Transporting students with disabilities. *School Business Affairs, 60*(4), 12–13, 15–17.

Bull, M.J., Stout, J., Doll, J.P., Stroup, K.B., & Rust, J. (1991). Safe transportation for infants with severe hydrocephalus. *Journal of Neuroscience Nursing, 23*(6), 369–373.

Bull, M.J., Weber, K., Derosa, G.P., & Stroup, K.B. (1989). Transporting children in body casts. *Journal of Pediatric Orthopedics, 9*(3), 280–284.

Carter, M., Carig, J., Hamilton, G., Redmon, H., & Mims, I. (1992, April). *Transportation: The neglected related service.* Paper presented at the 70th Annual Convention of the Council for Exceptional Children, Baltimore.

Consumer Reports. (1995). Child safety seats: Are they always safe? *Consumer Reports, 60*(9), 580–585.

Einstein, N. (1995). Guidelines for using transportation services. *Exceptional Parent, 25*(8), 68–69.

Einstein, N. (1996). Good news about wheelchairs and transportation. *Exceptional Parent, 26*(3), 57–58.

Everly, J.S., Bull, M.J., Stroup, K.B., Goldsmith, J., Doll, J.P., & Russell, R. (1993). A survey of transportation services for children with disabilities. *American Journal of Occupational Therapy, 47*(9), 804–810.

Feller, N., Gunnip, A., Stout, J., Bull, M.J., Stroup, K.B., & Stephanidis, J. (1986). A multidisciplinary approach to developing safe transportation for children with special needs. *Orthopedic Nursing, 5*(5), 25–27.

Kelly, M. (1993). Safe transport of technology-dependent children. *American Journal of Maternal/Child Nursing, 18*(1), 29–31.

Korn, G., & Korn, J.A. (1991). *The effective driver of handicapped students.* Kingston, NH: Safeway Training and Transportation Services, Inc.

Stewart, D.D. (1993). *Special care for transporting kids: Getting children with special needs to and from school safely: A manual for school transportation professionals.* Indianapolis, IN: Automotive Safety for Children's Program at Riley Hospital for Children.

Stout, J.D., Bandy, P., Feller, N., Stroup, K.B., & Bull, M.J. (1992). Transportation resources for pediatric orthopaedic clients. *Orthopedic Nursing, 11*(4), 26–30.

Stroup, K.B., Stout, J.D., Atkinson, B.L., Doll, J.P., & Russell, R. (1991). School bus safety. *Exceptional Parent, 21*(6), 80–87.

GUIDE TO TRANSPORTATION SAFETY PRODUCTS FOR CHILDREN WITH SPECIAL NEEDS

Vehicle restraints are now available for children with all kinds of special health care needs. Many under 50 pounds can use standard car seats. Use this guide in conjunction with the AAP Policy Statement, "Transporting Children with Special Needs," published in *Safe Ride News* (1993, Winter).

This list is adapted from materials of the National Easter Seal Society and the Automotive Safety for Children Program, Riley Hospital, Indianapolis, Indiana. It is not intended to be all-inclusive; inclusion does not imply product endorsement. Prices are subject to change.

Note: Products for children under 50 pounds are certified by manufacturers to meet FMVSS 213. Those for children over 50 pounds are not subject to any federal motor vehicle safety standard. Manufacturers of those listed here claim that their products pass tests similar to those for FMVSS 213.

LOW BIRTH WEIGHT INFANTS

Standard Safety Seats
Models without shields only
From: Retail outlets
Cost: $35–$70
Weight: Up to 20 lbs.
Height: Up to 26 inches
Comments: Blanket rolls at sides and between legs to provide positioning and support. Small harness dimensions recommended: 10" from buttocks to shoulder strap slots, 5.5" from crotch strap to buttocks.

Dyn-O-Mite
From: Evenflo Products
Cost: $21–$24.40
Weight: Up to 20 lbs.
Height: Up to 26 inches
Comments: Two harness positions accommodate growth, one-piece harness tie belt. In fully reclined position, use Dyn-O-Mite only with lap/shoulder belt wrapped around the back of the safety seat for added stability.

Dream Ride, D.R. Ultra
From: Cosco
Cost: $40
Weight: Up to 20 lbs.
Height: Up to 26 inches
Comments: Contact Sue Lindstrom to place order. Car bed converts to rear-facing infant safety seat.

INFANT/CHILD MUST LIE PRONE OR SUPINE

Dream Ride, D.R. Ultra
Comments: Use horizontal for preterm infant with potential breathing problems. (See above for information.)

Modified E-Z-On Vest
From: E-Z-On Products, Inc.
Cost: $80
Weight: Up to 100 lbs.
Height: Determined by length of vehicle seat.
Comments: Must have hip measurement to order vest. Sizes are for hips of 22–32 inches. Shoulder strap length adjustable on new models.

ORTHOPEDIC NEEDS REQUIRING CASTING

Spelcast Restraint
From: Snug Seat, Inc.
Cost: $250
Weight: Birth to 50 lbs. including cast
Height: Up to 40 inches
Comments: Appropriate for hip spica cast position. Convertible for rear or forward facing. Top tether recommended in forward-facing position.

Modified E-Z-On Vest
From: E-Z-On Products, Inc.
Cost: $70
Weight: Up to 100 lbs.
Height: Determined by height and length of vehicle seat.
Comments: Modified vest for child who must lie flat; requires full-width bench seat.

BEHAVIOR PROBLEMS

Regular E-Z-On Vest
From: E-Z-On Products, Inc.
Cost: $74.75
Weight: Up to 164 lbs.
Height: Determined by height of vehicle seat.
Comments: Top tether or Cam Wrap required sizes are for waists 22–43 inches. New styles with adjustable zippers and shoulder straps now available.

Besi Restraining Harness
From: Besi Manufacturing
Cost: $65
Size: Waist 22"–44"
Comments: Zipper inserts adjust sizes. School bus use only, with Cam Wrap. (Note: Another Besi product, Little People Restraint System, is not suitable.)

POOR TRUNK AND/OR HEAD CONTROL

Regular E-Z-On Vest
(see Behavior Problems; head control needed)

Besi Restraining Harness Seat
Comments: Head control is needed. (See Besi Restraining Harness above.)

Little Cargo Vest
From: Little Cargo, Inc.
Cost: $39.95
Weight: 25–40 lbs.
Height: Up to 40 inches
Comments: Head control is needed.

Standard Child Safety Seat
From: Retail outlets
Cost: Varies by product
Weight: Up to 40 lbs.
Height: Up to 40 inches
Comments: Blanket rolls at sides and between legs to provide positioning and support. Choose models with three recline positions. Use middle position for facing child with poor head control forward.

Columbia Positioning Seat
From: Columbia Medical
Cost: $599
Weight: 20–102 lbs.
Height: Up to 60 inches
Comments: Top tether strap (free) should be used for children over 60 lbs.

Ortho-Kinetics Travel Chair
From: Ortho-Kinetics
Cost: Varies with options
Weight: 15–90 lbs.
Height: 30–54 inches
Comments: Can be used in a bus with a Q-Straint or Kinedyne System tie-down system.

Carrie Car Seat
From: J.A. Preston
Cost: $932–$1,225
Weight: 20–130 lbs.
Height: 30–68 inches
Comments: Be sure model is approved for use in a motor vehicle. Tether required.

Kidster
From: Gunnell
Cost: $2,500
Weight: Up to 50 lbs.
Height: Customized to client
Comments: Wheel base has not passed dynamic crash testing.

Snug Seat I & II
From: Snug Seat, Inc.
Cost: $595–$750
Weight: Snug I: 15–40 lbs.
        Snug II: 20–70 lbs.
Height: Snug I: Child's head not to extend above seat back
       Snug II: Up to 60 inches
Comments: Snug I: Heavy duty mobility base is crash tested for vehicle use. Both seats for use facing forward only.

Gorilla
From: Snug Seat, Inc.
Cost: $495
Weight: 20–105 lbs.
Height: Child's head not to extend above seat back height
Comments: Side pads and seat extension.

Mulholland
From: Positioning Systems, Inc.
Cost: $2,500–$3,000
Weight: 6–50 lbs.
Height: Customized for client
Comments: Used as a car seat only up to 50 lbs. Base has not passed crash testing.

Sit'N'Stroll
From: Safeline Products
Cost: $149
Weight: Birth to 40 lbs.
Comments: Rear facing for infants up to 32 lbs. preferred position. Converts to stroller.

TECHNOLOGY DEPENDENT

Standard Safety Seats (with harness only)
From: Retail outlets
Comments: Seats with shields not recommended, could interfere with equipment. Secure ancillary equipment in motor vehicle.

BUS TRANSPORT

Carrie Bus Seat
From: J.A. Preston
Cost: Small $348.87, $464.14
Weight: 20–100 lbs.
Height: 30–58 inches
Comments: For use on the school bus seat. Lap belt and tether required.

Cruiser Transport

From: Convaid Products, Inc.

Cost: $808–$1,066

Comments: For children from ages 1–5. Crash tested facing forward with Q-Straint with positive lock. Accessories available.

Kid EZB (Bus Transport Model 4JB)

From: Kid-Care Mobility Products

Cost: $1,300–$1,900

Weight: Up to 35 lbs.

Age: Infant to age 7

Comments: Rear facing for infants to 20 lbs. Tilt and recline shell, and use tie-downs for infant facing rear of car. Tested forward facing with Q-Straint four-point tiedown and three-point restraint.

Kid-E-Plus (Kid Kart Model E05)

From: Kid-Care Mobility Products

Cost: $1,700

Weight: 20 (1 year)–50 lbs.

Height: Up to 40 inches

Comments: Crash tested in forward-facing position with Q-Straint with positive lock and three-point restraint system.

Kid-E-X (Kid Kart Model EX05)

From: Kid-Care Mobility Products

Cost: $1,400–$1,800

Weight: 50–90 lbs.

Height: 35–60 inches

Comments: Crash tested with Q-Straint with positive lock and three-point restraint system.

MANUFACTURERS

Besi Manufacturing
9445 Sutton Place
Hamilton, OH 45011
(800) 543-8222

Columbia Medical
Post Office Box 633
Pacific Palisades, CA 90270
(310) 454-6612

Convaid Products, Inc.
Post Office Box 2458
Ranchos Palos Verde, CA 90274
(800) 552-1020

Cosco
2525 State Street
Columbus, IN 47201
(800) 544-1108/(812) 372-0141

Evenflo Products
1801 Commerce Drive
Piqua, OH 45356
(800) 233-5921/(513) 773-3971

E-Z-On Products, Inc.
500 Commerce Way West, Suite 3
Jupiter, FL 33458
(800) 323-6589

Gunnell
8440 State Street
Millington, MI 48746
(800) 551-0055

Kid-Care Mobility Products
126 Rosebud, Suite 1
Belgrade, MT 59714
(800) 388-5278

Little Cargo, Inc.
100 North Broadway, Suite 2000
St. Louis, MO 63102
(800) 933-8580

Mulholland Positioning Systems, Inc.
215 North 12th Street
Post Office Box 391
Santa Paula, CA 93060
(805) 525-7165

Ortho-Kinetics
Springdale Road
Post Office Box 1647
Waukesha, WI 53187
(800) 824-1068

J.A. Preston
Post Office Box 89
Jackson, MI 49204
(800) 631-7277

Safeline Products
5335 West 48th Avenue
Denver, CO 80212
(800) 829-1625

Snug Seat, Inc.
Post Office Box 1141
Matthews, NC 28106
(800) 336-SNUG

Special Health Concerns

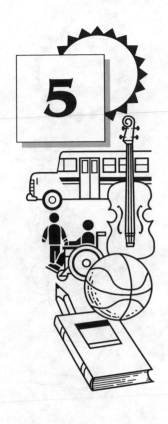

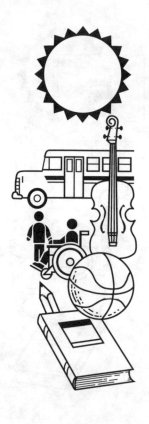

Universal Precautions and Infection Control in a School Setting

Richard G. Giardina and Christine E. Psota

A s a result of the increased prevalence of blood-borne illness and an inability to reliably identify all people with human immunodeficiency virus (HIV) or hepatitis B virus (HBV), the Centers for Disease Control and Prevention (CDC) recommends people understand and implement "universal blood and body fluid precautions"[1] (1987). These measures are intended to prevent transmission of HIV, HBV, and other blood-borne infections as well as to decrease the risk of exposure for health care providers and students.

UNIVERSAL PRECAUTIONS

Universal precautions pertain to blood and the following human body fluids: cerebrospinal fluid, synovial fluid, vaginal secretions, semen, pericardial fluid, pleural fluid, peritoneal fluid, amniotic fluid, any body fluid that is visibly contaminated with blood, and all body fluids in situations in which it is difficult or impossible to differentiate between body fluids. These precautions also apply to other body substances, such as sputum, feces, tears, vomit, nasal secretions, urine, and saliva, when blood is visible in these substances.

The Occupational Safety and Health Administration (OSHA) developed a standard for prevention of exposure to blood-borne pathogens (Occupational Exposure to Blood-Borne Pathogens, 1991). Full compliance with the standard was required as of July 6, 1992.

The standard applies to employees in all health care settings, including hospitals, clinics, dentists' and physicians' offices, blood banks, plasma centers, occupational health clinics, nursing homes, hospices, urgent care centers, clinical laboratories, mortuaries, and funeral homes.

---

[1]To assist hospitals in maintaining up-to-date isolation practices, in 1996 the CDC and the Hospital Infection Control Practices Advisory Committee (HICPAC) revised the *CDC Guideline for Isolation Precautions in Hospitals*. In the revised guideline, "universal precautions" has been renamed "standard precautions"; however, the concept of using personal protective equipment for the care of all patients regardless of their diagnosis or presumed infection status remains the same (Garner & Hospital Infection Control Practices Advisory Committee, 1996).

Although the OSHA standard does not generally apply to municipal or state governments, some states require schools to comply because these regulations set the standard for the safe handling of blood and body fluids. **We recommend that schools incorporate and/or adopt applicable sections of the OSHA standard into school policy.**

The standard mandates that employers provide the following:

- A written exposure control plan that identifies all job classifications that have risk of exposure to blood-borne illness
- Classes on how to prevent occupational exposure to blood-borne illness
- The procedure for evaluating exposure incidents
- A schedule for implementing all the provisions of the standard

For further information about the OSHA standard, contact your regional office of the U.S. Department of Labor, OSHA.

The most important step in preventing exposure to and transmission of any infectious agent is anticipating routine and emergent situations that would place a person in potential contact with infectious materials. **Diligent and proper hand washing is the most effective procedure to protect staff and other students from the transmission of infectious diseases.** The use of personal protective equipment (i.e., gloves, masks, protective eyewear, cover gowns) when having contact with blood or other potentially infectious material provides an additional measure of protection. Appropriate disposal of waste products and needles and proper cleanup and decontamination of spills and equipment are absolutely necessary steps in the control of infectious diseases. **To enhance protection of both the caregiver and the student, the health care provider must anticipate the tasks to be done, the risk involved, and the personal protective equipment needed.**

Hand Washing

Proper hand washing is crucial in preventing the spread of infection. Studies have demonstrated the role of the hands of caregivers in transmission of organisms (Garner & Favero, 1985). Proper hand washing requires

- The use of soap and water
- A vigorous rubbing together of all surfaces of lathered hands for at least 10 seconds
- A thorough rinsing under a stream of water
- Drying of hands
- Turning off the faucet with a dry paper towel
- Disposal of the paper towel

When soap and water are unavailable, a *waterless* skin antiseptic may be used as a temporary method. These products usually contain alcohol and may be irritating to the skin after prolonged use. A waterless product is not a substitute for the recommended handwashing procedure. Hand washing must be done as soon as feasible with soap and water, as described above.

Staff should always wash their hands under the following circumstances:

- Before and after contact with students
- After touching or cleaning inanimate objects contaminated with secretions, blood, or other potentially infectious material **even if gloves were worn**
- After cleaning up spills of blood or other potentially infectious material **even if gloves were worn**
- After contamination of the hands by secretions, blood, or other potentially infectious material **even if gloves were worn**
- After removal of gloves or other personal protective equipment
- Before taking breaks and at the end of the workday

**Hand washing is the most important procedure
for preventing infectious disease transmission.**

Personal Protective Equipment

The use of personal protective equipment is intended to reduce the risk of contact with blood and other potentially infectious materials for the caregiver and to control the spread of infectious agents from student to student. It is essential that appropriate personal protective equipment be used in a consistent manner to reduce the risk of exposure. The following items are considered personal protective equipment:

- Disposable gloves
- Protective eyewear (i.e., glasses with side shields)
- Masks
- A combination of eyewear and mask
- Laboratory coats
- Cover gowns

Gloves should be worn when direct care with a student involves possible contact with blood, mucous membranes, nonintact skin, and other potentially infectious material. When providing care for a student with diarrhea or cold or flu-like symptoms (e.g., cough, runny nose), it is suggested that gloves be worn when coming in contact with feces, respiratory secretions, or any item contaminated with these body substances.

If gloves are torn or in any way defective, they should be discarded. Gloves should be discarded after each use and not reused. Hands should be washed whenever gloves are removed. Gloves should be worn during the following times:

- When having contact with blood, other potentially infectious material, mucous membranes, and nonintact skin
- When changing diapers or assisting the student with cleansing after toileting or catheterization
- When changing dressings/bandages or sanitary napkins/tampons
- When providing mouth, nose, or tracheostomy care
- When the caregiver has broken skin on the hands or around the fingernails
- When cleaning up spills of secretions, blood, or other potentially infectious material
- When touching or cleaning items contaminated with secretions, blood, or other potentially infectious material

Laboratory coats or cover gowns should be worn to protect the caregiver's clothing when splattering of blood or other potentially infectious material is likely. Reusable coats or gowns should be laundered after each use and disposable ones discarded after each care session and never reused. In addition, protective eyewear and masks should be worn during procedures likely to generate splashes of blood or other potentially infectious material (i.e., mouth suctioning) into the nose, mouth, or eyes.

Absorbent underpads or other water barriers should be used to cover all work surfaces when gross contamination with blood or other potentially infectious material is likely. The barrier should be discarded after each care session and the work surface decontaminated.

In the event that cardiopulmonary resuscitation is necessary, a disposable mask with a one-way valve should be used. If this is unavailable, gauze or some other porous material may be placed over the mouth and mouth-to-mouth resuscitation given.

Disposal of Waste

Any disposable item (e.g., gloves or gauze; medical supplies, such as tubing or ostomy bags) contaminated with blood or other potentially infectious material during a care session should be discarded in sturdy plastic bags and tightly closed for transport. Federal, state, and local departments of public health regulations for containing, labeling, and transporting medical waste should be followed.

Needles, lancets, syringes, and other sharp objects should be placed into sealable puncture-proof containers immediately after use. To reduce the risk of an accidental needle stick or cut, needles should not be recapped, bent, broken, or removed from the syringe before disposal. Once the disposal container has been filled, it should be sealed and disposed according to federal, state, and local regulations for medical waste.

Body substances, such as urine, feces, and vomit, that have been collected in a potty or basin should be disposed of in the sanitary sewer (i.e., toilet). Care should be taken to minimize splashing when disposing of these substances. Gloves should be worn when performing disposal; when there is visible blood in these body substances, protective eyewear in combination with a mask also should be worn to prevent splashing to the nose, mouth, or eyes.

Cleanup of Spills

Spills of blood and other potentially infectious material should be cleaned up immediately. Gloves should be worn during cleaning. If splashing may occur, then protective eyewear in combination with a mask and cover gown should be worn. When the spill involves broken glass or sharp objects, the sharp pieces should be removed using a device, such as a dustbin and brush. Do not use your hands! The spill should be mopped up with paper towels or other absorbent material.

The area should then be decontaminated using a freshly made solution of 1-part liquid household bleach in 10-parts water. If the spill involves a large amount of blood or other potentially infectious material, flooding of the area with the bleach solution before cleaning up with disposable absorbent material is recommended.

All items contaminated during cleanup should be discarded into a waste receptacle designated for medical waste. Broken glass or sharp items should be placed in a sealable, puncture-proof container.

Routine cleaning of a bathroom, diaper-changing room, or nurse's examination room does not require any special cleaning method unless contamination with blood or other potentially infectious material occurs. If contamination does occur, the area should be decontaminated as outlined above.

Laundry

Gloves should be worn when handling laundry or clothing contaminated with blood or other potentially infectious material. All laundry that is to be transported to an outside laundry service must be placed in clearly labeled bags or containers designated for soiled laundry. Most laundry services have specific guidelines for containing, labeling, and transporting soiled laundry. If laundry is not sent to an outside service, it should be transported in a sealed bag and washed in hot water (at least 160° F) using ordinary laundry detergent (The APIC Curriculum for Infection Control Practice, 1983).

Accidental Exposure

Accidental exposure to blood and other potentially infectious material, as defined by OSHA, places all of the individuals in a school setting at risk of infection. If exposure to broken skin or to the eyes, nose, or mouth occurs,

- Wash the area immediately with soap and water.
- Notify each student's parents or guardian of the incident.
- Document the incident, describing in detail what occurred.
- Inform the appropriate school authorities.
- Contact a physician for further care as outlined by the OSHA regulations.

Pregnant Women

Pregnant women are at no higher risk of infection than are other health care providers. Because of the possibility of transmission of certain viral infections that can cause congenital diseases, however, pregnant women are at higher risk of an adverse outcome from an infection. The consistent use of universal precautions and hand washing greatly reduces the risk of exposure to blood and other potentially infectious material for all individuals.

REFERENCES

The APIC Curriculum for Infection Control Practice. (1983). Dubuque, IA: Kendall/Hunt Publishing.

Centers for Disease Control and Prevention. (1987). Recommendations for prevention of HIV transmission in health care settings. *Morbidity and Mortality Weekly Report, 36*(Suppl.), 3S–18S.

Garner, J.S., & Favero, M.S. (1985). *Guidelines for handwashing and hospital environmental control, 1985.* Atlanta, GA: Centers for Disease Control and Prevention.

Garner, J.S., & Hospital Infection Control Practices Advisory Committee. (1996). CDC guideline for isolation precautions in hospitals. *American Journal of Infection Control, 24,* 24–25.

Occupational exposure to blood-borne pathogens: Final rule. 29 CFR, § 1910.1030, *Federal Register 56*(235): 64004-64182, December 6, 1991.

SUGGESTED READINGS

American Federation of Teachers. (1992). *The medically fragile child in the school setting.* Washington, DC: Author.

Bradley, B. (1994). *Occupational exposure to bloodborne pathogens: Implementing OSHA standards in school settings.* Scarborough, ME: National Association of School Nurses, Inc.

RESOURCES

For additional information on compliance with OSHA Regulation 29 CFR 1910.1030, contact the local offices of the Occupational Safety and Health Administration listed.

Region I
(CT*, MA, ME, NH, RI, VT*)
133 Portland Street
1st Floor
Boston, MA 02114
(617) 656-7164

Region II
(NJ, NY*, PR, VI*)
20 Varick Street
Room 670
New York, NY 10014
(212) 337-2378

Region III
(DC, DE, MD*, PA, VA*, WV)
Gateway Building
Suite 2100
3535 Market Street
Philadelphia, PA 19104
(215) 596-1201

Region IV
(AL, FL, GA, KY*, MS, NC*, SC*, TN*)
1375 Peachtree Street, N.E.
Suite 587
Atlanta, GA 30367
(404) 347-3573

Region V
(IL, IN*, MI*, MN*, OH, WI)
230 South Dearborn Street
Room 3244
Chicago, IL 60604
(312) 353-2220

Region VI
(AR, LA, NM*, OK, TX)
525 Griffin Street
Room 602
Dallas, TX 75202
(214) 676-4731

Region VII
(IA*, KS, MO, NE)
911 Walnut Street
Room 406
Kansas City, MO 64106
(816) 426-5861

Region VIII
(CO, MT, ND, SD, UT*, WY)
Federal Building
Room 1576
1961 Stout Street
Denver, CO 80294
(303) 844-3061

Region IX
(American Samoa, AZ*, CA*, Guam, HI*, NV*, Trust Territories of the Pacific)
71 Stevenson Street
Room 415
San Francisco, CA 94015
(415) 744-6670

Region X
(AK*, ID, OR*, WA*)
1111 Third Avenue
Suite 715
Seattle, WA 98101-3212
(206) 442-5930

---

*These states and regions operate their own OSHA-approved job safety and health programs. (Connecticut and New York plans cover public employees only.) States with approved programs must have a standard that is identical with, or at least as effective, as the federal standard.

Alert: Latex Allergy

Ellen Meeropol

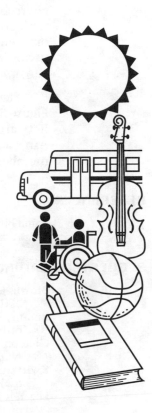

Latex is the sap from the *Hevea brasiliensis* tree. When chemicals are added to the sap to increase durability, strength, and elasticity, rubber is formed. Latex-containing items are found in many medical products used in the hospital, clinic, and school setting. Latex items also are commonly found in nonmedical objects used in the home, school, and community. The following items **may** contain latex:

Medical items:
- Gloves
- Catheters
- Tape or elastic bandages
- Occupational therapy elastic bands
- Wheelchair cushions or tires
- Crutch pads
- Intravenous set-up ports

Nonmedical items:
- Balloons
- Rubber balls or toys (e.g., Koosh ball)
- Baby bottle nipples or pacifiers
- Art supplies
- Condoms
- Diapers or elastic clothing

Allergic reactions to natural latex rubber frequently have been reported, particularly in children with chronic conditions, such as spina bifida, and urological anomalies; these children are often exposed to latex products. Health care workers and children with histories of multiple surgical procedures or many allergies also are at risk.

Allergic reactions to latex include watery eyes, wheezing, rash, hives, swelling, and, in severe cases, life threatening anaphylactic shock. Allergic responses can occur when latex-containing items touch the skin; touch mucous membranes, including mouth, urethra, rectum, or genitals; enter the bloodstream, through intravenous or intraoperative exposure; are inhaled, usually carried by the powder from latex gloves or balloons (the powder absorbs the latex protein and can cause reactions when in contact with a child's skin as well or when ingested on food handled by latex gloves); and come into contact with internal organs during surgery.

Alternative, nonlatex products for most of the previously mentioned items, usually made of vinyl, silicone, or plastic, are available. The alternative products are recommended for any individual who has a history of allergic reaction to latex and for individuals who are at risk for developing these allergies.

School personnel who use latex products should be aware of the possibility of allergic reactions in students with chronic conditions and in themselves. Communication with students and families about this allergy and documentation of the allergy are recommended. Individuals with allergies should discuss with their physician the possible use of Medic Alert tags, injectable epinephrine kits, and prophylactic medication before surgery or invasive testing.

Figure 5.1 is a list of latex products and alternatives in the hospital environment, and Figure 5.2 is a list of latex products and alternatives in the home and community. These lists are updated twice a year and are available from the Spina Bifida Association of America (1996). To safely manage a child with allergies to latex in the school setting, members of the child's health care team may be good resources.

REFERENCES

Spina Bifida Association of America. (1996). *Latex in the home and community.* Washington, DC: Author.

SUGGESTED READINGS

Brown, J.P. (1994). Latex allergy requires attention in orthopaedic nursing. *Orthopaedic Nursing, 13*(1), 7–11.

Emans, J.B. (1992). Allergy to latex in patients who have myelodysplasia: Relevance for the orthopaedic surgeon. *The Journal of Bone and Joint Surgery, 74-A*(7), 1103–1109.

Gleeson, R.M. (1995). Use of non-latex gloves for children with latex allergies. *Journal of Pediatric Nursing, 10*(1), 64–65.

Kwittkin, P.L., & Sweinberg, S.K. (1992). Childhood latex allergy: An overview. *American Journal of Asthma and Allergy for Pediatricians, 6,* 27–33.

Leger, R.R., & Meeropol, E. (1992). Children at risk: Latex allergy and spina bifida. *Journal of Pediatric Nursing, 7*(6), 371–376.

Meeropol, E., Frost, J., Pugh, L., Roberts, J., & Ogden, J.A. (1993). Latex allergy in children with myelodysplasia: A survey of Shriners Hospitals. *Journal of Pediatric Orthopaedics, 13,* 1–4.

Meeropol, E., Leger, R., & Frost, J. (1993). Latex allergy in patients with myelodysplasia and in healthcare providers: A double jeopardy. *Urologic Nursing, 13*(2), 39–44.

Nelson, L.P., Sopporowski, N., & Shusterman, S. (1994). Latex allergies in children with spina bifida: Relevance for the pediatric dentist. *Pediatric Dentistry, 16*(1), 18–22.

Romanczuk, A. (1993). Latex use with infants and children: It can cause problems. *The American Journal of Maternal/Child Nursing, 18,* 208–212.

Shaer, C., & Meeropol, E. (1995). Latex (natural rubber) allergy in spina bifida patients. *Spotlight Newsletter.*

Shapiro, E., Kelly, K.J., Setlock, M.A., Suwalski, K.L., & Meyers, P. (1992). Complications of latex allergy. *Dialogues in Pediatric Urology, 15*(3), 1–8.

Swartz, M.K., & Leger, R. (1992). Latex hypersensitivity. *Journal of Pediatric Health Care, 6*(6), 381–382.

Vessey, J.A., Holland, C.V., McNatt, S., McVay, C.J., & Williams, S.D. (1993). Latex allergy: A threat to you and your patients? *Pediatric Nursing, 19*(5), 517–520.

Frequently contain LATEX	Examples of LATEX-SAFE alternatives/barriers
Anesthesia, ventilator circuits, bags	Neoprene (Anesthesia Associates, Ohmeda adult), well-washed systems
Bandaids Bed protectors (washable rubber) Blood pressure cuff, tubing Bulb syringe	Active Strips (3M-latex in package), Snippy Band (Quantasia), Readi-Bandages Disposable underpads Cleen Cuff (Vital Signs), Dinamap (Critikon), nylon (PyMaH) PVC (Davol), Medline, Rusch
Casts: Delta-Lite Conformable (J&J) Catheters, condom Catheters, indwelling Catheters, leg bags, drainage systems Catheters, straight, coude Catheters, urodynamics Catheters, rectal pressure	Scotchcast soft cast, Delta-Lite S, Fiberglass, Fabric (J&J), Caraglas Ultra Clear Advantage (Mentor), ProSys NL (ConvaTec), Coloplast, Rochester Silicone (Argyle, Bard, Kendall, Rochester, Rusch, Vitaid) Velcro, nylon, PVC (Dale, Mentor), Bard systems Bard, Coloplast, Mentor, RobNel (Sherwood) Bard, Cook, Lifetech, Rusch Cook, Lifetech

Dressings: Dyna-flex (J&J), BDF Elastoplast
    Action Wrap, Coban (3M),
	Duoderm (Squibb), Reston foam (3M), Opsite, Venigard, Comfeel (Coloplast)
	    Xerofoam (Sherwood), PinCare (Hollister), Bioclusive, Montgomery straps
	    (J&J), Webrill (Kendall), Metalline, Selopor , Opraflex (Lohmann)
	NOTE: Steri-strips, Tegaderm, Tegasorb (3M) have latex in package

Elastic wrap: ACE, Esmarch, Zimmer
    Dyna-flex, Elastikon (J&J)
Electrode bulbs, pads, grounding
Endotracheal tubes, airways
Enemas, Ready-to-use (Fleet-latex valve)
	coNco All Cotton Elastic Bandages, Adban Adhesive Elastic Bandage,
	    X-Mark (Avcor), Comprilan (Jobst), Esmark (DeRoyal)
	Baxter, Dantec EMG, Conmed, ValleyLab, Vermont Med
	Berman, Mallinckrodt, Polamedco, Portex, Rusch, Sheridan, Shiley
	Glycerin, BabyLax (Fleet), Theravac, Bowel Management Tube (MIC)
	    cone irrigation set (Convatec)

G-tubes, buttons Gloves, sterile, clean, surgical	Silicone (Bard, MIC, Stomate), Rusch Vinyl, neoprene, polymer gloves: Allergard (J&J), dermaprene (Ansell), Neolon, SensiCare, Tru-touch (B-D), Nitrex, Tactyl 1,2 (SmartPractice), Duraprene, Triflex (Baxter)

IV access: injection ports, Y-sites, bags
    buretrol ports, PRN adapters, buretrol ports,
PRN adapters, needleless systems
	Cover Y-sites and do not puncture. Use stopcocks for meds. Flush tubing.
	    Do not puncture bag ports to add meds. Polymer injection caps (Braun),
	    Abbot nitroglycerin tubing; Walrus, Gemini (IMED), some Baxter systems,
	    Braun, Baxter buretrols, SAFSITE (Braun), Clave, Abbott needleless systems

OR masks, hats, shoe covers Oxygen masks, cannulas	Replace elastic bands with twill tape ties Remove elastic bands; check content of valves
Medication vial stoppers Moleskin	Eli Lilly, Fujisawa; if not certain, remove stopper adhesive felt (Acme)
Penrose surgical drains Pulse oximeters	Jackson-Pratt, Zimmer Hemovac Certain Oxisensor (Nellcor), cover digit with Tegaderm
Reflex hammers Respirators - tb (3M 9970) Resusitators, manual	Cover with plastic bag Advantage (MSA), HEPA-Tech (Uvex) Silicone: PMR 2 (Puriton Bennett), SPUR (Ambu), Vital Blue, Respironics, Laerdal, Armstrong, Rusch
Stethescope tubing Suction tubing Syringes, disposable	PVC tubing, cover with stockinette or ScopeCoat PVC (Davol, Laerdal, Mallinckrodt, Superior, Yankauer)., Medline, Ballard Draw up medication in syringe right before use; Terumo Medical, Abboject, Norm-Ject (Air-Tite), Abbott PCA, EpiPen, certain 1cc, 60 cc syringes (BD)
Tapes: adhesive, porous, pink, Waterproof (3M) Tourniquet Theraband, Therastrip, Theratube Tubing, sheeting	Dermaclear, Dermicel, Waterproof (J&J), Durapore, Microfoam, Micropore, Transpore (3M), Mastisol liquid adhesive Children's Med Ventures, Grafco, VelcroPedic, X-Tourn straps (Avcor) Exercise putty (Rolyan) plastic tubing -Tygon LR-40 (Norton), elastic thread, sheets (JPS Elastomerics)
Vascular stockings (Jobst)	Compriform Custom (Jobst)

Figure 5.1. Latex-containing items found in the hospital environmental and latex-safe alternatives and/or barriers for each. (Reprinted by permission of the Spina Bifida Association of America.)

Frequently contain LATEX	Examples of LATEX-SAFE alternatives/barriers
Art supplies: paints, glue, erasers, fabric paints	Elmers (School Glue, Glue-All, GluColors, Carpenters Wood Glue, Sno-Drift Paste), FaberCastel art erasers, Crayola Products (**except** for rubber stamps, erasers). Liquitex paints. Silly Putty
Balloons Balls: Koosh balls, tennis balls, bowling balls	Mylar balloons PVC (Hedstrom Sports Ball)
Carpet backing, gym floor, basement sealant Clothes: applique on Tees, elastic on socks, underwear, soles on sneakers, sandals Condoms, contraceptive diaphragm Crutches: tips, axillary pads, hand grips	Provide barrier - cloth or mat Cloth-covered elastic, neoprene (Decent Exposures, NOLATEX Industries) Polyurethane (Avanti), female condom (Reality) Cover with cloth, tape
Dental dams, cups, bands, root canal material Diapers, Incontinence pads, rubber pants	Wire springs, dental sealant (Delton) Huggies, First Quality, Gold Seal, Tranquility, Drypers, Attends (some)
Feeding nipples Food handled with latex gloves	selected Gerber, Evenflo, MAM, Ross, Mead Johnson nipples Synthetic gloves for food handling
NOTE: associated allergies are reported to kiwi, banana, avocado and other fruits	
Handles on racquets, tools	Vinyl, leather handles, or cover with cloth or tape
Infant toothbrush-massager	Soft bristle brush or cloth, Gerber/NUK
Kitchen cleaning gloves	PVC MYPLEX (Magla), cotton liners (Allerderm)
Newsprint, ads, coupons dusted with latex	
Pacifiers	Binky, Gerber, Infa, Kip, MAM, Childrens Medical Ventures
Rubber bands, bungee cords	Plasti bands
Toys - Stretch Armstrong, old Barbies	Jurassic Park figures (Kenner), 1993 Barbie, Disney dolls (Mattel), many toys by Fisher Price, Little Tikes, Playschool, Discovery, Trolls (Norfin)
Water toys & equipment: beach thongs, masks, bathing suits, caps, scuba gear, goggles Wheelchair cushions, tires	PVC, plastic Jay, ROHO cushions, Cover seats, Use leather gloves
Zippered plastic storage bags	Waxed paper, plain plastic bags

Latex free products for home and community can be ordered from:
- Alternative Resource Catalog (Latex Free Products for Daily Living) 708-503-8298
- NOLatex Industries 800-296-9185

Please note: This list is offered as a guideline to individuals, families and professionals by the Latex Committee of the Nursing Council, Spina Bifida Association of America, with contributions from North East Myelodysplasia Association and many individuals. It is very difficult to obtain full and accurate information on the latex content of products, which may vary between companies and product series. Checking with suppliers before use with latex allergic individuals is strongly recommended. The information in this list is constantly changing as manufacturers improve their products and as we learn more about latex allergy. For more information, or to share product content information, please contact the Spina Bifida Association of America.

Edited by Elli Meeropol RN MS & Amy Romanczuk RN MSN

Figure 5.2. Latex-containing items found in the home and community and latex-safe alternatives and/or barriers for each. (This list and that shown in Figure 5.1 are updated twice each year; for updated versions of these lists or more information about latex allergy, contact the Spina Bifida Association of America, 4590 MacArthur Boulevard, NW, Suite 250, Washington, DC 20007-4226 [800-621-3141].) (Reprinted by permission of the Spina Bifida Association of America.)

Human Immunodeficiency Virus and Acquired Immunodeficiency Syndrome

Andrea Rubin Hale

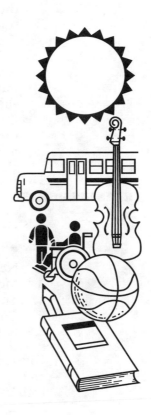

S ince the diagnosis of the first cases of acquired immunodeficiency syndrome (AIDS) in June of 1981, much has been learned about the course of this illness. It is now known that AIDS is the final stage of immune system breakdown in a person infected with the human immunodeficiency virus (HIV). HIV infects and destroys T helper cells, a type of white blood cell that is important in fighting infections. When enough T cells have been destroyed, the body's immune system is unable to fight off infections.

A person may carry HIV for many years before a diagnosis of AIDS is made. For this reason, it is more appropriate to refer to this illness as HIV infection or HIV disease than as AIDS. Once mild symptoms appear, early therapy may continue to delay the progression of the disease. Research continues to show that early treatment is beneficial.

SPECTRUM OF DISEASE

The spectrum of HIV disease consists of four phases:

1. ***Initial infection***   Initial infection occurs when a person is first infected with HIV. Adults may experience a flu-like syndrome approximately 3–12 weeks after infection. Antibody to HIV will be detected in the blood between 3 weeks and 6 months after infection. (Even when the antibody cannot be detected, the virus is present and can be transmitted to others.) In children infected perinatally, it is not always clear whether they were infected before birth, during delivery, or both. Evidence points toward all these possibilities and many studies are under way to examine this.

2. ***Asymptomatic HIV infection***   During this period, the person infected with HIV has no signs of clinical disease although the virus is present and may be multiplying. This period may last from months to years, although it appears to be shorter in children than in adults.

3. ***Symptomatic HIV infection***   During this period, symptoms may range from mild, such as swollen lymph nodes, liver, and spleen, to more severe, such as weight loss, vomiting, diarrhea, and persistent fever. During this phase, the virus is present in the body in increasing amounts; the T cells are destroyed by the multiplying HIV in the cells.

4. ***Acquired Immunodeficiency Syndrome (AIDS)*** The actual syndrome is defined by the occurrence of an otherwise unusual infection or cancer that indicates a severe immunodeficiency. These indicator illnesses include *pneumocystis carinii* pneumonia (PCP) and other uncommon infections, commonly called opportunistic infections because they take advantage of the body's weak immune system. Only the diagnosis of one of these "AIDS-defining illnesses" indicates the presence of this final phase of HIV infection. Once a person has had an AIDS-defining illness, that person's health may return to his or her "pre-AIDS" condition, but he or she will always have AIDS. Because unusual infections also occur in children with other immunodeficiencies (i.e., genetic immunodeficiency syndrome and acquired immunodeficiency from chemotherapy), these other causes of immunodeficiency should be ruled out. Other AIDS-defining illnesses in children include failure to thrive and HIV encephalopathy. HIV encephalopathy is caused by the presence of the virus in the brain and can lead to a variety of symptoms (e.g., loss of developmental milestones, delayed developmental progress, difficulties in motor function).

TRANSMISSIBILITY

It is known that HIV can be transmitted in the following ways:

1. Sexual contact with an infected person
2. Needles shared with an infected person
3. Mother-to-child infection during pregnancy, labor, or delivery
4. Transfusion of infected blood or blood products
5. Contact with blood across broken skin and/or mucous membranes
6. Breastfeeding

Given the widespread practice of screening blood donations, transfusions are considered an extremely unlikely transmission source. HIV cannot be transmitted by donating blood.

There is no evidence that HIV is transmitted via any sort of casual contact, including hand shaking; social kissing; hugging; or sharing drinking glasses, clothing, or linens. HIV is not transmitted via shared swimming pools or hot tubs; by touching telephones or doorknobs; or via insects or vaccines. Furthermore, there is no documented evidence of transmission between infected and uninfected family members who have routine, daily contacts, such as sharing silverware, bathrooms, or bedrooms. However, people with HIV should not share toothbrushes, razors, home intravenous infusion equipment, or any other object that may be contaminated with blood or body fluids with other household members.

POLICY AND PRACTICE CHANGES: TRENDS FOR THE FUTURE

Considerable variation exists among school systems in both policies and regulations and in roles, responsibilities, and collaboration among school nurses, health care educators, and other professionals with respect to issues surrounding HIV infection. An overview[1] of the evolution of policies and practices over time reflects substantial changes in the following five policy domains: confidentiality, universal precautions, public controversy, bereavement, and preparedness.

---

[1]The text in this overview on pages 84–85 is from Lavin, A.T., Porter, S., Shaw, D.M., Weill, K.S., Crocker, A.C., & Palfrey, J.S. (1994). School health services in the age of AIDS. *Journal of School Health, 64*(1), 28–30; reprinted by permission of *Journal of School Health,* American School Health Association, Kent, Ohio. This nonexclusive right to publish is in no way intended to be a transfer of copyright, and the American School Health Association maintains copyright ownership and authorization of the use of said material. This authorization in no way restricts republication of the material in any other form by the American School Health Association or others authorized by the American School Health Association.

Confidentiality

During the 1980s, confidentiality policies (when they existed) emphasized the rights of the institution and often permitted or required disclosure of a student's HIV infection to school authorities. Now, greater recognition exists of the rights of students and families to determine disclosure. The "best practices guidelines" in Figures 5.3 (on pp. 89–90) and 5.4 (on pp. 91–92) (Figure 5.4 is a Spanish translation of Figure 5.3) recommend eliminating the terms *need to know* and *right to know* and support transferring such information only at the discretion of a parent, guardian, and/or student. HIV infection probably will be viewed more broadly as a chronic illness without stigma, and confidentiality will remain at the discretion of the family in the future.

Universal Precautions

Universal precautions received little emphasis in school settings until the late 1980s. Despite increasing recognition of the urgent importance of these measures, which is reflected in explicit policies and in required training for school staff, considerable concern remains about inconsistent and inadequate implementation. With administrative support, schools should achieve full and adequate implementation in the future.

Public Controversy

Some communities have experienced public controversy over the actual or hypothetical presence of students and staff with HIV infection in school. The issue continues to receive sporadic attention from the U.S. media. Intensified efforts to educate students, staff members, families, and the public at large, coupled with strong leadership from school administrators and health care professionals, can relieve concerns and facilitate broad public acceptance.

Bereavement

Until the 1990s, most schools did not perceive a particular need to provide education and counseling related to bereavement. With the increasing incidence of AIDS-related deaths among students, families, and school personnel, many school districts have begun to recognize this emerging issue. Some have hired new staff or revised position descriptions to include bereavement counseling. All schools should anticipate the need for such counseling and develop appropriate resources.

Preparedness

Overall, in the mid-1980s, schools were not prepared to address issues presented by the AIDS epidemic. Schools are at various stages of developing and revising policies and programs and report a range of experiences with respect to students and staff with HIV infection. An apparent need exists for more communication and follow-through between HIV prevention education and those responsible for counseling and testing and for policies for students and staff with HIV infection. School nurses and educators would benefit from greater collaboration with respect to providing training in HIV issues in schools, thereby benefiting schools and students themselves.

Table 5.1 provides more information on changes in the five HIV policy domains.

SCHOOL ATTENDANCE

In the absence of blood exposure, HIV infection is not acquired through the types of contact that usually occur in a school setting, including contact with saliva and tears. Hence, children with HIV infection should not be excluded from school for the protection of other children or personnel. Specific recommendations[2] concerning school attendance of children and adolescents with HIV infection are the following:

---

[2] The text on pages 85–87 is from American Academy of Pediatrics. School attendance and education of children with HIV infection. In Peter G., ed. *1994 Red Book: Report of the Committee on Infectious Diseases.* 23rd ed. Elk Grove Village, IL: American Academy of Pediatrics; 1994: pp. 266–267.

- Most school-age children and adolescents infected with HIV should be allowed to attend school without restrictions, provided the child's physician gives approval.
- There may be a need for a more restricted school environment for some infected children, which should be evaluated on a case-by-case basis. Conditions that may pose an increased risk to others (e.g., aggressive biting behavior, the presence of exudation matter, weeping skin lesions that cannot be covered) must be considered.
- No one other than a child's parents or guardians and physician has an absolute need to know that a child has HIV infection. The number of personnel aware of a child's condition should be kept to the minimum needed to ensure proper care of that child. The child's parents or guardians have the right to determine whether to inform the school of the child's diagnosis. People involved in the care and education of a student with HIV infection must respect the student's right to privacy.
- All schools should adopt routine procedures for handling blood or blood-contaminated fluids, including the disposal of sanitary napkins, regardless of whether students with HIV infection are known to be in attendance. School health care workers, teachers, administrators, and other employees should be educated about procedures. The authors recommend using these procedures for all students and staff.
- Children infected with HIV develop progressive immunodeficiency, which may increase their risk of experiencing severe complications from infections such as vari-

Table 5.1. Changes in five HIV policy domains over time

Through 1989	1990–1993	1994 on
Confidentiality		
• Rights of the institution prevailed • Disclosure to authority expected and usual	• Greater recognition of the rights of the student and family to determine disclosure • *Pseudo-confidentiality*	• HIV infection perceived as a chronic illness, not prejudicial • No "need to know" • Sharing of information at discretion of parent, guardian, and student
Universal Precautions		
• Little emphasis on school settings	• Recognition of need for universal precautions • Explicit policies and training programs • Inconsistent implementation and administrative support	• Full implementation with administrative support • Occupational Safety and Health Administration regulations for school health area developed
Public Controversy		
• Public alarm • Objections to enrollment of student with HIV infection	• Admission of students secured by Section 504 of the Rehabilitation Act of 1973 (PL 93-112) and the Americans with Disabilities Act (PL 101-336) • Confusion regarding obligations for disclosure • Discussion regarding curriculum content	• Public concerns abated • Full inclusion of children in school setting
Bereavement		
• Unrecognized need with respect to AIDS	• Sporadic efforts in personal support	• Bereavement issues always included in health education
Preparedness		
• Staff uncertain, in denial • Spotty HIV education	• Incomplete involvement of school employees • Ongoing need for school and community education, more energetic efforts	• Training materials validated • Training for teachers provided uniformly and in greater depth

From Lavin, A.T., Porter, S., Shaw, D.M., Weill, K.S., Crocker, A.C., & Palfrey, J.S. (1994). School health services in the age of AIDS. *Journal of School Health, 64*(1), 30; adapted by permission of *Journal of School Health,* American School Health Association, Kent, Ohio. This nonexclusive right to publish is in no way intended to be a transfer of copyright, and the American School Health Association maintains copyright ownership and authorization of the use of said material. This authorization in no way restricts republication of the material in any other form by the American School Health Association or others authorized by the American School Health Association.

cella, tuberculosis, measles, cytomegalovirus, and herpes simplex virus. Although risk of exposure to or infection with these viruses should not routinely preclude school attendance, a child's physician should be made aware of infectious outbreaks so that regular assessment of the school environment and its impact on the child's health can be made.

- Routine screening of school children for HIV infection is not recommended.

As the incidence of HIV infection increases, the school population of children with this disease will increase. With the advent of new drug therapy, children are surviving longer, resulting in an increasing number of children with HIV infection entering school. An understanding of the effect of chronic illness and the recognition of neurodevelopmental problems in these children is essential to provide appropriate educational programs. The American Academy of Pediatrics Task Force on Pediatric AIDS (1994) has made the following recommendations regarding the education of children with HIV infection:

- All children with HIV infection should receive an appropriate education that is adapted to their evolving special needs. The spectrum of needs differs with the stage of the disease.
- HIV infection should be treated like other chronic illnesses that may require special education and other related services.
- Continuity of education must be ensured whether at school or at home.
- Because of the stigma that exists with this disease, maintaining confidentiality is essential. Disclosures of information should be made only with the informed consent of a student's parents or legal guardians and age-appropriate assent of the student.

HEALTH CARE PLAN CONSIDERATIONS

The following is a list of considerations for the school nurse when developing a health care plan for a child with HIV infection in school:

1. Meet with the family or guardian(s) of the child and, if the family requests, the child's primary health care providers. Keeping in mind that the family may choose not to disclose the diagnosis, discuss the following:
   - Child's current health status
   - Medications, including when and how medication should be given, potential side effects of the medication, and if the medication is experimental or part of an experimental protocol
   - What the child knows about the diagnosis (This is a good time to discuss when and if the parent or guardian intends to share information about the diagnosis and what school personnel should say if faced with specific questions. Include a discussion regarding what the student knows about the medications he or she takes.)
   - Outbreaks of illness about which the family must be informed
   - Any special dietary restrictions or other health care needs
   - Student's participation in self-care

2. Secure medical information records in a locked cabinet. Other students and staff should **never** have access to confidential medical information.

3. Be aware of changes in health and treatment.

4. Provide a forum for students, families, and staff to discuss chronic illness, coping, grief, and bereavement.

5. Review guidelines in this chapter on Universal Precautions and Infection Control in a School Setting (pp. 74–78) and Alert: Latex Allergy (pp. 79–82). Anticipating the tasks to be performed, the risk involved, and the personal protective equipment needed will enhance protection of caregivers and students. Of potential concern is the possibility of an allergy to either latex or the powder found within the gloves, which is often first noted with repeated wearing of gloves when using universal pre-

cautions. Because gloves are necessary for protection from infected blood and body fluid, a substitute (e.g., lambskin, powder-free gloves) should be used.

WHEN A CHILD IS ENROLLED IN A CLINICAL TRIAL

As more children are enrolling in experimental drug studies, it is becoming more likely for a child who is participating in a clinical trial to be in school. The following steps ensure that the drug is being given legally and properly and that any possible side effects are noted:

- After obtaining the parents' or guardian's permission, contact the research staff at the hospital (usually a doctor or nurse), and request information about the study, drug, side effects, and medication administration. Ask for a copy of the protocol being used or, if it is not possible to obtain one, request a brief written summary of the study to keep in the child's file.
- Determine whether the drug is Food and Drug Administration approved. Check with the state department of public health regarding the regulations for administering experimental medications in the school.
- Arrange an appropriate time with the child to administer the medication.
- Keep parents informed of the child's health status during the day and of any problems with medication administration. Document any missed doses. This information will be collected by the research center.

SUMMARY

This chapter has addressed key issues in ensuring that children and youth with HIV and AIDS begin or continue their education. Understanding facts about the disease spectrum and transmissibility of the disease lays a foundation for everyone who serves these students and their families. Continued support is needed for children and youth involved in clinical trials because new treatment information emerges from participation. Through everyone's best efforts, constructive local, state, and national policy and practice changes occur. The Best Practice Guidelines provide direction for communities that are committed to combining objective information with the respect and confidentiality that all students and families deserve.

**SUPPORTS FOR CHILDREN WITH HIV INFECTION IN SCHOOL
BEST PRACTICES GUIDELINES**

I. PREPARATION OF THE SCHOOL SETTING

1. An *advisory committee on HIV-related issues* shall be established for the school district and commissioned by the superintendent. Membership shall be comprised of health professionals (e.g., community physicians, school nurses, and other child and adolescent health workers), parents, teachers, students, persons with HIV infection, attorneys, advocates, and persons representing diversity in the community. At regular meetings, matters shall be discussed concerning HIV that relate to administrative practices, legal and policy questions, educational programs, universal infection control standards, and student welfare. Consultants shall be used as appropriate.

2. The school district shall adopt *policy statements of relevance to students with HIV infection*, in collaboration with the advisory committee. These shall conform with state and federal laws and regulations and draw on state-of-the-art medical and scientific information from appropriate government sources, model documents from national organizations, research studies, and expert consultation. It may be helpful to use public hearings to gain input into these matters. The policy statements shall then be disseminated to all administrative levels; made available to staff, students, parents, and community leaders; and included in student and parent handbooks. They shall be reviewed at yearly intervals.

3. *Staff education and inservice training* concerning the issues of HIV infection, including transmission, prevention, civil rights, mental health, and death and bereavement, shall be carried out at least annually for all school personnel, including the school board. The program content shall be determined by a multidisciplinary team of appropriate individuals that shall include families of children with HIV infection and also persons with HIV infection. It shall aim to affect staff members' knowledge, feelings, attitudes, behavior, and acceptance of people who are HIV positive. For new employees, this education shall be built into the orientation program and offered within three months of hire. Teachers responsible for instruction of students regarding HIV infection shall receive specific inservice training.

4. *Universal precautions relating to blood-borne infections,* as adapted for schools, shall be in effect. School clinics and nursing offices shall follow OSHA guidelines for health care facilities. It is the responsibility of the school district to ensure adequate gloves, bleach, sinks, and disposal containers. There shall be systems of quality assurance or monitoring to document compliance with universal precautions in all school settings. These matters shall be featured in the staff education program.

5. The school district shall provide *education relating to the prevention of HIV infection for students in grades K–12* within the context of a quality comprehensive school health program. Delivered by trained teachers, health educators, and nurses, it shall be developmentally, culturally, and linguistically appropriate. It shall actively promote abstinence as the best protection, and shall also offer explicit information about the use and availability of condoms. Acknowledgment shall be given to the special needs of adolescents regarding emerging sexual orientation. An additional effect of this effort should be to enhance understanding of the needs of students, staff, and others who are infected with HIV.

II. THE ENROLLMENT PROCESS

6. The parent, guardian, or student shall decide *whether or not to inform the school system* about HIV status or other health conditions. They may support the transfer of this information by another professional or person, including a personal physician or a case manager, but only in the context of strict informed consent procedures. It shall be recognized that disclosure of HIV status often involves revealing related facts, such as medication, parent condition, transmission, and other matters. Under no circumstances shall parents, guardians, or students be required by school personnel to obtain HIV testing or to release information about HIV test results on the student or other family members.

(continued)

Figure 5.3. Supports for children with HIV infection in school best practices guidelines. (From Crocker et al. [1994]. Supports for children with HIV infection in school: Best practices guidelines. *Journal of School Health, 64*[1], 33–37; reprinted by permission of *Journal of School Health,* American School Health Association, Kent, Ohio. This nonexclusive right to publish is in no way intended to be a transfer of copyright, and the American School Health Association maintains copyright ownership and authorization of the use of said material. This authorization in no way restricts republication of the material in any other form by the American School Health Association or others authorized by the American School Health Association.)

Figure 5.3. *(continued)*

7. Few, if any, personnel in the school or school district shall ***receive information about the HIV status*** of a student. Determination of those who are to be informed is the prerogative of the parents, guardian, or student, and shall be made in the setting of consideration about special health care or social services that are needed while the student is in school. The terms "need to know" and "right to know" are usually not applicable for school staff, and are best eliminated. Specific release of information by the family as they wish it is obviously acceptable, but such material should then be treated confidentially regarding further dissemination.

8. ***Information about a student's HIV status*** shall not be included in the educational record, usual school health records, or any other records that are accessible to school staff beyond those the parents, guardian, or student has determined should know. Documentation about specific health care given by school nurses, counselors, clinicians, or other personnel to students with HIV infection shall be put in special health records kept in locked files. If the child changes schools, a plan for the transfer of these records shall be developed with the family and student.

III. ASSURANCE OF APPROPRIATE SERVICES

9. The ***design of an individual student's program*** shall be based on educational needs and not the status regarding HIV infection. The curriculum and other activities of a student with HIV infection shall be modified only as required per developmental and/or personal health needs. Exclusion or segregation of students solely on the basis of HIV infection is never appropriate.

10. ***In-school health services*** shall be provided as needed, including special regimens required because of HIV infection, but the origin of these programs shall not be identified at the classroom level. Specific "health care plans" may be formulated by school health personnel for students with symptomatic HIV infection. Notification for families about the presence of other communicable diseases at school (e.g., chicken pox) that place students at risk shall be forwarded universally. Particular notification will be given to families who have informed key school personnel about HIV infection. School nurses, and others with appropriate training, shall participate in counseling for students regarding HIV matters, including the availability of testing. They shall establish quality linkages with youth-serving HIV programs in the community that can provide culturally sensitive, age-appropriate medical, mental health, social, and drug treatment services.

IV. OTHER ELEMENTS

11. School administrators shall provide culturally sensitive information, technical assistance/consultation, and access to resources on HIV issues to the ***school's parents and families*** through PTAs and other parent organizations. Appropriate issues for discussion include prevention, confidentiality, classroom educational services and related supports, and community resources.

12. Relevant to existing federal and state statutes, teachers, school health professionals, and other qualified employees shall have the ***right to employment and confidentiality*** regardless of their own HIV status or other health conditions. If they choose to disclose their HIV status to students or other staff this shall not have ramifications regarding employment.

**APOYOS PARA NIÑOS CON EL VIRUS DEL SIDA (HIV) EN LA ESCUELA
PAUTAS PARA LAS MEJORES PRACTICAS**

I. PREPARACION DEL AMBIENTE ESCOLAR

1. Se establecerá un *comité consultivo en cuestiones relacionadas al Virus del SIDA (HIV)* para el distrito escolar, y éste será nombrado por el Superintendente. El número de miembros deberá incluir profesionales de salud (médicos de la comunidad, enfermeras escolares y otros trabajadores de salud para niños y adolescentes), padres, maestros, estudiantes, personas con el Virus del SIDA (HIV), abogados, defensores y personas representantes de diversidad en la comunidad. Se discutirán, en reuniones regulares, asuntos concernientes al Virus del SIDA (HIV) que tengan que ver con prácticas administrativas, cuestiones legales y de reglas de procedimiento, programas educacionales, modelos universales de control de infección y bienestar estudiantil. Se usarán consultores según sea apropiado.

2. El distrito escolar deberá adoptar *declaraciones de reglas de procedimiento relevantes a estudiantes con Virus del SIDA (HIV)*, en colaboración con el comité consultivo. Estas declaraciones deberán estar de acuerdo con leyes y regulaciones estatales y federales y deben utilizar las informaciones médicas y científicas más avanzadas de apropiadas fuentes de gobierno, documentos modelos de organizaciones nacionales, estudios de investigación y consulta con expertos. Las audiencias públicas podrían servir de ayuda para obtener contribuciones de ideas y opiniones sobre estos asuntos. Las declaraciones de reglas de procedimientos deberán ser diseminadas después a todos los niveles administrativos, estar disponibles al personal, estudiantes, padres, y líderes de la comunidad y ser incluídas en manuales para estudiantes y padres. Estas serán repasadas anualmente.

3. *Educación del personal y entrenamiento en el trabajo* sobre los problemas de infección del Virus del SIDA (HIV), incluyendo transmisión, prevención, derechos civiles, salud mental, muerte y aflicción por muerte, deberán ser aplicados por lo menos anualmente para todo el personal de la escuela, incluyendo a la junta escolar. El contenido del programa deberá ser determinado por un equipo multidisciplinario de individuos adecuados que deberán incluir a familias de niños con infección del Virus del SIDA (HIV) y también a personas con infección del Virus del SIDA (HIV). Este equipo deberá aspirar a afectar, en los miembros del personal, el conocimiento, los sentimientos, las actitudes, el comportamiento y la aceptación de personas que tienen el Virus del SIDA (HIV). Para nuevos empleados, esta educación deberá ser incluída en el programa de orientación y ofrecida dentro de los tres primeros meses de empleo. Los maestros responsables de la instrucción de estudiantes acerca de la infección del Virus del SIDA (HIV) deberán recibir entrenamiento específico mientras trabajan.

4. *Precauciones universales relacionadas a las infecciones que se transmiten por la sangre*, como han sido adaptadas para la escuela, deberán ser puestas en vigor. Clínicas escolares y oficinas de enfermería deberán seguir las pautas de OSHA para centros de cuidado de salud. El distrito escolar tiene la responsabilidad de asegurar guantes adecuados, lejía, fregaderos y envases de recolección. Deberá haber sistemas para asegurar la calidad o vigilación para documentar si se está de acuerdo con precauciones universales en todos los ambientes escolares. Estos asuntos deberán ser incluídos en el programa de educación del personal.

5. El distrito escolar deberá proveer *educación relacionada a la prevención de infección del Virus del SIDA (HIV) para estudiantes en los grados K a 12,* dentro del contexto de un programa escolar de salud completo y de calidad. Enseñada por maestros adiestrados, educadores de salud y enfermeros, esta educación deberá ser apropiada al desarrollo, la cultura y la lingüística. Deberá promover activamente la abstinencia como la mejor protección, y también deberá ofrecer información explícita sobre el uso y la disponibilidad de condones. Se deberán reconocer las necesidades especiales de los adolescentes en cuanto a la orientación sexual en boga. Un efecto adicional de este esfuerzo debería poner enfasis en la comprensión de las necesidades de los estudiantes, del personal y de otros que están infectados con el Virus del SIDA (HIV).

(continuado)

Figure 5.4. Supports for children with HIV infection in school best practices guidelines—Spanish version. (From Crocker et al. [1994]. Supports for children with HIV infection in school: Best practices guidelines. *Journal of School Health, 64*[1], 33–37; reprinted by permission of *Journal of School Health,* American School Health Association, Kent, Ohio. This nonexclusive right to publish is in no way intended to be a transfer of copyright, and the American School Health Association maintains copyright ownership and authorization of the use of said material. This authorization in no way restricts republication of the material in any other form by the American School Health Association or others authorized by the American School Health Association.)

Figure 5.4. *(continuado)*

II. EL PROCESO DE MATRICULACION

6. El padre, la madre, el guardián o el estudiante debe decidir *si informarle o no al sistema escolar* sobre el estado de Virus del SIDA (HIV) u otras condiciones de salud. Ellos podrán apoyar la transferencia de esta información por otro profesional o persona, incluyendo un médico personal o un administrador del caso, pero sólo en el contexto de procedimientos de autorización informativos y estrictos. Se deberá reconocer que la notificación del estado de Virus del SIDA (HIV) a menudo trae consigo la notificación de hechos relacionados, como medicamentos, condiciones de los padres, transmisión y otros asuntos. De ninguna manera el personal de la escuela puede exigirle a los padres, guardianes o estudiantes que obtengan pruebas de Virus del SIDA (HIV) o que den a conocer información sobre resultados del examen del Virus del SIDA (HIV) del estudiante u de otros miembros de la familia.

7. Pocos, si alguno, de los miembros del personal de la escuela o del distrito escolar *recibirán información sobre el estado de Virus del SIDA (HIV)* de un estudiante. La determinación de quienes serán informados es la prerrogativa de los padres, del guardián o del estudiante, y deberá ser hecha dentro del marco de consideraciones sobre cuidados especiales de salud o servicios sociales que son necesarios mientras el estudiante está en la escuela. Los términos "necesidad de saber" y "derecho de saber" no son aplicables normalmente al personal de la escuela, y es mejor que se eliminen. La divulgación específica de información por la familia, según ella desee, es claramente aceptable, pero tal material deberá entonces ser tratado con confidencialidad en cuanto a divulgación futura.

8. *Información sobre el estado de Virus del SIDA (HIV) de un estudiante* no deberá ser incluída en el archivo educacional, en los archivos normales de salud de la escuela o en otros archivos que sean accesibles al personal de la escuela que no sea aquél que los padres, guardián o estudiante ha determinado que pueden saber. Documentación sobre cuidados de salud específicos provistos por enfermeros escolares, consejeros, doctores clínicos u otro miembro del personal a estudiantes con infección del Virus del SIDA (HIV) debe ser puesta en archivos especiales de salud guardados bajo llave. Si el niño cambia de escuela, se deberá desarrollar, con la familia y estudiante, un plan para la transferencia de estos archivos.

III. ASEGURAR LOS SERVICIOS APROPIADOS

9. El *diseño del programa de un estudiante* deberá estar basado en las necesidades educacionales y no en el estado de infección del Virus del SIDA (HIV). El plan de estudios y otras actividades de un estudiante que tenga infección del Virus del SIDA (HIV) deberán ser modificados sólo cuando las necesidades de desarrollo y/o de salud personal lo requieran. La exclusión o la segregación de estudiantes únicamente por razones de infección del Virus del SIDA (HIV) nunca es apropiada.

10. *Servicios de salud en la escuela* deberán ser provistos según sea necesario, incluyendo regímenes especiales que se requieren por la infección del Virus del SIDA (HIV), pero el origen de estos programas no deberá ser identificado a nivel del salón de clases. "Planes de cuidado de salud" específicos pueden ser formulados por el personal de salud de la escuela para estudiantes con infección sintomática del Virus del SIDA (HIV). La notificación para familias sobre la presencia de otras enfermedades contagiosas en la escuela (ej., varicela), que ponen en riesgo a los estudiantes, deberá ser transmitida universalmente. Se le dará notificación particular a familias que han informado a personal clave de la escuela sobre infección del Virus del SIDA (HIV). Enfermeros escolares, y otros con entrenamiento apropiado, deberán participar en consejería para estudiantes sobre asuntos del Virus del SIDA (HIV), incluyendo la disponibilidad de exámenes para hacerse la prueba. Ellos deberán establecer enlaces de calidad con programas de Virus del SIDA (HIV) en la comunidad que sirven a la juventud y que dan servicios culturalmente sensibles, apropiados médicamente a la edad, de salud mental, sociales y de tratamiento de drogas.

IV. OTROS ELEMENTOS

11. Los administradores escolares deberán proveer información que sea culturalmente sensible, asistencia/consulta técnica y acceso a recursos sobre asuntos del Virus del SIDA (HIV) para *los padres y familias de la escuela* a través de Asociaciones de Padres y Maestros (PTAs) y otras organizaciones de padres. Puntos apropiados para discutir incluyen prevención, confidencialidad, servicios educacionales y asistencias relacionadas para el salón de clases, y recursos en la comunidad.

12. Pertinente a estatutos federales y estatales existentes, maestros, profesionales de salud en la escuela y otros empleados calificados deberán tener el *derecho a empleo y confidencialidad*, sin importar cual sea su estado de Virus del SIDA (HIV) o sus otras condiciones de salud. Si ellos deciden revelar su estado de Virus del SIDA (HIV) a estudiantes u otros miembros del personal, esto no debiera tener ramificaciones respecto a empleo.

REFERENCES

American Academy of Pediatrics. (1994). In G. Peter (Ed.), *1994 red book: Report of the Committee on Infectious Diseases* (23rd ed., pp. 266–267). Elk Grove Village, IL: Author.

Americans with Disabilities Act (ADA) of 1990, PL 101-336, 42 U.S.C. § 12101 *et seq.*

Crocker, A.C., Lavin, A.T., Palfrey, J.S., Porter, S.M., Shaw, D.M., & Weill, K.S. (1994). Supports for children with HIV infection in school: Best practices guidelines. *Journal of School Health, 64*(1), 33–37.

Lavin, A.T., Porter, S., Shaw, D.M., Weill, K.S., Crocker, A.C., & Palfrey, J.S. (1994). School health services in the age of AIDS. *Journal of School Health, 64*(1), 28–30.

Rehabilitation Act of 1973, PL 93-112, 29 U.S.C. § 701 *et seq.*

SUGGESTED READINGS

American Bar Association. (1989). *AIDS and persons with developmental disabilities: The legal perspective.* Washington, DC: Author.

American Bar Association. (1991). *AIDS/HIV and confidentiality: Model policy and procedures.* Washington, DC: Author.

Bogden, J.F., Fraser, K., Vega-Matos, C., & Ashcroft, J. (1996). *Someone at school has AIDS: A complete guide to education policies concerning HIV infection.* Alexandria, VA: National Association of State Boards of Education.

Bradley, B.J. (1994). *HIV infection in the school setting: A guide for school nursing practice.* Kent, OH: American School Health Association.

Brainerd, E.F. (1989). HIV in the school setting: The school nurse's role. *Journal of School Health, 59*(7), 316–317.

Crocker, A.C., Cohen, H.J., & Kastner, T.A. (Eds.). (1992). *HIV infection and developmental disabilities: A resource for service providers.* Baltimore: Paul H. Brookes Publishing Co.

Fahrner, R., & Benson, M. (1996). HIV infection and AIDS. In P. Jackson & J. Vessey (Eds.), *Primary care: The child with a chronic condition* (2nd ed., pp. 463–484). St Louis: Mosby-Yearbook.

Gross, E.J., & Passannante, M. (1993). Educating school nurses to care for HIV-infected children in school. *Journal of School Health, 63*(7), 307–311.

Hein, K., & DiGeronimo, T.F. (1989). *AIDS: Trading fears for facts (a guide for teens).* Mount Vernon, NY: Consumers Union.

Katsiyannis, A. (1992). Policy issues in school attendance of children with AIDS: A national survey. *Journal of Special Education, 26*(2), 219–226.

Kirp, D.L. (1989). *Learning by heart: AIDS and schoolchildren in America's communities.* New Brunswick, NJ: Rutgers University Press.

Lipson, M. (1993). What do you say to a child with AIDS? *Hastings Center Report, 23*(2), 6–12.

Majer, L.S. (1992). HIV-infected students in school: Who really "needs to know?" *Journal of School Health, 62*(6), 243–245.

Massachusetts Nurses Association Parent Child Health Council. (1994). *Children and adolescents with HIV/AIDS: A nursing resource.* Boston: Author.

Melchiono, M., Lauerman, J.F., & Palfrey, J.S. (1990). *Reaching out to at-risk youth.* Boston: Children's Hospital.

National Pediatric HIV Resource Center. (1993). *Nursing care plan: The child/adolescent with HIV infection in school.* Washington, DC: Author.

Rand, T.H., & Meyers, A. (1993). Role of the general pediatrician in the management of human immunodeficiency virus infection in children. *Pediatrics in Review, 14*(10), 371–379.

Reeder, J.M., & Killen, A.R. (1994). Nurse's knowledge, attitudes about HIV, AIDS: A replication study. *American Operating Room Nursing Journal, 59*(2), 450–466.

Sterken, D.J. (1995). HIV/AIDS in the classroom: Ethical and legal issues surrounding the education of the HIV-infected child. *Journal of Pediatric Health Care, 9*(5), 205–210.

Useful Documents

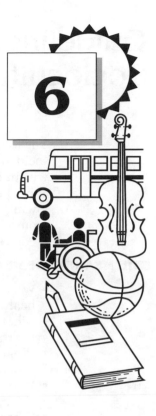

This chapter includes useful documents that represent different assessment tools, which can be used to help create a foundation for a student's individualized health care plan (IHCP).

The first two documents provided are the Guidelines for Analysis of Sociocultural Factors in Health and Bloch's Ethnic/Cultural Assessment Guide. These documents are useful for gathering unique cultural information about a student. Specific information gleaned from these two documents can be used to make IHCP interventions culturally relevant for the student.

The next form is a blank IHCP Checklist, a tool that can be used to document a plan of care for the child with special health care needs. It is based on a health assessment of the student by the school nurse in collaboration with the family, physician, and student. An IHCP outlines the student's current health status and specific issues related to his or her health care. IHCPs foster consistency in health care across all environments. (See Chapter 3 for a detailed description of each section.) Some or all of the blank IHCP pages may be used.

The Checklist of Items for Consideration in Developing Individualized Education Plans (IEP) for Students with Physical Disabilities or Special Health Needs then helps in the identification of important elements when developing an educational plan. The General Classroom Inclusion Checklist assists school staff and families in examining domains that are important but often overlooked in including students in typical classroom routines. In addition to the tools mentioned above, Additional Considerations for Education Planning and Programs, located at the end of this chapter, identifies strategies in the key areas of social participation, communication, and accommodation.

Guidelines for Analysis of Sociocultural Factors in Health

The following guidelines[1] for analyzing factors that affect health include a broad range of sociocultural, psychological, and behavioral guidelines for assessing medical systems within different cultural contexts. A working knowledge of sociocultural factors that affect health is an essential tool for health educators and educators in general. The following assessment questions, which are divided into groups, are offered in the spirit of promoting better cross-cultural understanding.

THE MEANING OF HEALTH IN A COMMUNITY

- What do people in the community generally consider a state of "wellness" or "good health"? A state of "illness" or "poor health"?
- What conditions of the body are considered normal and abnormal?
- Do these definitions vary with different groups within the community?
- What do people want out of life?
- When is life worth living?
- When does it become better to die?
- What priority does the value of "good health" have within the community?
- Where does "good health" fit within the hierarchy of values or goals in the community?
- What general changes in the quality of life do individuals or groups in the community desire, if any?
- How can health-related changes fit in with these general goals?
- What beliefs do people have concerning the organs and systems of the body and how they function?
- What are people's beliefs concerning "prevention of illness"?
- Do they feel it is possible? In what types of cases?
- Are there any particular methods people use to help maintain their own health or that of others?
- What are people's attitudes toward vaccinations, immunizations, various screening tests, and other preventive health measures?
- Are illnesses within the culture divided into those considered "physical" and "mental" (or "emotional")?
- If so, which illnesses are considered to be physical and which mental? Which a combination of the two?
- What types of mental illness, if this is a category used within the culture, are generally thought to exist by various members of the community?
- Are there any conditions that may be considered "mental illness" by outsiders, but that community members feel are normal?
- What mental illnesses identified by Western medical science are common or of importance in the community?

---

[1]The guidelines in this section are taken from Office of International Health. (1978). *Guidelines for analysis of socio-cultural factors in health*. Rockville, MD: Author; adapted by permission.

- Do various members of the community have knowledge of the occurrence of each of these illnesses, either by name or symptoms?
- Are any "diseases" of malnutrition common in the local community?
- Who is affected?
- What are the local beliefs about the causes of these diseases? Possible prevention and treatment?

THE MEANING OF MENTAL HEALTH

- What is its traditional or local name (if any)?
- What is its Western medical name (if any)?
- What are its symptoms? Its cause(s)?
- What type(s) of individual(s) does the mental illness usually affect?
- Can it be prevented, and if so, how?
- How is it diagnosed? Treated? Cured?
- What types of practitioners or other individuals are best able to prevent, diagnose, and/or treat the mental illness?
- What methods generally are used by each?
- What are the typical attitudes toward this mental illness and the person who has it?
- Are there any special taboos or other beliefs connected with the mental illness?
- In situations in which members of the community have migrated recently from another cultural area, is mental illness caused or influenced by the culture conflicts experienced during the period of readjustment?
- To what extent has this been a factor in the illnesses of particular immigrant patients?
- What are the typical community attitudes toward mental illness?
- How are the people with mental illnesses treated and cared for by their families? Others in the community?
- What are the attitudes of community members toward receiving various types of help for their mental or emotional problems?
- Are certain types of treatment more acceptable within the culture? More likely to be successful?

THE MEDICAL BELIEF SYSTEM

- What general beliefs do various community people have concerning cause, prevention, diagnosis, and treatment of disease?
- Are there any special "theories of disease" to which certain people adhere?
- What is the general understanding of and attitudes toward Western medical explanations and practices?
- What specific types of disease or sickness traditionally are thought to exist by various members of the community?
- What diseases identified by Western medical science are common or of importance in the area?
- Do various members of the community have knowledge of the occurrence of each of these diseases either by name or symptoms? For each disease identified by community members,

  - What is its traditional or local name (if any)?
  - What is its Western medical name (if any)?
  - What are its symptoms? Its cause(s)?
  - What type(s) of person(s) does the disease usually affect?
  - Can it be prevented, and if so, how?
  - How is it diagnosed? Treated? Cured?
  - What types of practitioners or other individuals are best able to prevent, diagnose, and/or treat the disease?
  - What methods generally are used by each?
  - What are typical attitudes toward this disease and the people who have it?
  - Are there any special taboos or other beliefs connected with the disease?

- What types of accidents are common in the community?
- Who typically has various accidents? When? Where?
- What beliefs are common concerning the causes of various types of accidents? Their prevention?
- How are various injuries treated?
- What types of physical disabilities are common within the community?
- What types of physical conditions do the local people consider disabilities?
- What do people feel may be the cause of various disabilities?
- Do people believe various abnormalities can be prevented? If so, how?
- What types of treatment are common?
- What types of efforts are made toward rehabilitation, if any?
- What are the typical attitudes toward people with disabilities in various ways?
- Are they treated in any way differently from other members of the community?
- What are the attitudes of people of various ages, sexes, ethnic groups, and religions about the body? About discussion of the body? About self-examination?
- Which areas of the body are considered private?
- What are the local attitudes about display of various parts of the body?
- Are there any taboos or restrictions on who can see a woman's or a man's body?
- What are the consequences of violations of the taboo?
- What remedies or rituals should follow violation of the taboo, if any?
- What are the attitudes toward examination of the body by medical personnel of various sexes, ages, and statuses?
- Do feelings of modesty make certain people uncomfortable or embarrassed in certain medical situations?
- What might the health care worker do to lessen embarrassment?

BELIEFS ABOUT DYING

- What are the local attitudes and practices surrounding dying?
- Are there any special omens or signs portending death?
- Are special measures taken to ward off death?
- Where and how do people want to die?
- Are there types of deaths or places one might die that are particularly feared or disliked?
- What roles do various family and community members play when people are dying?
- Are any special rituals or ceremonies performed when someone is dying?
- What happens when people die?
- What are the practices concerning mourning, preparation of the body, the funeral, and burial?
- Do the practices vary depending on the age, sex, religion, ethnic group, or social status of the deceased?
- Are there any later observations of the death or further rites connected with it?
- When family and/or friends receive news of a death, how do they react?
- How is grief manifested within the culture?
- What are the usual ways of dealing with grief?
- What role should a friend, health worker, or others play in case of a death? When, if ever, does one offer condolences? What other actions may be expected?
- How do people normally feel about the subject of death?
- Are there any special taboos concerning death (i.e., mention of death or the dead; contact with the dead body, the place of death, or the deceased's possessions)?
- Are the dead believed to have any influence on those still living?
- How do (or should) beliefs about death and dying affect health program routines?
- What roles do family, friends, and others like to play during the death of a family member in a health facility?
- How may attitudes toward death affect the functioning of local health program workers?

FAMILY AND PERSONAL HYGIENE

- What are people's beliefs and attitudes concerning the benefits of various hygienic practices? Their possible effect on health?
- How may living conditions and resources available in the area influence habits of personal hygiene?
- What would be the attitudes of people toward possible changes in hygienic practices?
- What are local attitudes and practices concerning washing various parts of the body?
  - Washing clothes?
  - Caring for teeth?
  - Wearing shoes?
- Are there any problems of body pests or parasites? What is done about them?
- Which hygienic practices promoted either by the outside health worker or the local culture seem to have a real effect on health?

ATTITUDES ABOUT PREGNANCY AND CHILDBIRTH

- How does a woman determine she is pregnant?
- Do women of various groups follow any special practices during pregnancy? Follow any special taboos? Eat or not eat certain foods? Follow any rituals? Take any special treatments or medicines? Change sexual practices? Change work patterns?
- Are certain conditions recognized as dangerous during pregnancy? What is done about them?
- What sources of advice and care are sought during pregnancy?
- Are certain traditional or Western health practitioners consulted by various women during pregnancy? Who are they? What do they do?
- Are there any special beliefs concerning forces (both animate and inanimate) that may have an influence on an unborn baby?
- What effects may these forces have?
- Is protection of any kind sought against forces that may be harmful?
- What are considered abnormal signs during pregnancy? Why?
- What is done about them?
- In what settings do various women in the community give birth?
- Who is present during the delivery in each setting, and what role does each person play?
- What methods of delivery are used?
- What sanitary precautions are taken?
- What methods are used to cut and treat the umbilical cord?
- What is done with the placenta?
- What is done when various complications arise?
- Are any special customs or rituals followed concerning delivery or birth?
- Are there any special attitudes toward or customs concerning twins? Multiple births?
- What is done in the case of maternal or infant death during childbirth?
- What if the baby is stillborn?
- Is infanticide practiced? In what cases?
- Does a child's sex make a difference?
- What are the local attitudes toward this practice?

ATTITUDES ABOUT CHILD CARE

- Do mothers follow any special practices after the birth of a child? Change work schedules in any way? Change eating habits? Take any special medicines? Perform or take part in any special rituals or ceremonies? Go through a period of confinement?
- How do mothers and/or other relevant people care for infants and children of various ages?
- How are infants and children cleaned? Fed? Watched? Toilet trained? Disciplined? Taught various skills? Cared for when ill?

- What happens if the mother is working? Ill? Absent? Dead?
- Who babysits for the mother? Under what circumstances?
- Are there any child care practices hazardous to the health of the child?
- How is food allocated in families when it is scarce?

SEXUAL BEHAVIOR

- How is knowledge concerning sex acquired by growing children?
- What are the attitudes toward sex education of various types?
- How easily will various people discuss sexual topics?
- Is male or female circumcision practiced? Why? At what age?
- What methods and rituals (if any) are followed?
- Does the procedure ever cause infection or other harm to the health of those circumcised?
- What are the social and cultural beliefs and practices concerning menstruation?
- Are there any special rites, rituals, or taboos that must be observed during this period? Special measures to relieve cramps or problems of irregularity?
- What are the social and cultural beliefs and practices surrounding sexual intercourse (e.g., premarital sex play, obtaining a lover, techniques of coitus, reasons for intercourse, sexual restrictions or abstentions, extramarital intercourse, sexual aberrations in adulthood, concealment of the sexual organs)?
- What are the social and cultural beliefs and practices surrounding conception (e.g., theories of conception, development and feeding of the fetus, determining the sex of the offspring, barrenness and sterility)?
- How is menopause experienced within the culture?
- What are its symptoms?
- What meaning does it have?
- Are there special cures for related problems?
- What forms of homosexuality and bisexuality are common within the culture, if any? What are the local attitudes toward homosexuality? Bisexuality?

UNDERSTANDING THE PSYCHOLOGICAL AND SOCIOCULTURAL MAKEUP OF A COMMUNITY

- What is the history of the community?
- From where does the culture come?
- What is the basic worldview? How was earth created, and who or what maintains the earth and all power within it?
- To what extent is the worldview influenced by religion?
- What are the major religious groups in the community?
- Are there certain religious groups that may be difficult to identify because they operate in secret?
- For each religious group,

  - How is it organized?
  - Who are its members within the community?
  - The size of the membership?
  - Requirements for membership?
  - Social characteristics of the members (e.g., sex, age, social class)?
  - What are the group's general beliefs, values, and practices?
  - Does the religion have any organized theology?
  - What role does the group play in overall community life?
  - What is the general history of the group and its role in the community?

- Who are the leaders of the religious groups within the community?
- What roles do they play within their religious group and the wider community?
- How do the various religious groups relate to each other?
- What conflicts exist?
- Are there areas of cooperation?

- How much overlap is there between the systems of religion and medicine within the community?
- What involvement do various religious groups and their leaders have in the area of health and illness?
- Do the religious groups hold special beliefs concerning what or who causes various illnesses and whether and how these illnesses can be prevented, diagnosed, and treated?
- The cause(s) of death and whether and how death might be prevented?
- Do any of the leaders or followers in the religious groups play roles in the prevention, diagnosis, and/or treatment of illness?
- How do the religious groups in the community affect the secular practice of medicine?
- How do they affect the health beliefs and practices of their followers?
- How do they affect the utilization of health care facilities?
- How do they affect the organization and practice of medical care?
- Do any of the beliefs and practices of various religious groups conflict with the philosophy or procedures of the health program?
- Should any special effort be made to discourage religious beliefs or practices that may be detrimental to health?
- Do any of the religious beliefs and practices of various religious groups complement each other?
- What rituals and ceremonies are observed by each religious group in the community?
- Are there religious rituals or ceremonies marking stages in the life cycle such as birth, entrance into adulthood, marriage, and death?
- Are there certain general rituals or ceremonies observed by all or part of the religious community?
- What are the major events in the "church calendar"?
- Who participates and how?
- Do some of these rituals or ceremonies affect the health or health care of the religious group's members?
- How could the operation of the health program be adapted to take into account important rituals and the needs of patients or other community members participating in them?
- Is the health care program or other health care facilities operated or strongly influenced by certain religious groups?
- To what extent does religious affiliation influence the type of care given? To what extent does religious affiliation affect the type of clientele that will use a particular facility?
- What is the attitude of the government and local community toward religiously affiliated health care facilities?
- Do governmental and community attitudes affect the delivery of health care in these organizations?
- What are the religious backgrounds and/or current religious affiliations of health care providers?
- How does religion influence their work?
- Are there religious obligations that may interfere with a health care provider's job?
- Are there religious attitudes that may influence the care a worker provides?
- Should any adaptations be made within the health care program to accommodate religious obligations, beliefs, and practices of the health care provider?
- What are the current relationships between various health care providers and religious leaders and healers?
- Could these relationships be improved?
- Could (and should) various religious leaders and healers be involved in health program activities? Would they be willing to use their influence in ways that might benefit the health program?
- Are there any current conflicts between religious groups that would affect how the health program should relate to various religious leaders and their groups?

UNDERSTANDING BEHAVIORAL FACTORS

- What indications may the people give of fear, pain, and discomfort?
- How do people's nonverbal gestures and facial and body expressions vary from those to which health care providers are accustomed?
- What is the meaning of silence in various situations?
- How is one expected to act during various types of silence?
- How do members of the culture typically use their language when trying to persuade or explain things to others?
- Do they use logical explanations, stories, or proverbs? Hold debates? Appeal to certain values?
- Could the health care provider use similar techniques when communicating with people?
- How can health-related explanations be adapted so they will be related to things people are familiar with in daily life?
- How does one show disapproval? Disagreement? Frustration? Is direct criticism and complaint accepted within the culture?
- If not, what ways are accepted culturally for expressing negative feelings?
- How is affection displayed? What about anger, embarrassment, and other emotions?
- When can various emotions be displayed, and with whom?
- What are the cultural norms concerning raised voices, arguments, sarcasm, swearing, and expression of humor?
- How are "calls for help" (especially medical) made within the culture?
- What signs, besides the verbal ones, do people give when they feel they need treatment?

UNDERSTANDING THE ROLE OF AN INVESTIGATOR

- What are your own attitudes, beliefs, and practices concerning health, illness, and medical care? (Answer for yourself and your culture the questions that have been posed.)
- Examine your beliefs and practices. Which seem scientifically justified and which seem simply a part of your "cultural baggage" and not useful or desirable within the local culture?
- What areas of agreement and disagreement can you find between your attitudes, beliefs, and practices and those of other health care providers or community members?
- Do certain areas of disagreement or conflict cause problems within the program?
- How should change take place? (These same questions should be applicable to professionals and administrators.)
- Is the culture one in which things are changing fast, or one in which things pretty much stay the same?
- Has the rate of change varied?
- What is the culture's view concerning the desirability of change?
- Are the people change oriented, or do they tend to be conservative and tradition minded?
- How is the general orientation toward change likely to affect efforts to promote changes in health beliefs and practices?
- What changes in health beliefs and practices do the people themselves want?
- What beliefs and practices in the health area are beneficial to health? Have no effect on health? Are harmful to health? Should harmful beliefs and practices be changed?
- What are the functions of various beliefs and practices?
- How are various beliefs and practices linked to one another?
- What meaning do they have to those who practice them?
- Do the individual beliefs and practices link together to form a meaningful whole?
- Are suggestions for changing of certain health beliefs and practices realistic, considering the total situation? What is the place of the belief or practice within the culture?

- What effects or repercussions may certain changes in health beliefs and practices have in other areas of life?
- When proposing changes in health beliefs and practices, is it possible to develop innovations that fit easily within the existing culture? Emphasize continuity with old traditions?
- If certain health beliefs and practices are influenced by religion, will this affect the ease with which they might be changed?
- What changes might be expected in the organization and influence of various religious groups in the community?
- What might be the effect of these changes on health and health care?

UNDERSTANDING HOW THE COMMUNITY OPERATES

- How does information usually spread from one place to another within the community?
- What are the important formal channels of communication?
- What are the important informal channels of communication?
- Who do the channels reach and how effective are they?
- What are the patterns of interaction within the community?
- Where do people usually gather? Are these important places of communication?
- Who are important opinion leaders and "communicators" within the community?
- Who has the greatest authority in the health area?
- Why are various leaders influential?
- What effect does the authority of various leaders have on the acceptance of their messages?
- What channels of communication do these leaders use?
- What channels of communication between the health care program and community are currently being used? Are there certain difficulties that might be traced to lack of effective communication in some fields? Are there segments of the population that are not being reached?
- Could other means of communication be developed and used?
- Is there an active grapevine between the program and the community?
- Could distortions be minimized by better communication at certain points?
- Could certain channels of communication already in operation within the community be used by the health program itself?
- Would certain community leaders and other communicators be willing to transmit messages between the program and their constituents?

UNDERSTANDING THE RELATIONSHIP BETWEEN
THE COMMUNITY AND THE HEALTH CARE AND EDUCATION PROGRAM

- What are the attitudes of outside staff toward community members?
- What are the community's attitudes toward staff members coming from outside the local area?
- Does it vary depending on the area from which the staff member comes? With the staff member's position? Personality?
- How does the population feel toward outsiders and foreigners in general?
- How may these feelings affect specific attitudes toward the health worker?
- What might be the reasons for these feelings?
- How long do outside staff members usually remain in their positions in the local health care program?
- Are there any difficulties in community and patient relations caused by the short-term nature of some of the contracts?
- Do the outside staff members' lifestyles and physical living conditions tend to integrate or separate them from the local community?
- Should any changes be made?

- How will attempts by outside staff members to adjust to or imitate local behavior patterns be seen by the local population?
- To what extent should outsiders try to adopt or at least show appreciation of local customs?
- How do the community and staff make their opinions about the health program known?
- How are suggestions and complaints registered and handled?
- If the present system is inadequate, what new ways to handle suggestions and complaints could be developed?
- Do certain complaints mask hidden areas of concern? What can be done about the underlying causes of difficulty?

POSSIBLE PROGRAM PROBLEMS

- What community members are ignored by the services?
- Do certain people act as "gatekeepers," controlling communication within the program between patients and staff?
- How must information be altered if focused at various levels within the population?
- Are there traditional channels of communication through which information flows from the leaders down to the population and is simplified in the process?
- Could the health care provider use any of these channels?
- Are there any problems among staff that arise because of racial prejudice or discrimination?
- What is program policy toward the hiring of members of various ethnic groups?
- Within the program itself, what percentage of various ethnic or national groups are in positions of power and authority?
- What may account for differences?
- Are changes needed?
- What techniques might be used within the health care program to begin working on problems of racial prejudice and discrimination among the staff itself?
- With what community groups or people can the health care provider communicate most easily? Least easily?
- Do tendencies to interact with certain people more often cause distortions in the way in which the health care worker perceives the community? How can distortion be lessened?
- What means of communication are being used currently among staff and patients within the health care program?
- Is communication adequate? If not, what adjustments might be made?
- Are there ways to check for areas where understanding is poor and eliminate them?
- Can you identify possible barriers to effective staff–patient communication within the program? (Barriers may be caused by differences in cultural beliefs, practices, and values or differences of social and economic status, education, sex, or age.) What might be done to overcome these barriers?
- Do any typical difficulties seem to arise among health care providers of differing ages, sexes, religious affiliations, education levels, health care program statuses, or health care disciplines?
- Do any difficulties arise because health care providers of various cultures have differing attitudes about roles they should play?
- Are there any basic clashes of personality among staff members? What seem to be the causes of disagreement or dislike?
- What can be done to emphasize or broaden positive aspects of staff interrelations and lessen difficulties and misunderstandings?
- What means of communication are used currently among staff members within the health care program?
- Is communication adequate? If not, what new means for facilitating communication might be used?

- What means of communication between the health care program and its sponsoring and/or supervising organization(s) are currently being used?
- How effective is communication?
- If poor, how could it be improved?

Bloch's Ethnic/Cultural Assessment Guide

Data category	Guideline questions/instructions	Data collected
CULTURAL		
Ethnic origin	Does the patient identify with a particular group (e.g., Puerto Rican, African)?	
Race	What is the patient's racial background (e.g., black, Filipino, American Indian)?	
Place of birth	Where was the patient born?	
Relocations	Where has he lived (country, city)? During what years did patient live there and for how long? Has he moved recently?	
Habits, customs, and beliefs	Describe habits, customs, values, and beliefs patient holds or practices that affect his attitude toward birth, life, death, health and illness, time orientation, health care system, and health care providers. What is degree of belief and adherence by patient to his overall cultural system?	
Behaviors valued by culture	How does patient value privacy, courtesy, respect for elders, behaviors related to family roles and sex roles, and work ethic?	
Cultural sanctions and restrictions	Sanctions—What is accepted behavior by patient's cultural group regarding expression of emotions and feelings, religious expressions, and response to illness and death?	
	Restrictions—Does patient have any restrictions related to sexual matters, exposure of body parts, certain types of surgery (e.g., hysterectomy), discussion of dead relatives, and discussion of fears related to the unknown?	

From Bloch, B. (1983). Bloch's ethnic/cultural assessment guide. In M. Orque, B. Bloch, & M. Monrroy (Eds.), *Ethnic nursing care: A multicultural approach* (pp. 63–69). St. Louis, MO: C.V. Mosby; reprinted by permission of B. Bloch.

Data category	Guideline questions/instructions	Data collected
Language and communication process	What are some overall cultural characteristics of patient's language and communication process?	
Language(s) and/or dialect(s) spoken	Which language(s) and/or dialect(s) does patient speak most frequently? Where? At home or work?	
Language barriers	Which language does patient predominantly use in thinking? Does patient need bilingual interpreter in client–professional interactions? Is patient able to read and/or write in English?	
Communication process	What are rules (linguistics) and modes (style) of communication process (e.g., "honorific" concept of showing "respect or deference" to others using words only common to specific ethnic/culture group)?	
	Is there need for variation in technique of communicating and interviewing to accommodate patient's cultural background (e.g., tempo of conversation, eye or body contact, topic restrictions, norms of confidentiality, and style of explanation)?	
	Are there any conflicts in verbal and nonverbal interactions between patient and professional?	
	How does patient's nonverbal communication process compare with other ethnic/cultural groups, and how does it affect patient's response to health care?	
	Are there any variations between patient's interethnic/interracial communication process or intracultural/intraracial communication process (e.g., between ethnic minority patient and white middle-class professional, or ethnic minority patient and ethnic minority professional; beliefs, attitudes, values, role variations, stereotyping [perception and prejudice])?	
Healing beliefs/Cultural healing system	What cultural healing system does the patient adhere to (e.g., Asian healing system, Raza/Latina Curanderismo)? What religious healing system does the patient predominantly adhere to (e.g., Seventh Day Adventist, West African voodoo, Fundamentalist sect, Pentecostal)?	

Data category	Guideline questions/instructions	Data collected
Cultural health beliefs	Is illness explained by the germ theory, presence of evil spirits, imbalance between "hot" and "cold" (yin and yang in Chinese culture), or disequilibrium between nature and man?	
	Is good health related to success, ability to work or fulfill roles, reward from God, or balance with nature?	
Cultural health practices	What types of cultural healing practices does the patient practice? Does he/she use healing remedies to cure *natural* illnesses caused by the external environment (e.g., massage to cure *empacho* [a ball of food clinging to stomach wall], wearing of talismans or charms for protection against illness)?	
Cultural healers	Does patient rely on cultural healers (e.g., medicine man, Curandero, Chinese herbalist, hougan [voodoo priest], spiritualist, minister)?	
Nutritional variables or factors	What nutritional variables or factors are influenced by the patient's ethnic/cultural background?	
Characteristics of food preparation and consumption	What types of food preferences and restrictions, meanings of foods, style of food preparation and consumption, frequency of eating, time of eating, and eating utensils are culturally determined for patient? Are there any religious influences on food preparation and consumption?	
Influences from external environment	What modifications, if any, did the patient's ethnic group make in its food practices in white dominant American society? Are there any adaptations of food customs and beliefs from rural setting to urban setting?	
Patient education needs	What are some implications of diet planning and teaching to patient who adheres to cultural practices concerning foods?	

SOCIOLOGICAL

Economic status	Who is principal wage earner in patient's family? What is total annual income (approximately) of family? What impact does economic status have on life-style, place of residence, living conditions, and ability to obtain health services?	

Data category	Guideline questions/instructions	Data collected
Educational status	What is highest education level obtained? Does patient's educational background influence his ability to understand how to seek health services, literature on health care, patient teaching experiences, and any written material patient is exposed to in health care setting (e.g., admission forms, patient care forms, teaching literature, and lab test forms)? Does patient's educational background cause him to feel inferior or superior to health care personnel in health care settings?	
Social network	What are patient's social networks (kinship, peer, cultural healing networks)? How do they influence health or illness status of patient?	
Family as supportive group	Does patient's family feel need for continuous presence in patient's clinical setting (is this an ethnic/cultural characteristic)? How is family valued during illness or death? How does family participate in patient's nursing care process (e.g., giving baths, feeding, using touch as support [cultural meaning], supportive presence)? How does ethnic/cultural family structure influence patient response to health or illness (e.g., roles, beliefs, strengths, weaknesses, and social class)? Are there any key family roles characteristic of a specific ethnic/cultural group (e.g., grandmother in some black and American Indian families), and can these key persons be a resource for health personnel? What role does family play in health promotion or cause of illness (e.g., would family be intermediary group in patient interactions with health personnel and make decisions regarding his care)?	
Supportive institutions in ethnic/cultural community	What influence do ethnic/cultural institutions have on patient receiving health services (i.e., institutions such as Organization of Migrant Workers, NAACP, Black Political Caucus, churches, schools, Urban League, community clinics)?	

Data category	Guideline questions/instructions	Data collected
Institutional racism	How does institutional racism in health facilities influence patient's response to receiving health care?	

PSYCHOLOGICAL

Self-concept (identity)	Does patient show strong racial/cultural identity? How does this compare to that of other racial/cultural groups or to members of dominant society?	
	What factors in patient's development helped to shape his self-concept (e.g., family, peers, society labels, external environment, institutions, racism)?	
	How does patient deal with stereotypical behavior from health professionals?	
	What is impact of racism on patient from distinct ethnic/cultural group (e.g., social anxiety, noncompliance to health care process in clinical settings, avoidance of utilizing or participating in health care institutions)?	
	Does ethnic/cultural background have impact on how patient relates to body image change resulting from illness or surgery (e.g., importance of appearance and role in cultural group)?	
	Any adherence or identification with ethnic/cultural "group identity" (e.g., solidarity, "we" concept)?	
Mental and behavioral processes and characteristics of ethnic/cultural group	How does patient relate to his external environment in clinical setting (e.g., fears, stress, and adaptive mechanisms characteristic of a specific ethnic/cultural group)? Any variations based on the life span?	
	What is patient's ability to relate to persons outside of his ethnic/cultural group (health personnel)? Is he withdrawn, verbally or nonverbally expressive, negative or positive, feeling mentally or physically inferior or superior?	
	How does patient deal with feelings of loss of dignity and respect in clinical setting?	
Religious influences on psychological effects of health/illness	Does patient's religion have a strong impact on how he relates to health/illness influences or outcomes (e.g., death/chronic illness, cause and effect of illness, or adherence to nursing/medical practices)?	

Data category	Guideline questions/instructions	Data collected
	Do religious beliefs, sacred practices, and talismans play a role in treatment of disease?	
	What is role of significant religious persons during health/illness (e.g., ministers, priests, monks, imams)?	
Psychological/ cultural response to stress and discomfort of illness	Based on ethnic/cultural background, does patient exhibit any variations in psychological response to pain or physical disability of disease processes?	

BIOLOGICAL/PHYSIOLOGICAL
(consideration of *norms* for different ethnic/cultural groups)

Racial-anatomical characteristics	Does patient have any distinct racial characteristics (e.g., skin color, hair texture and color, color of mucous membranes)? Does patient have any variations in anatomical characteristics (e.g., body structure [height and weight] more prevalent for ethnic/cultural group, skeletal formation [pelvic shape, especially for obstetrical evaluation], facial shape and structure [nose, eye shape, facial contour], upper and lower extremities)?	
	How do patient's racial and anatomical characteristics affect his self-concept and the way others relate to him?	
	Does variation in racial-anatomical characteristics affect physical evaluations and physical care, skin assessment based on color, and variations in hair care and hygienic practices?	
Growth and development patterns	Are there any distinct growth and development characteristics that vary with patient's ethnic/cultural background (e.g., bone density, fatfolds, motor ability)? What factors are important for nutritional assessment, neurological and motor assessment, assessment of bone deterioration in disease process or injury, evaluation of newborns, evaluation of intellectual status or capacity, assessment of sensory/motor sensory development in children? How do these differ in ethnic/cultural groups?	

Data category	Guideline questions/instructions	Data collected
Variations in body systems	Are there any variations in body systems particular to distinct ethnic/cultural group (e.g., gastrointestinal disturbance with lactose intolerance, nutritional intake of cultural foods causing adverse effects on gastrointestinal tract and fluid and electrolyte system, variations in chemical and hematological systems [certain blood types prevalent in particular ethnic/cultural groups])?	
Skin and hair physiology, mucous membranes	How does skin color variation influence assessment of skin color changes (e.g., jaundice, cyanosis, ecchymosis, erythema, and its relationship to disease processes)?	
	What are methods of assessing skin color changes (comparing variations and similarities between different ethnic groups)?	
	Are there conditions of hypopigmentation and hyperpigmentation (e.g., vitiligo, mongolian spots, albinism, discoloration caused by trauma)? Why would these be more striking in some ethnic groups?	
	Are there any skin conditions more prevalent in a distinct ethnic group (e.g., keloids in blacks)?	
	Is there any correlation between oral and skin pigmentation and their variations among distinct racial groups when doing assessment of oral cavity (e.g., leukoedema is normal occurrence in blacks)?	
	What are variations in hair texture and color among racially different groups? Ask patient about preferred hair care methods or any racial/cultural restrictions (e.g., not washing "hot-combed" hair while in clinical setting, not cutting very long hair of Raza/Latina patients).	
	Are there any variations in skin care methods (e.g., using Vaseline on black skin)?	
Diseases more prevalent among ethnic/cultural group	Are there any specific diseases or conditions that are more prevalent for a specific ethnic/cultural group (e.g., hypertension, sickle cell anemia, G6-PD, lactose intolerance)?	

Data category	Guideline questions/instructions	Data collected
	Does patient have any socioenvironmental health conditions common among ethnic/cultural groups (e.g., lead paint poisoning, poor nutrition, overcrowding; alcoholism resulting from psychological despair and alienation from dominant society, rat bites, poor sanitation)?	
Diseases ethnic/ cultural group has increased resistance to	Are there any diseases that patient has increased resistance to because of racial/cultural background (e.g., skin cancer in blacks)?	

Individualized Health Care Plan

INDIVIDUALIZED HEALTH CARE PLAN CHECKLIST

Preparation for Entry:

☐ Home Visit/Assessment _____
(date)

☐ Health History _____
(date)

☐ Planning Meetings _____   _____   _____
(date)   (date)   (date)

☐ Staff Training Meetings _____   _____   _____
(date)   (date)   (date)

☐ Educational Team Meetings _____   _____   _____
(date)   (date)   (date)

Health Care Plan Included in:

☐ Student Record _____
(date)

☐ Individualized   ☐ Individualized Student
Education Program _____   Accommodation Plan _____
(date)   (date)

Health Care Plan

☐ Health Assessment _____
(date)

☐ Physician's Order   ☐ Health Care
for Medications _____   Procedure _____
(date)   (date)

☐ Student-Specific   ☐ Procedural
Procedural Guidelines _____   Skills Checklist _____
(date)   (date)

☐ Problems/Goals/Actions _____
(date)

Emergency Plan

☐ School _____
(date)

☐ In Transit _____
(date)

☐ Health Care Plan Reviewed by Physician _____
(date)

☐ Signed by Parent, Education Administrator,
School Nurse/Health Care Coordinator _____
(date)

Children and Youth Assisted by Medical Technology in Educational Settings (2nd ed.) © 1997 Paul H. Brookes Publishing Co., Baltimore.

_____
(School Nurse/Health Care Coordinator)

_____
(Education Coordinator)

INDIVIDUALIZED HEALTH CARE PLAN

Student Information:

_____   _____
(Name)   (Birthdate)

_____   _____
(Parent/Guardian)   (Address)

Mother/Guardian: _____   _____
                        (Home telephone)   (Work telephone)

Father/Guardian: _____   _____
                        (Home telephone)   (Work telephone)

_____   _____
(School)   (Grade/Class)

Language(s) spoken; student: _____   Caregiver(s): _____

Immunizations: _____   _____
(date and type)

_____   _____

_____   _____

_____   _____

_____   _____

Primary Physician: _____   Telephone: _____

Specialty Physicians:

_____   Telephone: _____

_____   Telephone: _____

_____   Telephone: _____

_____   Telephone: _____

_____   Telephone: _____

In Emergency, Notify:

Name: _____   Telephone: _____   Relationship: _____

Name: _____   Telephone: _____   Relationship: _____

Children and Youth Assisted by Medical Technology in Educational Settings (2nd ed.) © 1997 Paul H. Brookes Publishing Co., Baltimore.

Name: _____   Date: _____

IMPORTANT PERSONNEL

School contacts:

_____   _____
_____   _____
_____   _____
_____   _____
_____   _____

	Training
Direct caregivers:	Student-specific	General
_____	_____	_____
	(date)	(date)
_____	_____	_____
	(date)	(date)

Substitute caregivers/back-up staff:

_____	_____	_____
	(date)	(date)
_____	_____	_____
	(date)	(date)
_____	_____	_____
	(date)	(date)
_____	_____	_____
	(date)	(date)

Student-specific training done by:

_____   _____
                                                 (date)

General staff training done by:

_____   _____
                                                 (date)

Peer awareness training done by:

_____   _____
                                                 (date)

Children and Youth Assisted by Medical Technology in Educational Settings (2nd ed.) © 1997 Paul H. Brookes Publishing Co., Baltimore.

Name: _____   Date: _____

BACKGROUND INFORMATION

Brief health history: _____
_____
_____
_____
_____
_____

Special health care needs of the student: _____
_____
_____
_____
_____
_____
_____
_____

Other considerations: _____
_____
_____

Student participation in care: _____
_____
_____
_____

Baseline status (i.e., skin color, activity/energy level, blood pressure, pulse, temperature, respirations): _____
_____
_____
_____
_____

Medication (dose, route, time): _____
_____
_____
_____
_____

Diet: _____
_____

Allergies: _____

Transportation needs: _____
_____

What is the transportation emergency communication system: _____
_____

Children and Youth Assisted by Medical Technology in Educational Settings (2nd ed.) © 1997 Paul H. Brookes Publishing Co., Baltimore.

Name: _____ Date: _____

PROCEDURE INFORMATION SHEET

Procedure: _____

Frequency: _____ Times: _____

Position of student during procedure: _____

Ability of the student to assist/perform procedure: _____
_____

Suggested setting for procedure: _____

Equipment (include make and model when applicable):

Daily: _____   Emergency: _____
_____   _____
_____   _____
_____   _____
_____   _____
_____   _____

Checked by: _____   Checked by: _____

Storage: _____   Storage: _____

Maintenance: _____   Maintenance: _____

Home care company: _____   Home care company: _____

Child-specific techniques and helpful hints: _____
_____
_____
_____
_____
_____
_____

Procedural considerations and precautions: _____
_____
_____
_____
_____
_____
_____

Children and Youth Assisted by Medical Technology in Educational Settings (2nd ed.) © 1997 Paul H. Brookes Publishing Co., Baltimore.

Name: _____ Date: _____

POSSIBLE PROBLEMS

Observation	Reason	Action

Name: _____

School Nurse: _____

Date: _____

Individualized Health Care Plan

Date	Health Need/Nursing Diagnosis	Goals	Action/Intervention	Evaluation

Children and Youth Assisted by Medical Technology in Educational Settings (2nd ed.) © 1997 Paul H. Brookes Publishing Co., Baltimore.

Date	Health Need/Nursing Diagnosis	Goals	Action/Intervention	Evaluation

Daily Log

Name: _____ School: _____

Procedure(s): _____

Parent: _____ Telephone number: _____

Date/time	Procedure notes	Observations	Name

EMERGENCY PLAN

Name: _____   **Date:** _____

Child-specific emergencies:

If you see this	Do this

If an emergency occurs:

1. Stay with child.
2. Call or designate someone to call the nurse.
   - State who you are.
   - State where you are.
   - State the problem.
3. The school nurse will assess the child and decide whether the emergency plan should be implemented.
4. If the school nurse is unavailable, the following staff members are trained to initiate the emergency plan:

_____

_____

_____

_____

Emergency Telephone Procedure

Name: _____   Date: _____

1. **Dial 911 and/or designated emergency response team.**

2. **State who you are:** "I am _____ , a nurse/teacher/paraprofessional in the _____ school."

3. **State where you are.**
   School name: _____
   Address: _____
   City: _____

4. **State what is wrong with student.**

5. **Give specific directions** (e.g., which school entrance should be used, location of student).

6. **Do not hang up.** Ask for the information to be repeated and provide any other necessary information. Hang up only when all information has been received and is correct.

7. **Notify people.**
   a. School principal or school official in charge of the building at that time: _____
   (telephone number)
   b. School back-up personnel: _____
   (telephone number)

8. **State the following:**
   "Emergency plan for _____ is in effect."
   "The student is located _____ ."

9. **Do the following:**
   a. Meet the emergency response team.
   b. Direct emergency response team to the emergency area.
   c. Call parents and other necessary individuals (including physician).

An adult should be designated to accompany student in the ambulance.

Hospital that the student should be transported to: _____ .

Children and Youth Assisted by Medical Technology in Educational Settings (2nd ed.) © 1997 Paul H. Brookes Publishing Co., Baltimore.

EMERGENCY INFORMATION

Name: _____ Birthdate: _____

Address: _____ Telephone number: _____

Mother/Guardian: _____

    Home telephone number: _____ Work telephone number: _____

Father/Guardian: _____

    Home telephone number: _____ Work telephone number: _____

Other contact: _____ Telephone number: _____

Health insurance: _____ Telephone number: _____

Emergency numbers:

Emergency medical response team: _____ Telephone number: _____

Fire: _____ Telephone number: _____

Police: _____ Telephone number: _____

Home care company: _____ Telephone number: _____

Ambulance: _____ Telephone number: _____

Gas company: _____ Telephone number: _____

Electric company: _____ Telephone number: _____

Preferred hospital:

_____ Telephone number: _____

Local hospital emergency room:

_____ Telephone number: _____

Primary physician: _____ Telephone number: _____

Dentist: _____ Telephone number: _____

Specialists:

_____ Telephone number: _____

_____ Telephone number: _____

_____ Telephone number: _____

_____ Telephone number: _____

_____ Telephone number: _____

Children and Youth Assisted by Medical Technology in Educational Settings (2nd ed.) © 1997 Paul H. Brookes Publishing Co., Baltimore.

Parent Authorization for Specialized Health Care

We (I), the undersigned, who are the parents/guardians of

_____
(name)   (birthdate)

request that the following health care service(s) _____

_____

_____

_____

_____

_____

be administered to our child. We understand that a qualified designated person(s) will be performing the above-mentioned health care service. It is our understanding that in performing this service, the designated person(s) will be using a standardized procedure that has been approved by our physician.

_____
(name)   (address)   (telephone number)

We will notify the school immediately if the health status of _____
changes, we change physicians, or there is a change or cancellation of the procedure.

We understand that the above procedure should be scheduled before or after school hours whenever possible.

Signature of parents/guardians: _____

_____

Address: _____

Telephone numbers: _____ _____
                              (home)   (work)

_____ _____
                              (home)   (work)

Date: _____

This authorization form is from Pupil Personnel Services. (1983). *Recommended practices and procedures manual.* Chicago: Illinois State Department of Education; adapted by permission.

Children and Youth Assisted by Medical Technology in Educational Settings (2nd ed.) © 1997 Paul H. Brookes Publishing Co., Baltimore.

PHYSICIAN'S ORDER FOR SPECIALIZED HEALTH CARE PROCEDURE

Student's name: _____ Birthdate: _____ Physician's Name (Print): _____

Address: _____ Address: _____

Telephone: _____

☐ I have reviewed and approve the Health Care Plan as written

☐ I have reviewed and approve the Health Care Plan with the indicated changes/suggestions

Signature: _____ Date: _____

Procedures:

Name	Frequency	Indications	Date of Order	Expiration Date

Children and Youth Assisted by Medical Technology in Educational Settings (2nd ed.) © 1997 Paul H. Brookes Publishing Co., Baltimore.

PHYSICIAN'S ORDER FOR MEDICATION ADMINISTRATION

Student's name: _____ Birthdate: _____ Physician's Name (Print): _____

Address: _____ Address: _____

Telephone: _____

☐ I have reviewed and approve the Health Care Plan as written

☐ I have reviewed and approve the Health Care Plan with the indicated changes/suggestions

Signature: _____ Date: _____

Medications:

Name	Dose/Frequency	Time	Route	Date of Order	Expiration Date

Children and Youth Assisted by Medical Technology in Educational Settings (2nd ed.) © 1997 Paul H. Brookes Publishing Co., Baltimore.

SAMPLE SINGLE MEDICATION ORDER FORM
TO BE COMPLETED BY A LICENSED PRESCRIBER

Student name: _____ Birthdate: _____

Address: _____ Grade: _____
                (street)   (city/town)

Name of licensed prescriber: _____ Title: _____

Business telephone number: _____

Emergency telephone number: _____

Medication: _____

Route of administration: _____ Dosage: _____

Frequency: _____ Time(s) of administration: _____

(Please note: *Whenever possible, medication should be scheduled at times other than school hours.*)

Specific directions or information for administration: _____

Date of order: _____ Discontinuation date: _____

Diagnosis[1]: _____

Any other medical condition(s)[1]: _____

Optional Information

1. Special side effects, contraindications, or possible adverse reactions to be observed: _____

   _____

   _____

2. Other medication being taken by the student: _____

   _____

   _____

3. The date of the next scheduled visit or when advised to return to prescriber: _____

   _____

4. Consent for self-administration (provided the school nurse determines it is safe and appropriate):

   Yes _____ No _____

                                               _____

                                             Signature of licensed prescriber

                                             Date: _____

[1]if not in violation of confidentiality.

From Goodman, I.F., & Sheetz, A.H. (Eds.). (1995). *The comprehensive school health manual.* Boston: School Health Unit, Bureau of Family and Community Health, Massachusetts Department of Public Health; reprinted by permission.

Children and Youth Assisted by Medical Technology in Educational Settings (2nd ed.) © 1997 Paul H. Brookes Publishing Co., Baltimore.

Name: _____ Date: _____

HEALTH CARE PLAN

Written and submitted by: _____
                                          (school nurse)   (date)

Reviewed and signed by:

Parent/Guardian and Student _____
                                             (name)   (date)

                                               _____
                                             (name)   (date)

Education Administrator: _____
                                             (name)   (date)

Reviewed and/or
signed by physician: _____
                                             (name)   (date)

Next review and revision of health care plan: _____
                                                            (date)

Health care plan should be revised according to student's specific needs.

Children and Youth Assisted by Medical Technology in Educational Settings (2nd ed.) © 1997 Paul H. Brookes Publishing Co., Baltimore.

Checklist of Items for Consideration in Developing Individualized Education Plans (IEP) for Students with Physical Disabilities or Special Health Needs

The following checklist contains items often identified by parents and professionals as important components of appropriate educational plans. Not all items will be important to all students; some students may have needs that are not reflected here. We invite your comments and suggestions for additions that can be included in future revisions.

TRANSPORTATION

☐ Regular bus
☐ Van
☐ Wheelchair car
☐ Special equipment
☐ Seat belt
☐ Car seat
☐ Other _____

☐ Special Assistance
  ☐ To and from home to vehicle
  ☐ To and from school to vehicle
  ☐ Aide
  ☐ Positioning
  ☐ Other _____

NOTES: _____

_____

ACCESSIBILITY

☐ Use of elevators
☐ Bathrooms
☐ Classrooms
☐ Gym
☐ Cafeteria
☐ Library

☐ Vocational areas
☐ Auditorium (stage)
☐ Administrative offices
☐ Locker location
☐ Other _____

NOTES: _____

_____

THERAPIES

☐ Occupational therapy
☐ Physical therapy
☐ Speech therapy

☐ Other _____
☐ Other _____
☐ Other _____

NOTES: _____

_____

SELF-HELP SKILLS

☐ Eating
☐ Dressing
☐ Toileting
☐ Student needs:
  ☐ Assistance
  ☐ Training

☐ Grooming
  ☐ Bathing/washing
  ☐ Tooth brushing
☐ Other _____

NOTES: _____

_____

From Anderson, B. (1980). *Checklist of items for consideration in developing individualized education plans (IEP) for students with physical disabilities or special health needs.* Boston: Federation for Children with Special Needs, Collaboration Among Parents and Health Professionals (CAPP) Project; reprinted by permission.

CURRICULUM

☐ Materials to be modified
    ☐ Taped
    ☐ Written in large print
    ☐ Computer software
    ☐ Other _____
☐ Timelines set
☐ Responsibility assigned

☐ Methods to be adapted
    ☐ Timelines for completing tasks/assignments/tests
    ☐ Written *and* spoken
    ☐ Use of computer

NOTES: _____

_____

CLASSWORK

☐ Backup tutoring
    ☐ Regularly scheduled
    ☐ As needed

☐ Make-up assistance
    ☐ Regularly scheduled
    ☐ As needed

NOTES: _____

_____

PHYSICAL EDUCATION

☐ Regular program
☐ Modified regular program
☐ Adaptive physical education program
☐ Other _____

☐ Special equipment
☐ Special staff
☐ Other _____
☐ Other _____

NOTES: _____

_____

ENRICHMENT CLASSES/ACTIVITIES

☐ Art
☐ Music
☐ Computer
☐ Other _____

☐ Modifications needed
    ☐ Special equipment
    ☐ Special staff
    ☐ Other _____

NOTES: _____

_____

EQUIPMENT NEEDED

☐ Typewriter
☐ Computer
☐ Special grip pencils

☐ Communication devices
☐ Extra set of books for home
☐ Other _____

NOTES: _____

_____

MEDICATIONS

☐ Who administers:
    ☐ Student
    ☐ Nurse
    ☐ Teacher
    ☐ Backup person
☐ Side effects implications for
    ☐ Regular school schedule
    ☐ Test schedule
    ☐ Special events/activities

☐ Storage
☐ Recordkeeping, logs
☐ Instructions on self-administering for student

NOTES: _____

_____

SPECIAL HEALTH NEEDS AT SCHOOL

☐ Regular basis   ☐ Specify
☐ As needed   ☐ Who
☐ Use of bathroom as needed   ☐ What
☐ Other _____   ☐ Backup person

NOTES: _____

_____

SPECIAL SUPPLIES OR EQUIPMENT

☐ Storage   ☐ At school only
☐ Whose responsibility   ☐ Shared between home and school

Other considerations: _____

NOTES: _____

_____

BACKUP MEDICAL SUPPORT:

List specific health-related emergencies that may occur: _____

_____

_____

_____

Who to contact _____

Where to go _____

What to do in an emergency _____

_____

_____

NOTES: _____

_____

MOBILITY

☐ Need for assistance   ☐ Proximity considerations for developing schedule
☐ Regular method/person   ☐ Classrooms
☐ Backup person   ☐ Lunchroom
☐ Use of elevator   ☐ Gym
☐ Other _____   ☐ Other _____

NOTES: _____

_____

POSITIONING

☐ Wheelchair   ☐ Aids
☐ Car   ☐ Prone board
☐ Classroom   ☐ Back supports
☐ Gym   ☐ Other _____
☐ Lunch   ☐ When _____
☐ Other _____

NOTES: _____

_____

STAMINA

☐ Scheduling concerns   ☐ Identifiable signs of fatigue
☐ Length of day   ☐ Whose responsibility
☐ Effect on testing, especially timed ones   ☐ Whose authority
☐ Breaks/rest periods   ☐ Role of student
    ☐ As needed
    ☐ Regularly scheduled

NOTES: _____

_____

FIRE SAFETY

☐ Plan
☐ Who is responsible
☐ Backup person

NOTES: _____

_____

FIELD TRIPS

☐ Early notification
☐ Transportation

☐ Aide
☐ Other _____

NOTES: _____

_____

EXTRACURRICULAR ACTIVITIES/PROGRAMS (This is a Section 504 issue)

☐ Special learning opportunities
    ☐ Drivers education
    ☐ Work experience
    ☐ Job placement programs
    ☐ Other _____
☐ Extended day programs
☐ Clubs

☐ Sports programs
☐ Social events
☐ Transportation
☐ Aide
☐ Accessibility

NOTES: _____

_____

HOME/HOSPITAL TUTORING

☐ Needed now
☐ Possibly needed later
☐ Outline plan (even if tentative)

NOTES: _____

_____

General Classroom Inclusion Checklist

Directions: Record a "y" for yes and an "n" for no on the blank preceding each item. If the answer to any of the items is "no" your team may wish to consider whether any changes should be made and what those changes might be.

Going with the Flow:

____ Does the student enter the classroom at the same time as classmates? _____

____ Is the student positioned so that she or he can see and participate in what is going on? _____

____ Is the student positioned so that classmates and teachers may interact easily with him or her (e.g., without teacher between the student and his or her classmates, not isolated from classmates)? _____

____ Does the student engage in classroom activities at the same time as classmates? _____

____ Does the student make transitions in the classroom at the same time as classmates? _____

____ Is the student involved in the same activities as his or her classmates? _____

____ Does the student exit the classroom at the same time as classmates? _____

Acting Cool:

____ Is the student actively involved in class activities (e.g., asks or responds to questions, plays a role in group activities)? _____

____ Is the student encouraged to follow the same classroom and social rules as classmates (e.g., hugs others only when appropriate, stays in seat during instruction)? _____

____ Is the student given assistance only as necessary (assistance should be phased out as soon as possible)? _____

____ Is assistance provided for the student by classmates (e.g., transitions to other classrooms, within the classroom)? _____

____ Are classmates encouraged to provide assistance to the student? _____

____ Are classmates encouraged to ask for assistance from the student? _____

____ Is assistance provided for the student by classroom teachers? _____

____ Does the student use the same or similar materials during classroom activities as his or her classmates (e.g., popular actors on notebooks, school mascot on folders)? _____

Talking Straight:

____ Does the student have a way to communicate with classmates? _____

____ Do classmates know how to communicate with the student? _____

____ Does the student greet others in a manner similar to that of his or her classmates? _____

____ Does the student socialize with classmates? _____

____ Is this facilitated? _____

____ Does the student interact with teachers? _____

____ Is this facilitated? _____

____ Do teachers (e.g., classroom teachers, special education support staff) provide the same type of feedback (e.g., praise, discipline) for the student as for his or her classmates? _____

____ If the student uses an alternative communication system, do classmates know how to use it? _____

____ If the student uses an alternative communication system, do teachers know how to use it? _____

____ Is the system always available to the student? _____

Looking Good:

____ Is the student given the opportunity to attend to his or her appearance as classmates do (e.g., check appearance in mirror between classes)? _____

____ Does the student have accessories that are similar to his or her classmates (e.g., backpacks, friendship bracelets, hair jewelry)? _____

____ Is the student dressed similarly to classmates? _____

____ Is clothing needed for activities age appropriate (e.g., napkins instead of bibs, "cool" paint shirts)? _____

____ Are personal supplies or belongings carried or transported discreetly? _____

____ Is the student's equipment (e.g., wheelchair) kept clean? _____

Given the opportunity (and assistance as needed):
____ Is the student's hair combed?
____ Are the student's hands clean and dry?
____ Does the student change clothing to maintain a neat appearance?
____ Does the student use chewing gum, breath mints, breath spray?

From Vandercook, T., & York, J. (1990). A team approach to program development and support. In Stainback, W., & Stainback, S. (Eds.), *Support networks for inclusive schooling: Interdependent integrated education* (pp. 117–118). Baltimore: Paul H. Brookes Publishing Co.; adapted by permission.

Additional Considerations for Education Planning and Programs

Actively involve the family and student when considering the following:

Social Issues:

Minimize the effect of equipment and caregivers in classroom.

Maximize social opportunities in the classroom and school.

Ensure student participation in social activities outside school, field trips, and extracurricular activities.

Plan for accessibility of above-mentioned activities.

Review plan of disability/diversity awareness in school for classmates/peers.

Develop strategies that encourage classmates to maintain contact with student at home or in hospital.

Ensure privacy for health care procedures.

Be sensitive to and address comments peers may make about student appearances/body functions/abilities.

Identify if siblings/relatives attend the same school and consider their desired level of involvement with the student.

Communication:

Establish ongoing means of communication among school staff, student, and family (i.e., communication book, regular phone calls, periodic meetings).

Identify how student communicates with peers, teachers, and other school staff (i.e., sign language, symbol or object boards, computers, communicative behaviors).

Consider and analyze challenging behaviors to identify the student's intent and purpose.

Review plans for interpreters.

Teach classmates about other languages and communication systems/methods (e.g., American Sign Language, signed English, communication board).

Accommodations:

Secure and maintain needed assistive technology (e.g., assistive listening devices, hearing aids, Brailler, closed-caption television, augmentative communication devices) with training provided as needed.

Plan instruction with a focus on postschool outcomes.

Teach skills in the context of naturally occurring activities and daily routines.

When appropriate, make outlines and teacher and/or student notes available.

Be aware of changes in student's energy level and maximize use of student's energy by

- Reducing amount of class and homework assignments
- Arranging for classmates to take notes
- Arranging for rest time during school day
- Arranging most complex subjects during periods of alertness
- Arranging nontimed tests and alternative exam methods

Seat student close to teacher if vision or hearing problems exist.

Adapt classroom furnishings to meet student needs (e.g., desk to fit wheelchair/wagon use, if age appropriate, for transporting children or equipment to recess/classrooms).

Have mat or cot available for rest time, if needed.

Plan for and identify functional back-up equipment.

Integrate universal precautions principles into classroom routine.

Identify and offer school support services to student (i.e., guidance/transition counselor, peer tutor/mentor, teacher aide).

If health condition affects student's ability to write, consider using note takers, tape recorders, and computers or reducing amount of written schoolwork.

Evaluate performance and review work after long absences.

Develop mechanisms to address academic participation during absences, if appropriate.

- Arrange time for makeup work and tests.
- Arrange home tutoring.
- Consider extended school year or summer program.

Provide systemwide alternatives to measuring student's progress (e.g., portfolio assessment).

Provide related services (e.g., physical therapy, occupational therapy, speech therapy) within the general education setting (e.g., in class, during physical education).

Make individual support systems available (e.g., peer tutors/buddies, mentors).

Include disability-specific consultants to assist school personnel with respect to curricular modifications, assistive technology, and support services.

Use existing disability-specific guidelines when developing services for students.

GUIDELINES FOR CARE

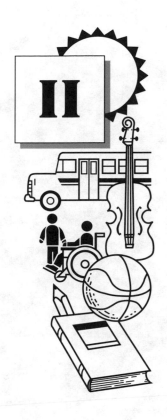

TUBE FEEDING

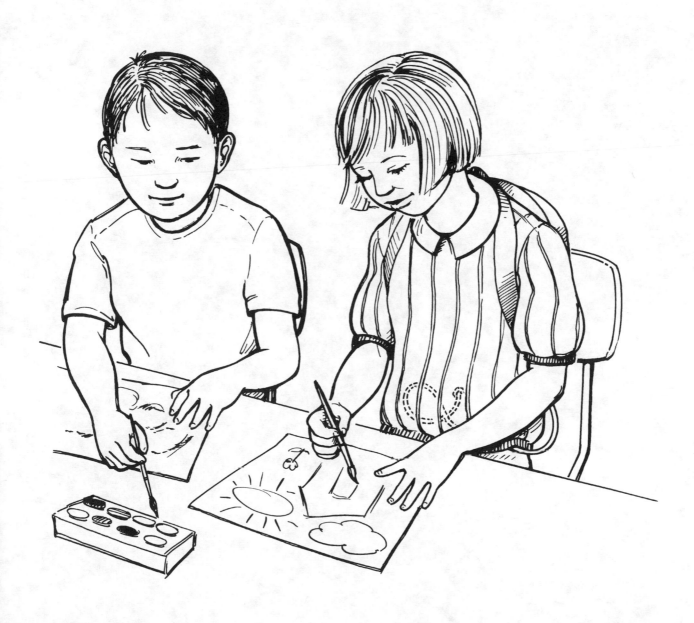

GASTROINTESTINAL SYSTEM

STRUCTURE AND FUNCTION

The gastrointestinal system breaks down food into basic nutrients that can feed the cells of the body. Functionally, the gastrointestinal tract is divided into two parts: upper and lower.

The upper gastrointestinal tract is where digestion and absorption of most of the nutrients occur. The mouth, throat, esophagus, stomach, and small intestine are components of this part of the digestive tract.

The *mouth* is where processing of food starts. Chewing is important because digestion is more effective with smaller particles. The food is swallowed and passes through the throat, then through the esophagus.

The *esophagus* is a straight tube approximately 10 inches in length in an adult. It extends from the base of the throat behind the trachea to the stomach.

The *stomach* is a curved, pouch-like organ that is located under the diaphragm in the upper left portion of the abdomen. The stomach partially digests food and regulates passage of food into the intestine.

The *small intestine* is approximately 12 feet long in an adult. The duodenum, jejunum, and ileum are parts of the small intestine. Food passes from the stomach through the small intestine, where most digestion and absorption of nutrients take place.

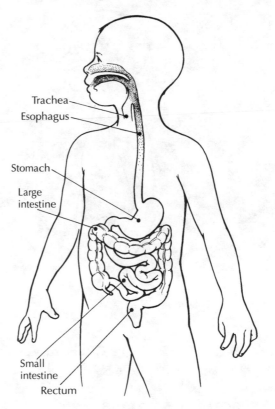

The lower gastrointestinal tract consists of the *large intestine*, where water is reabsorbed and undigested food is consolidated into fecal waste.

The large intestine extends from the end of the small intestine to the *rectum*. The *anus* is the opening to the outside of the body.

FUNCTION

Digestion takes place in two ways:

- *Mechanical*: Chewing and stomach contractions break down food.
- *Chemical*: Food is broken down by digestive acids and enzymes.

The digested food is absorbed through the lining of the intestine and then enters the bloodstream, where it is carried to the cells and tissues throughout the body.

Gastrostomy Tube

PURPOSE

A gastrostomy is a surgical opening into the stomach through the surface of the abdomen.

The gastrostomy tube (G-tube) is a flexible catheter held in place by a balloon or a widened flat "mushroom" at the tip of the tube inside the stomach. The tube remains in place at all times and is closed between feedings to prevent leakage of stomach contents. G-tubes cause no discomfort.

The G-tube may be used to administer food and fluids directly into the stomach. This method is used to bypass the usual route of feeding by mouth when

- There is an obstruction of the esophagus (i.e., food pipe).
- Swallowing is impaired, and the student is at risk for choking/aspiration.
- The student has difficulty taking enough food by mouth to maintain adequate nutrition.

A student may receive a G-tube feeding by either the *bolus* or *continuous (slow-drip)* method. A bolus is a specific amount of feeding given at one time (over 20–30 minutes). A slow drip is a feeding that is given slowly over a number of hours, running continuously.

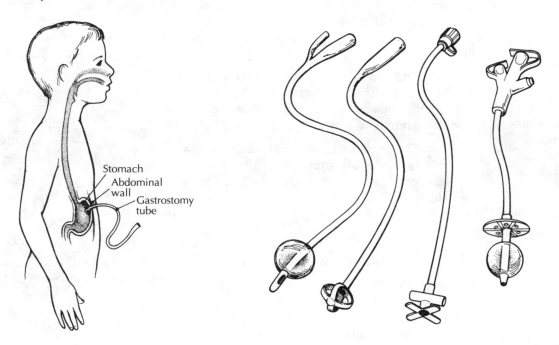

Stomach
Abdominal wall
Gastrostomy tube

The G-tube may be used to drain abdominal contents or to release air or gas when venting is required.

SUGGESTED SETTINGS

There are no restrictions as to where a student may be fed. The setting should be clean and appropriate to the student's need/desire for privacy. The student may be fed with other students or, if he or she prefers, in a private setting (e.g., the health room). Some students receive feedings every 2–3 hours. These students may have their feedings administered in the classroom. They need to remain stationary and should be able to continue sedentary school activities (e.g., reading, doing art, singing, working on a computer, learning social studies).

Some students do not require feedings during the school hours. Their G-tubes are used to supplement oral intake of food and fluids or are used when the student is ill or when oral intake is not adequate.

For students whose G-tubes require venting or drainage, the procedures should be done in the health room or another private area. These procedures may be done after each feeding or according to physicians' orders.

G-tubes usually are covered by clothing. Students with G-tubes should be able to participate in all school activities, but participation in physical education should be determined on an individual basis and may require modification of activities.

SUGGESTED PERSONNEL AND TRAINING

A health assessment needs to be completed by the school nurse. State nurse practice regulations should be consulted for guidance on delegating health care procedures.

A G-tube feeding may be administered by the school nurse, parent, teacher, student's aide, or other staff person with proven competency-based training in appropriate techniques and problem management. The student should be encouraged to assist with the G-tube feeding as much as possible.

School personnel who have regular contact with a student who has a G-tube should receive general training that covers the student's specific health care needs, potential problems, and how to implement the established emergency plan.

The basic skills checklist on pages 319–323 can be used as a foundation for competency-based training in appropriate techniques. It outlines specific procedures step by step. Once the procedures have been mastered, the completed checklist serves as documentation of training.

THE INDIVIDUALIZED HEALTH CARE PLAN: ISSUES FOR SPECIAL CONSIDERATION

Each student's IHCP must be tailored to the individual's needs. The following section covers the procedure for G-tube care and possible problems and emergencies that may arise. It is essential to review it before writing the IHCP.

A sample plan is included in Chapter 6. It may be copied and used to develop a plan for each student. For a student with a G-tube, the following items should receive particular attention:

- Size and type of feeding device
- Type of portable pump
- Type of feeding the student is receiving (e.g., bolus/continuous drip; liquid formula-puréed/liquified food from home)
- Activity level after feeding
- Positioning during and after feeding
- Determining the need to measure gastric residuals
- Determining the need to vent the G-tube
- Patency of gastrostomy tract and time frame for reinsertion should the G-tube fall out
- Monitoring concerns (e.g., vomiting, abdominal distension, pain)
- Amount of food or drink a student can take by mouth
- Amount of oral stimulation during feeding, as ordered
- Medications and schedule for administering
- Student-specific guidelines for feeding administration during transport
- Latex allergy alert (see Chapter 5)
- Universal precautions (Anticipating the tasks to be done, the risk involved, and the personal protective equipment needed will enhance protection of both the caregiver and student.)
- Manufacturer's specific directions

PROCEDURE FOR GASTROSTOMY TUBE FEEDING— BOLUS METHOD

PROCEDURE

1. Wash hands.

2. Assemble equipment:

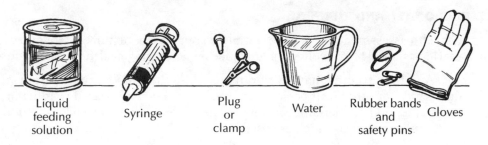

Liquid feeding solution   Syringe   Plug or clamp   Water   Rubber bands and safety pins   Gloves

- Liquid feeding solution/formula at room temperature

- 60-ml or -cc catheter–tipped syringe or other container for feeding
- Clamp or cap for end of tube (optional)
- Water (if prescribed)
- Rubber bands and safety pins
- Gloves (optional)

3. Explain the procedure to the student at his or her level of understanding. Encourage the student to participate as much as possible.

4. Position student.

5. Wash hands. Put on gloves.
6. Remove cap or plug from G-tube and insert a catheter-tipped syringe into the end of feeding tube.
7. Unclamp the tubing and gently draw back on the plunger to remove any liquid or medication that may be left in the stomach (i.e., residuals). Return residuals to stomach (if ordered).

8. Clamp the tubing, disconnect the syringe, and remove plunger from syringe.
9. Reinsert catheter tip of syringe into tubing.

POINTS TO REMEMBER

Anticipating the tasks to be done, the risk involved, and the personal protective equipment needed will enhance protection of both the caregiver and student.

Identify size and type of G-tube. Some students get cramps if the feeding solution is too cold. Shake can well to mix. Check expiration date.

Used to flush tubing after feeding.
Used to secure G-tube to clothing.

By encouraging the student to assist in the procedure, the caregiver helps the student achieve maximum self-care skills.

Student may be sitting or lying on right side with head elevated at a 30-degree angle. When positioning student, make sure clamp is not pressing on skin. Tubing may be pinned to shirt. Remember to unpin G-tube before proceeding with feeding.

G-tube is still clamped. Do not pull on tubing.

Note the amount that was withdrawn from the feeding tube. Adjust the feeding volume according to physician's orders if a residual is present. If the residual is greater than recommended, hold feeding, wait 30–45 minutes, and check again. Some students may not need to have residuals checked.

Syringe should be held 6 inches above level of stomach or at prescribed height.

10. Unclamp tube, and allow bubbles to escape.
11. Pour feeding/fluid into syringe and allow to flow in by gravity.

If medications are prescribed, administer before or after feeding, according to student-specific recommendations. If a container other than a syringe is used for the feeding, unclamp tubing and allow to flow in by gravity, using the same procedure.

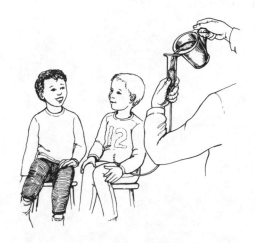

Be alert to any changes in the student's tolerance of the feeding. Nausea/vomiting, cramping, or diarrhea may indicate that the feeding is being given too quickly or the formula is too cold.

12. Continue to pour feeding into syringe as contents empty into stomach.

Depending on the age and capabilities of the student, have him or her assist with the feeding by holding syringe or pouring fluid into it. Keep syringe partially filled to prevent air from entering stomach.

13. Raise or lower syringe or container to adjust flow to prescribed rate.
14. When feeding is completed, pour prescribed amount of water into syringe, and flush tubing.

This will clear tubing of feeding and medication.

15. Vent G-tube if ordered. (Open G-tube to air.)

Venting allows drainage of fluid or release of gas bubbles in the stomach. Some students may have problems with gas otherwise.

16. Clamp tubing, remove barrel of syringe, and reinsert cap into end of tubing.

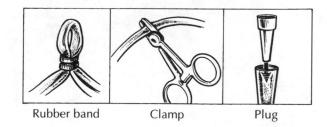

Rubber band   Clamp   Plug

17. Apply dressing, if needed, using universal precautions described in Chapter 5.
18. Remove gloves. Wash hands.
19. Make sure tubing is secure and tucked inside clothing, not inside diaper or underpants.

Tubing may be pinned or taped to shirt if parent follows this practice.

20. Refer to student-specific guidelines regarding position and activity after feeding.

21. Wash syringe and other reusable equipment in soapy water. Rinse thoroughly, dry, and store in a clean area.

Most open formula is good for 48 hours. The exceptions are some elemental formulas that are good for only 24 hours. Open formula should be stored in clean plastic containers, labeled correctly (not the original can) in the refrigerator. Formula should be discarded after 48 hours.

22. Document feeding/medication, residual amount, and feeding tolerance on log sheet.

Report to family any change in the student's usual pattern.

PROCEDURE FOR GASTROSTOMY TUBE FEEDING— SLOW-DRIP METHOD OR CONTINUOUS FEEDING BY PUMP

PROCEDURE

1. Wash hands.

2. Assemble equipment:

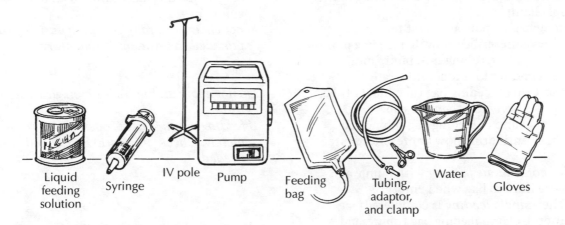

Liquid feeding solution · Syringe · IV pole · Pump · Feeding bag · Tubing, adaptor, and clamp · Water · Gloves

- Liquid feeding solution/formula at room temperature

- 60-ml or -cc catheter–tipped syringe
- Feeding pump and IV stand (optional)

- Clamp or cap for end of tube (optional)
- Water (if prescribed)
- Feeding bag and tubing
- Rubber bands and safety pins
- Gloves (optional)

3. Explain the procedure to the student at his or her level of understanding. Encourage the student to participate as much as possible.

4. Position student.

5. Wash hands. Put on gloves.

6. Remove cap or plug from G-tube and insert a catheter-tipped syringe into the end of feeding tube.

POINTS TO REMEMBER

Anticipating the tasks to be done, the risk involved, and the personal protective equipment needed will enhance protection of both the caregiver and student.

Identify size and type of G-tube. Some students get cramps if the feeding solution is too cold. Shake can well to mix. Check expiration date.

Feeding pumps have alarms. Become familiar with meanings of alarms and how to respond to them.

Used to flush tubing after feeding.

Used to secure G-tube to clothing.

By encouraging the student to assist in the procedure, the caregiver helps the student achieve maximum self-help skills.

Student may be sitting or lying on right side with head elevated at a 30-degree angle. When positioning student, make sure clamp is not pressing on skin. Remember to unpin G-tube before proceeding with feeding.

G-tube is still clamped. Do not apply undue traction or pull on gastrostomy tubing.

7. Unclamp the tubing and gently draw back on the plunger to remove any liquid or medication that may be left in the stomach (i.e., residuals). Look at amount in tube and push fluid slowly back into stomach.

Note the amount that was withdrawn from the feeding tube. Adjust the feeding volume according to physician's orders if a residual is present. If the residual is greater than recommended, hold feeding, wait 30–45 minutes, and check again. Some students may not need to have residuals checked.

8. Clamp the gastrostomy tubing. Disconnect the syringe.
9. Pour feeding/fluids into feeding bag and run feeding through bag and tubing to the tip. Clamp.
10. Hang bag on pole at height required to achieve prescribed flow. If a feeding pump is used, place tubing into pump mechanism and set for proper flow rate.
11. Insert tip of feeding bag tube into G-tube, tape securely. Unclamp G-tube.
12. Open clamp of feeding bag tubing and adjust until drips flow at prescribed rate.

If medication is prescribed, administer before or after feeding, according to student-specific guidelines.

School activities may continue during feeding provided the student is sedentary.

Do not apply undue traction on gastrostomy tubing.

If feeding pump is used, open clamp completely. Check flow periodically and adjust if needed.

13. For *continuous feeding* with pump, add more fluid to bag when empty.
14. When *single feeding* is completed (bag empty), clamp feeding bag tubing, and clamp G-tube.

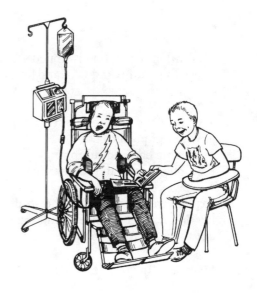

Be alert to any unusual changes in the student's tolerance of the feeding. Nausea/vomiting, cramping, or diarrhea may indicate that the feeding is being given too quickly or formula is too cold.

15. Disconnect feeding bag from G-tube.
16. Unclamp G-tube and flush with water if ordered, using a syringe.
17. Vent G-tube if indicated. (Open G-tube to air.)
18. Clamp and cap G-tube.

This clears the tube of any feeding fluid.

Some students may have gas otherwise.

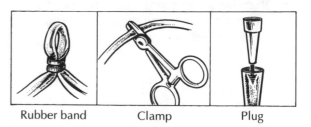

Rubber band   Clamp   Plug

19. Apply dressing, if needed, using universal precautions described in Chapter 5.
20. Remove gloves and wash hands.
21. Make sure tubing is secure and tucked inside clothing, not inside diaper or underpants.

Tubing may be pinned or taped to shirt.

22. Refer to student-specific guidelines regarding position and activity after feeding.

The feeding tube may be disconnected while the student is being transported to and from the school program.

23. Wash syringe and other reusable equipment in soapy water. Rinse thoroughly, dry, and store in a clean area.

Most open formula is good for 48 hours. The exceptions are some elemental formulas that are good for only 24 hours. Open formula should be stored in clean plastic, labeled containers (not the original can) in the refrigerator. Formula should be discarded after 48 hours.

24. Document feeding and/or medication, residual volumes, and feeding tolerance in log.

Report to family any change in the student's usual pattern.

Possible Problems that Require Immediate Attention

Observations

Color changes/breathing difficulty

Reason/Action

This may be due to aspiration of feeding into lungs. Stop feeding immediately. Call nurse if not present. Assess situation. If problem continues, institute emergency plan and notify family.

Possible Problems that Are Not Emergencies

Observations

Nausea and/or cramping

Reason/Action

Check rate of feeding—it may need to be decreased.

Check temperature—formula may be too cold: stop feeding, let feeding get to room temperature, then administer. If problem continues, notify school nurse, family, and physician.

Vomiting

If all the above have been checked, stop feeding, call school nurse or family. Remove residual if ordered.

Blocked gastrostomy tubing

May be due to inadequate flushing or very thick fluid. Squeeze or roll gastrostomy tubing with fingers moving slowly down toward student's stomach. Try a catheter-tipped syringe filled with warm water, held high to facilitate movement of fluid. Try to draw back plunger of syringe. If blockage remains, contact school nurse or family.

Redness/irritation/bleeding/drainage

Make sure tubing is not being pulled. Check G-tube site for leakage.

Clean stoma site if leakage of food/fluid/ medication comes in contact with skin.

Refer to student- or equipment-specific guidelines for cleaning instructions.

Notify school nurse and family of gastrostomy site problems.

G-tube falls out

The G-tube may need to be reinserted immediately if a student's tract closes quickly. Cover the site with a dry dressing or large bandage. Notify family.

General Information Sheet

Students with Gastrostomy Tubes

Dear (teacher, lunch aide, bus driver):

_____ [Student's name] has a condition that requires a gastrostomy tube (G-tube). This is a simple and safe way of giving food, medicines, and fluids directly into the stomach because the student is unable to take these by mouth.

The gastrostomy is a surgical opening into the stomach. A flexible rubber tube (i.e., the G-tube) is put into the surgical opening. It is held in place from the inside of the stomach, as well as from the outside, at all times. The tube is clamped or capped between feedings to prevent leakage. This tube does not normally cause the student discomfort and is covered by clothing.

The student may receive feedings or medication through the G-tube as needed during the schoolday in the classroom, the lunchroom, or the health office. Unless he or she has a condition that otherwise would interfere with participation in physical education or other activities, there is no reason why he or she cannot participate fully. Special consideration may be needed, however, for field trips or other activities during which the student may not be able to receive a regularly scheduled feeding.

The following staff members have been trained to deal with any problems that may arise with this student:

_____

_____

_____

For more information about G-tubes or the student's needs, consult the school nurse or family.

SKIN-LEVEL GASTROSTOMY INDWELLING FEEDING DEVICE

PURPOSE

A gastrostomy is a surgical opening into the stomach through the surface of the abdomen. The skin-level gastrostomy feeding device is a "T"-shaped plastic device held in place by a mushroom-shaped dome or fluid-filled balloon inside the stomach. The device remains in place at all times and is capped by an attached safety plug between feedings. In addition, the dome has an antireflux valve to further prevent leakage of stomach contents. A feeding is administered by inserting a small tube into the device. When the feeding is complete, the tube is removed and the safety plug closed.

The gastrostomy device may be used to administer food, fluids, and/or medications directly into the stomach. This method is used to bypass the usual route of feeding by mouth when

- There is an obstruction of the esophagus (i.e., food pipe).
- Swallowing is impaired, and the student is at risk for choking/aspiration.
- The student has difficulty taking enough food by mouth to maintain adequate nutrition.

A student may receive a gastrostomy feeding by either *bolus* or *continuous, or slow-drip*, method. A bolus is a specific amount of feeding given at one time (over 20–30 minutes). A slow drip, or continuous, feeding is given slowly over a number of hours.

The gastrostomy device also may be used to drain abdominal contents or to release air or gas when venting is required. This is done by inserting a special adaptor or tube to open the antireflux valve.

SUGGESTED SETTINGS

There are no restrictions as to when a student may be fed. The student may be fed with other students or, if he or she prefers, in a more private setting (e.g., the health room). Some students receive feedings every 2–3 hours. These students may have their feedings administered in the classroom. They need to remain stationary and should be able to continue sedentary school activities (e.g., reading, doing art, singing, working on the computer, learning social studies).

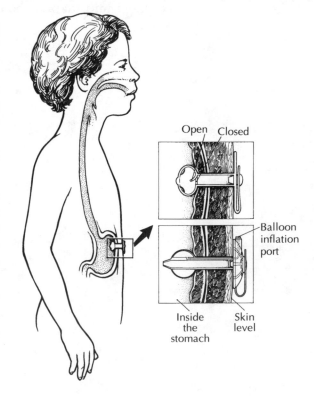

Open   Closed

Balloon inflation port

Inside the stomach

Skin level

Some students do not require feedings during the school hours. Their devices are used to supplement oral intake of food and fluids or are used when the student is ill or oral intake is not adequate.

For students whose gastrostomy devices require venting or drainage, the procedures should be done in the health room or another private area. These procedures may be done after each feeding or according to physicians' orders.

Gastrostomy devices usually are covered by clothing. Students with these devices should be able to participate in all school activities, but participation in physical education should be determined on an individual basis and may require modification of activities.

SUGGESTED PERSONNEL AND TRAINING

A health assessment must be completed by the school nurse. State nurse practice regulations should be consulted for guidance on delegating health care procedures.

A gastrostomy device feeding may be administered by the school nurse, parent, teacher, student's aide, or other staff person with proven competency-based training in appropriate techniques and problem management. The student should be encouraged to assist with the feeding as much as possible.

School personnel who have regular contact with a student who has a skin-level gastrostomy feeding device should receive general training that covers the student's specific health care needs, potential problems, and how to implement the established emergency plan.

The basic skills checklist on pages 324–326 can be used as a foundation for competency-based training in appropriate techniques. It outlines specific procedures step by step. Once the procedures have been mastered, the completed checklist serves as documentation of training.

THE INDIVIDUALIZED HEALTH CARE PLAN: ISSUES FOR SPECIAL CONSIDERATION

Each student's IHCP must be tailored to the individual's needs. The following section covers the procedure for skin-level gastrostomy device care and possible problems and emergencies that may arise. It is essential to review it before writing the IHCP.

A sample plan is included in Chapter 6. It may be copied and used to develop a plan for each student. For a student with a skin-level gastrostomy device, the following items should receive particular attention:

- Size and type of feeding device
- Type of portable pump
- Type of feeding the student is receiving (e.g., bolus/continuous drip)
- Activity level after feeding
- Positioning during and after feeding
- Determining the need to measure gastric residuals
- Determining the need to vent the gastrostomy device (familiarity with student-specific device and venting method)
- Patency of gastrostomy tract and time frame for reinsertion of the device should it fall out
- Monitoring concerns regarding feeding (e.g., vomiting, abdominal distension, pain)
- Amount of food and fluid a student can take by mouth
- Amount of oral stimulation during feeding, as ordered
- Procedure should tube come out
- Student-specific guidelines for feeding administration during transport
- Latex allergy alert (see Chapter 5)
- Universal precautions (Anticipating the tasks to be done, the risk involved, and the personal protective equipment needed will enhance protection of both the caregiver and student.)
- Manufacturer's specific directions

Procedure for Skin-Level Gastrostomy Device Feeding— Bolus Method

PROCEDURE

1. Wash hands.

2. Assemble equipment:

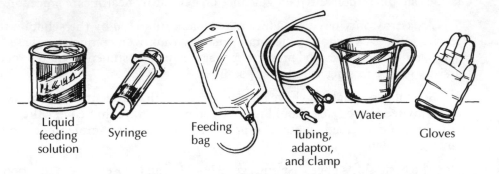

Liquid feeding solution   Syringe   Feeding bag   Tubing, adaptor, and clamp   Water   Gloves

- Liquid feeding solution/formula at room temperature

- 60-ml or -cc catheter–tipped syringe or other container for feeding (e.g., bottle, bag)
- Adaptor with tubing and clamp

- Water (if prescribed)
- Gloves (optional)
3. Explain the procedure to the student at his or her level of understanding. Encourage the student to participate as much as possible.
4. Position student.

5. Wash hands. Put on gloves.

POINTS TO REMEMBER

Anticipating the tasks to be done, the risk involved, and the personal protective equipment needed will enhance protection of both the caregiver and student.

Identify size and type of gastrostomy device. Some students get cramps if the feeding solution is too cold. Be sure to shake cans of formula well and note expiration date.

The adaptor will vary with the size of the device.
Used to flush tubing after feeding.

By encouraging the student to assist in the procedure, the caregiver helps the student achieve maximum self-help skills.

Student may be sitting or lying on right side with head elevated at a 30-degree angle.

6. Remove plunger from syringe and attach the adaptor to feeding syringe.
7. Open safety plug from device and insert adaptor and tubing into device.

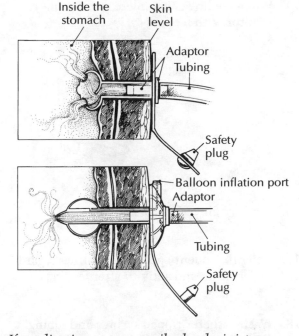

Inside the stomach
Skin level
Adaptor
Tubing
Safety plug

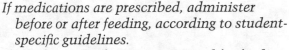

Balloon inflation port
Adaptor
Tubing
Safety plug

8. Clamp or pinch off tubing.

If medications are prescribed, administer before or after feeding, according to student-specific guidelines.

If another type of container is used for feeding solution, unclamp tubing and allow to flow in by gravity.

9. Pour feeding into syringe.
10. Elevate syringe and unclamp tubing.

11. Continue to pour feeding into syringe as contents empty into stomach.

Syringe should be held 6 inches above level of stomach or at prescribed height.

Depending on the age and capabilities of the student, have him or her assist with the feeding by holding syringe or pouring fluid into it. Keep syringe partially filled to prevent air from entering stomach.

12. Raise or lower syringe or container to adjust flow to prescribed rate.

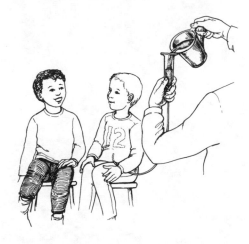

Be alert to any changes in the student's tolerance of the feeding. Nausea/vomiting, cramping, or diarrhea may indicate that the feeding is being given too quickly or the formula is too cold.

13. Flush tubing and device with water, if ordered.

This will clear device of feeding and medication. After flushing, lower the syringe below stomach level to facilitate burping.

14. When feeding is complete, remove the adaptor with feeding syringe.

15. Close safety plug.

 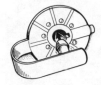

16. Remove gloves. Wash hands.

17. Refer to student-specific guidelines regarding position and activity after feeding.

18. Wash catheter-tipped syringe and tubing with warm water and mild soap. Rinse, dry, and store in clean area.

Most open formula is good for 48 hours. The exceptions are some elemental formulas that are good for only 24 hours. Open formula should be stored in clean plastic containers, labeled correctly, (not the original can) in the refrigerator. Formula should be discarded after 48 hours.

19. Document feeding/medication, residual amount, and feeding tolerance on log sheet.

Report to family any change in the student's usual pattern.

Procedure for Skin-Level Gastrostomy Device Feeding—Slow-Drip Method/Continuous Feeding by Pump

PROCEDURE

1. Wash hands.

2. Assemble equipment:

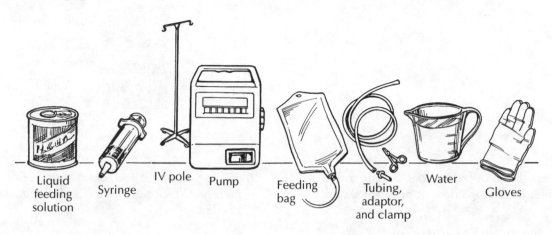

Liquid feeding solution   Syringe   IV pole   Pump   Feeding bag   Tubing, adaptor, and clamp   Water   Gloves

- Liquid feeding solution/formula at room temperature

- 60-ml or -cc catheter–tipped syringe
- Feeding pump and IV stand (optional)
- Adaptor with tubing and clamp

- Water (if prescribed)
- Feeding bag
- Gloves (optional)

3. Explain the procedure to the student at his or her level of understanding. Encourage the student to participate as much as possible.

4. Position student.

5. Wash hands. Put on gloves.
6. Attach the adaptor to feeding bag tubing.

7. Pour feeding/fluids into feeding bag and run feeding through bag and tubing to the tip. Clamp.

POINTS TO REMEMBER

Anticipating the tasks to be done, the risk involved, and the personal protective equipment needed will enhance protection of both the caregiver and student.

Identify size and type of gastrostomy device. Some students get cramps if the feeding solution is too cold.

The adaptor will vary with the size of the device.
Used to flush tubing after feeding.

By encouraging the student to assist in the procedure, the caregiver helps the student achieve maximum self-care skills.

Student may be sitting or lying on right side with head elevated at a 30-degree angle.

If medication is prescribed, administer before feeding.
School activities may continue during feeding provided the student is sedentary.

8. Hang bag on pole at height required to achieve prescribed flow. If a feeding pump is used, place tubing into pump mechanism and set for proper flow rate.

9. Open safety plug and insert tubing into device.

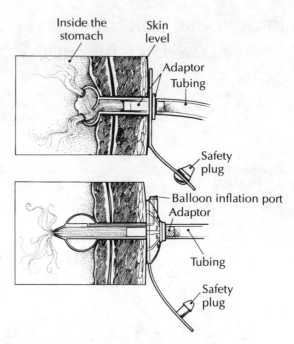

Inside the stomach

Skin level

Adaptor
Tubing

Safety plug

Balloon inflation port
Adaptor

Tubing

Safety plug

10. Open clamp of feeding bag tubing and adjust until drips flow at prescribed rate.

If feeding pump is used, open clamp completely. Check flow periodically and adjust if needed.

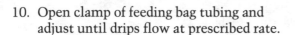

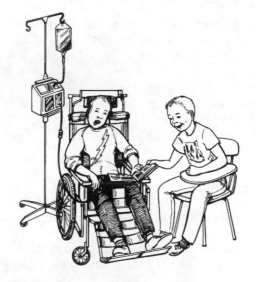

Be alert to any unusual changes in the student's tolerance of the feeding. Nausea/vomiting, cramping, or diarrhea may indicate that the feeding is being given too quickly or formula is too cold.

11. For continuous feeding with pump, add more fluid to bag when empty.

12. When single feeding is completed (bag empty), clamp feeding bag tubing.

13. Flush device with water if ordered.

14. Remove adaptor and tubing from device.

Check rate and flow periodically and adjust if needed.

This clears the device of any feeding fluid. After flushing, lower the syringe below the stomach level to facilitate burping.

15. Close safety plug.

 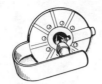

16. Remove gloves. Wash hands.

17. Refer to student-specific guidelines regarding position and activity after feeding.

18. Wash feeding bag, tubing, and syringe in soapy water. Rinse, dry, and store in a clean area.

Most open formula is good for 48 hours. The exceptions are some elemental formulas that are good for only 24 hours. Open formula should be stored in clean plastic containers labeled correctly (not the original can) in the refrigerator. Formula should be discarded after 48 hours.

19. Document feeding/medication, residual amount, and feeding tolerance on log sheet.

Report to family any change in the student's usual pattern.

Possible Problems that Require Immediate Attention

Observations

Color changes/breathing difficulty

Reason/Action

This may be due to aspiration of feeding into lungs. Stop feeding immediately. Call nurse if he or she is not present. Assess situation. If problem continues, institute emergency plan and notify family.

Possible Problems that Are Not Emergencies

Nausea and/or cramping

Check rate of feeding—it may need to be decreased.

Check temperature—feeding may be too cold: Stop feeding, let feeding get to room temperature, then administer. If problem continues, notify school nurse, family, and physician.

Vomiting

If all of the above have been checked, stop feeding, and call school nurse or family.

Blocked gastrostomy device

May be due to inadequate flushing or very thick fluid. Flush with warm water after feeding or medication. If blockage remains, contact family.

Bleeding/drainage/redness/irritation

Check skin around gastrostomy device site daily. Clean stoma site if leakage of food/fluid/medication comes in contact with skin.

Refer to student-specific guidelines for cleaning instruction.

Turn device in a complete circle with each cleaning.

Dry stoma well; open to air to facilitate drying.

Leaking of stomach contents

May be due to a problem with the antireflux valve (sticking or broken). Clean skin and notify family.

Gastrostomy device falls out

This is not an emergency. Save the device in a clean gauze or container for reinsertion. In some students, whose tracts may close quickly, the gastrostomy device may need to be inserted within 1–2 hours. Cover gastrostomy site with bandage or clean dressing. Contact family and/or school nurse.

General Information Sheet

Students with Skin-Level Gastrostomy Feeding Devices

Dear (teacher, lunch aide, bus driver):

_____ [Student's name] has a condition that requires a gastrostomy feeding device. This is a simple and safe way of giving food, medicines, and fluids directly into the stomach because the student is unable to take these by mouth.

The gastrostomy is a surgical opening into the stomach. A skin-level gastrostomy feeding device is put into the surgical opening. It is held in place from the inside of the stomach and is capped between feedings to prevent leakage. This gastrostomy device does not normally cause the student discomfort and is covered by clothing.

The student may receive feedings or medication through the gastrostomy feeding device as needed during the schoolday in the classroom, the lunchroom, or the health office. Unless he or she has a condition that otherwise would interfere with participation in physical education or other activities, there is no reason why he or she cannot participate fully. Special consideration may be needed, however, for field trips or other activities during which the student may not be able to receive a regularly scheduled feeding.

The following staff members have been trained to deal with any problems that may arise with this student:

_____

_____

_____

For more information about skin-level gastrostomy devices or the student's needs, consult the school nurse or family.

NASOGASTRIC TUBE

PURPOSE

A nasogastric tube (NG-tube) is a rubber or plastic tube that passes through a nostril, down into the throat and esophagus (i.e., food pipe), and into the stomach. It is used to give liquids, medication, and feedings when a person is unable to take these by mouth. Some students will have a tube inserted for each feeding. Others will have a tube in place for several weeks.

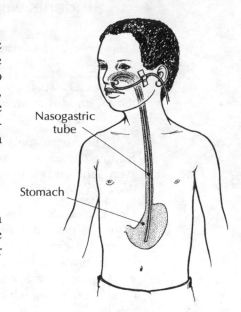

Nasogastric tube

Stomach

SUGGESTED SETTINGS

The student may be fed in the lunchroom with the other students or in the health room. The NG-tube should be inserted in the health room or in another private setting.

SUGGESTED PERSONNEL AND TRAINING

A health assessment must be completed by the school nurse. State nurse practice regulations should be consulted for guidance on delegating health care procedures.

A registered nurse with proven competency-based training in appropriate techniques and problem management should do the nasogastric tube feedings. Any school personnel who have regular contact with a student with an NG-tube must receive general training that covers the student's specific health care needs, potential problems, and how to implement an established emergency plan.

The basic skills checklist on pages 328–332 can be used as a foundation for competency-based training in appropriate techniques. It outlines specific procedures step by step. Once the procedures have been mastered, the completed checklist serves as documentation of training.

THE INDIVIDUALIZED HEALTH CARE PLAN: ISSUES FOR SPECIAL CONSIDERATION

Each student's IHCP must be tailored to the individual's needs. The following section covers the procedure for NG-tube care and possible problems and emergencies that may arise. It is essential to review it before writing the IHCP.

A sample plan is included in Chapter 6. It may be copied and used to develop a plan for each student. For a student with an NG-tube, the following items should receive particular attention:

- Size and type of feeding device
- Type of feeding student is receiving (e.g., bolus/continuous drip)
- Proper placement of the NG-tube
- Method of securing the NG-tube
- Activity level after feeding
- Positioning during and after feeding
- Determining the need to measure gastric residuals
- Latex allergy alert (see Chapter 5)
- Universal precautions (Anticipating the tasks to be done, the risk involved, and the personal protective equipment needed will enhance protection of both the caregiver and student.)

PROCEDURE FOR CHECKING PLACEMENT
OF THE NASOGASTRIC TUBE

PROCEDURE

1. Wash hands.

2. Assemble equipment:

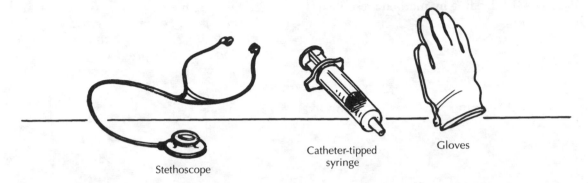

Stethoscope   Catheter-tipped syringe   Gloves

- Stethoscope
- 60-cc catheter–tipped syringe
- Gloves (optional)
3. Explain procedure at the student's level of understanding.

4. Position student.
5. Wash hands and put on gloves.
6. Unclamp or remove cap from NG-tube.
7. Connect 60-cc catheter–tipped syringe to the end of NG-tube.
8. Place a stethoscope over the mid-left abdomen and gently push in 5–10 cc of air with syringe.

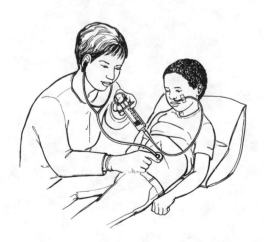

POINTS TO REMEMBER

Anticipating the tasks to be done, the risk involved, and the personal protective equipment needed will enhance protection of both the caregiver and student.

By encouraging the student to assist in the procedure, the caregiver helps the student achieve maximum self-care skills.

A whooshing sound should be heard if NG-tube is placed properly.
*If NG-tubing does not appear to be in place, **do not give feeding**. Replacement or repositioning of the NG-tube should only be done by a nurse with appropriate training and if ordered by the student's physician. (Check student-specific guidelines.)*

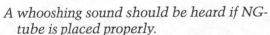
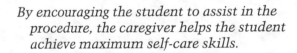

9. If ordered, gently draw back on the plunger to remove any liquid or medication that may be left in the stomach (i.e., residuals).

Refer to physician's orders. Note the amount that was withdrawn from the feeding tube and return the contents to the stomach (if ordered). Adjust the feeding volume according to physician's orders if a residual is present. If the residual is greater than recommended, hold feeding, wait 30–45 minutes, and check again. Some students may not need to have residuals checked.

10. Close the tubing, disconnect the syringe, and remove plunger from syringe.
11. Proceed with feeding by method prescribed for student.

Feedings are usually bolus (feeding given over a short period of time by gravity) or slow drip (feeding given by pump or over a long period of time by gravity).

PROCEDURE FOR NASOGASTRIC TUBE FEEDING—BOLUS METHOD

PROCEDURE

1. Wash hands.

2. Assemble equipment:

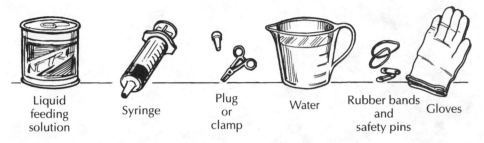

Liquid feeding solution • Syringe • Plug or clamp • Water • Rubber bands and safety pins • Gloves

- Liquid feeding solution/formula at room temperature

- 60-ml or -cc catheter–tipped syringe
- Clamp or cap for end of tube (optional)
- Water (if prescribed)
- Rubber bands and safety pins
- Stethoscope
- Gloves (optional)

3. Explain procedure at the student's level of understanding. Position student.

4. Wash hands. Put on gloves.
5. Check placement of NG-tube. (Refer to pp. 167–168.)

6. Remove cap or plug from NG-tube. Insert catheter-tipped syringe into the end of feeding tube. If ordered, gently draw back on the plunger to remove any liquid or medication that may be left in the stomach (i.e., residuals). Note the amount that was withdrawn from the feeding tube and return the contents to the stomach (if ordered).

7. Close the tubing, disconnect the syringe, and remove plunger from syringe. Attach syringe without plunger to NG-tube.

POINTS TO REMEMBER

Anticipating the tasks to be done, the risk involved, and the personal protective equipment needed will enhance protection of both the caregiver and student.

Identify size and type of NG-tube. Shake can well to mix. Note expiration date. Some students may get cramps if feeding solution is too cold.

Used to flush tubing after feeding.
Used to secure NG-tube to clothing.

Student may be sitting or lying on right side with head elevated at a 30-degree angle. Make sure tubing is secured according to student-specific guidelines.

Always check placement before giving a feeding or medication. Do not apply undue traction or pull on NG-tubing.
Some students do not need to have residuals checked. Refer to physician's orders. Adjust the feeding volume according to physician's orders if a residual is present. If the residual is greater than recommended, hold feeding, wait 30–45 minutes, and check again.

Syringe should be held 6 inches above level of head or at prescribed height.

8. Pour feeding/fluid into syringe and allow to flow in by gravity.

Be alert to any changes in the student's tolerance of the feeding. Nausea/vomiting, cramping, or diarrhea may indicate that the feeding is being given too quickly or formula is too cold.

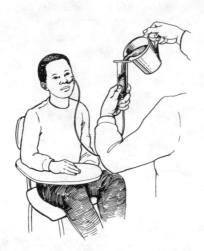

9. Continue to pour feeding into syringe as contents empty into stomach.

Depending on the age and capabilities of the student, have him or her assist with the feeding by holding syringe or pouring fluid into it.

10. Raise or lower syringe to adjust flow to prescribed rate.
11. When feeding is completed, pour prescribed amount of water into syringe, and flush tubing.

This will clear tubing of feeding and medication.

12. Clamp tubing; remove barrel of syringe and reinsert cap into end of tubing.

13. Make sure tubing is securely attached to cheek.

Make sure NG-tubing is not pulling on nose or causing discomfort.

14. Remove gloves and wash hands.
15. Refer to student-specific guidelines regarding position and activity after feeding.
16. Wash catheter-tipped syringe with warm water and mild soap, rinse thoroughly, dry, and store in clean area.

Most open formula is good for 48 hours. The exceptions are some elemental formulas that are good for only 24 hours. Open formula should be stored in clean plastic, labeled containers (not the original can) in the refrigerator. Formula should be discarded after 48 hours.

17. Document feeding/medication, residual amount, and feeding tolerance on log sheet.

Report to family any changes in student's usual pattern.

PROCEDURE FOR NASOGASTRIC TUBE FEEDING—
SLOW-DRIP AND/OR CONTINUOUS FEEDING

PROCEDURE

1. Wash hands.

2. Assemble equipment:

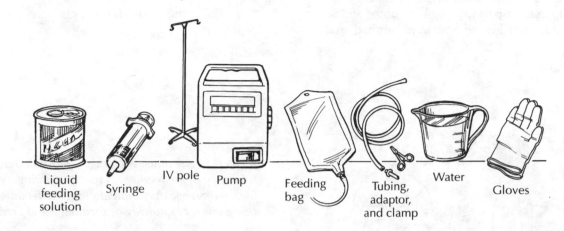

Liquid feeding solution   Syringe   IV pole   Pump   Feeding bag   Tubing, adaptor, and clamp   Water   Gloves

- Liquid feeding solution/formula at room temperature

- 60-ml or -cc catheter–tipped syringe
- Feeding pump and IV stand (optional)
- Water (if prescribed)
- Clamp or cap for end of tube (optional)
- Feeding bag
- Rubber bands and safety pins
- Stethoscope
- Gloves (optional)

3. Explain procedure at the student's level of understanding. Position student.

4. Wash hands. Put on gloves.

5. Check placement of NG-tube. (Refer to pp. 167–168.)

6. Remove cap or plug from NG-tube and insert a catheter-tipped syringe. If ordered, gently draw back on the plunger to remove any liquid or medication that may be left in the stomach (i.e., residuals). Note the amount that was withdrawn from the feeding tube and return the contents to the stomach (if ordered).

POINTS TO REMEMBER

Anticipating the tasks to be done, the risk involved, and the personal protective equipment needed will enhance protection of both the caregiver and student.

Identify size and type of NG-tube. Some students may get cramps if feeding solution is too cold. Shake can well to mix. Check expiration date.

Used to flush tubing after feeding.

Used to secure NG-tube to clothing.

By encouraging the student to assist in the procedure, the caregiver helps the student achieve maximun self-care skills. Student may be sitting or lying on right side with head elevated at a 30-degree angle. When positioning student, make sure NG-tube is secured according to student-specific guidelines.

Always check placement before giving a feeding or medication.

Do not apply undue traction or pull on nasogastric tubing. Some students may not need to have residuals checked. Refer to physician's orders. Adjust the feeding volume according to physician's orders if a residual is present. If the residual is greater than recommended, hold feeding, wait 30–45 minutes, and check again.

7. Close the nasogastric tubing. Disconnect the syringe.
8. Pour feeding/fluids into feeding bag and run feeding through bag and tubing to the tip. Clamp.
9. Hang bag on pole at height required to achieve prescribed flow. If a feeding pump is used, place tubing into pump mechanism and set for proper flow rate.
10. Insert tip of feeding bag tube into NG-tube, tape securely. Unclamp NG-tube.
11. Open clamp of feeding bag tubing and adjust until drips flow at prescribed rate.

If medication is prescribed, administer before or after feeding according to student-specific guidelines.
School activities may continue during feeding provided the student is sedentary.

If feeding pump is used, open clamp completely.

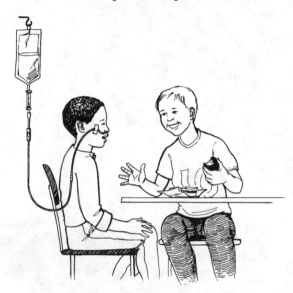

Be alert to any unusual changes in the student's tolerance of the feeding. Nausea/vomiting, cramping, or diarrhea may indicate that the feeding is being given too quickly or formula is too cold.

12. For *continuous feeding with a pump*, add more fluid to bag when empty.

Check rate and flow periodically and adjust if needed. Check for residual as ordered.

13. When *single feeding* is completed (bag is empty), clamp feeding bag tubing, and clamp NG-tube.
14. Disconnect feeding bag from NG-tube.
15. Unclamp NG-tube and flush with water, if ordered, using a syringe.

This clears the tubing of any feeding fluid.

16. Clamp and cap NG-tube.
17. Make sure tubing is securely attached to cheek.
18. Remove gloves and wash hands.
19. Refer to student-specific guidelines regarding position and activity after feeding.

The feeding tube may be disconnected while the student is being transported to and from the school program.

20. Wash feeding bag and syringe in soapy water. Rinse thoroughly, dry, and store in a clean area.

Most open formula is good for 48 hours. The exceptions are some elemental formulas that are good for only 24 hours. Open formula should be stored in clean plastic containers (not the original can), labeled, in the refrigerator. Formula should be discarded after 48 hours.

21. Document feeding/medication, residual volumes, and feeding tolerance on log sheet.

Report to family any changes in the student's usual pattern.

Possible Problems that Require Immediate Attention

Observations	Reason/Action
Gagging, choking	*This may be due to improper NG-tube placement.*
	Follow steps for checking NG-tube placement.
	If NG-tube is not in proper position, remove tube or follow student-specific guidelines for repositioning.
Color changes/breathing difficulty *when not receiving feeding*	*Color changes or breathing difficulty are not always related to NG-tube feeding. In addition to checking NG-tube placement, it is important to carefully assess the student for other problems.*
Color changes/breathing difficulty *while receiving feeding*	***STOP FEEDING IMMEDIATELY**. This may be due to improper NG-tube placement. Follow steps for checking NG-tube placement. Carefully assess the student for other problems.*
	This may be due to aspiration of feeding into lungs.
Respiratory distress continues	*Call for help and initiate emergency plan.*
Nausea and/or cramping	*Check rate of feeding—rate may need to be decreased. Check temperature—feeding may be too cold: stop feeding, let feeding get to room temperature, then administer. If problem continues, notify school nurse and family.*
Vomiting	*Stop feeding and refer to student-specific guidelines.*
	Vomiting may not be due to NG feeding. It is important to carefully assess the student for other problems.
NG-tube falls out	*Notify family, school nurse, and physician.*

General Information Sheet

Students with Nasogastric Tubes

Dear (teacher, lunch aide, bus driver):

_____ [Student's name] has a condition that requires a nasogastric tube (NG-tube). This is a simple and safe way of giving food, medicines, and fluids directly into the stomach because the student is unable to take these by mouth. The NG-tube is a soft rubber or plastic tube that is put into a nostril and down the food pipe into the stomach.

The tube is held to the skin by tape, so it will not usually come out, and is clamped between feedings to prevent leakage. Once it is in place, the NG-tube should not cause the student any discomfort. The student may receive feedings or medication through the NG-tube as needed during the schoolday in the health office, the lunchroom, or the classroom. Usually he or she will be able to participate in physical education or other activities. Special consideration may be needed, however, for field trips or other activities during which the student may not be able to receive a regularly scheduled feeding.

The following staff members have been trained to deal with any problems that may arise with this student:

_____

_____

_____

For more information about NG-tubes or the student's needs, consult the school nurse or family.

JEJUNOSTOMY TUBE

PURPOSE

A jejunostomy is a surgical opening into the jejunum (i.e., the small intestine between the duodenum and the ileum) through the surface of the abdomen. The jejunostomy tube (J-tube) is a flexible, rubber or latex catheter that is held in place on the abdominal wall with tape or is fed through the gastrostomy site through the intestine down to the jejunum and taped to the G-tube. The tube remains in the small intestine at all times and must not move in or out. The J-tube causes no discomfort when in place.

The jejunostomy tube may be used to administer food and fluids directly into the jejunum. This method is used to bypass the usual route of feeding by mouth and stomach when

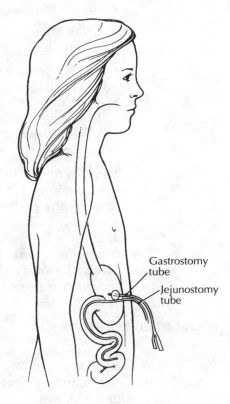

Gastrostomy tube

Jejunostomy tube

- There is blockage in the upper esophagus and/or stomach.
- The student is at risk for aspiration and gastroesophageal reflux.
- The student has difficulty taking enough food by mouth or gastrostomy feedings to maintain adequate nutrition.
- The student has intestinal pseudo-obstruction or short bowel syndrome.
- The student has had major stomach surgery or a problem with stomach emptying.
- The student has a depressed gag reflex.

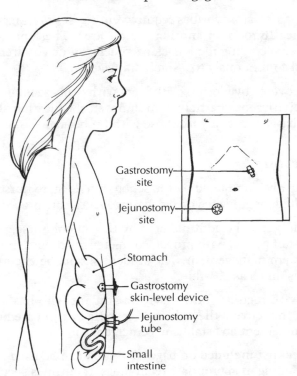

Gastrostomy site

Jejunostomy site

Stomach

Gastrostomy skin-level device

Jejunostomy tube

Small intestine

A student receives jejunal feeding by continuous drip method slowly over a number of hours. The continuous drip method is preferred over the bolus method to prevent giving a large volume of feeding over a short period of time.

In addition to J-tubes, gastrostomy skin-level feeding devices and nasojejunal tubes also are placed surgically to provide direct jejunal feeding.

Factors affecting selection of these devices are the student's age, the size of the device, and whether the student is allergic to the material of the device. Some students may have a G-tube and a J-tube in the same stoma. There may be two distinctly separate tubes or one tube with several identified ports. Some students may have a gastrostomy device and a jejunostomy device and will have two distinct abdominal stoma sites. In most cases, the gastrostomy device will be vented for comfort, and in many situations, the venting is continuous.

The gastrojejunal tube is a single tube with three limbs, including

- A jejunal feeding port (i.e., the opening of the tubing into the jejunum)
- A gastric port (i.e., the opening of the tubing into the stomach)
- A balloon inflation limb (holds the tube in place)

There is one abdominal stoma (gastrostomy), and the device passes through the gastrostomy and stomach and into the jejunum. Other students may have an NG-tube or other small tube inserted through the gastrostomy stoma alongside the G-tube and into the jejunum.

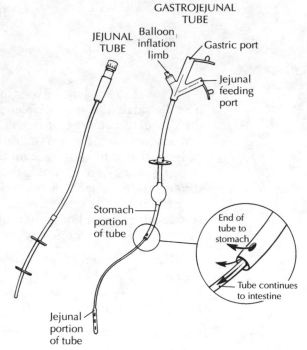

SUGGESTED SETTINGS

There are no restrictions as to where a student may be fed. The student may be fed with other students, or, if the student prefers, in a more private setting (e.g., health room). Some students receive feedings every 2–3 hours. These students may have their feedings administered in the classroom. They may need to remain stationary and should be able to continue sedentary school activities (e.g., reading, doing art, singing, working on a computer, learning social studies). Some students do not require feedings during school hours.

For students whose gastrostomy tubes require venting or draining, the procedures should be done in the health room or another private area. These procedures may be done after each feeding or according to physician's orders. Some children may have the gastrostomy tube vented continuously to a small drainage bag.

J-tubes usually are covered by clothing. Students with J-tubes should be able to participate in all school activities, but participation in physical education should be determined on an individual basis (especially for those with J-tubes taped to G-tubes).

SUGGESTED PERSONNEL AND TRAINING

A health assessment must be completed by the school nurse. State nurse practice regulations should be consulted for guidance on delegating health care procedures.

A jejunostomy feeding may be administered by the school nurse, parent, teacher, student's aide, or other staff person with proven competency-based training in appropriate techniques and problem management. The student should be encouraged to assist with the J-tube feeding as much as possible.

School personnel with regular contact with a student who has a J-tube should receive general training that covers the student's specific health care needs, potential problems, and how to implement an established emergency plan.

The basic skills checklist included on pages 333–334 can be used as a foundation for competency-based training in appropriate techniques. It outlines specific procedures step by step. Once the procedures have been mastered, the completed checklist serves as documentation of training.

THE INDIVIDUALIZED HEALTH CARE PLAN: ISSUES FOR SPECIAL CONSIDERATION

Each student's IHCP must be tailored to the individual's needs. The following section covers the procedure for J-tube care and possible problems and emergencies that may arise. It is essential to review it before writing the IHCP.

A sample plan is included in Chapter 6. It may be copied and used to develop a plan for each student. For a student with a J-tube, the following items should receive particular attention:

- Type of feeding the student is receiving
- Activity level after feeding
- Positioning during and after feeding
- Determining the need for venting G-tube during jejunostomy feeding (or continuously)
- Students who experience moderate to severe gastroesophageal reflux may need to receive their medications (except antacids) through the J-tube (only if specified in physician's orders in advance)
- Patency of jejunostomy tract and time frame for reinsertion should the tube fall out or come out of position (If medications are given through the J-tube, it is imperative to flush the tube before and after medication administration in order to maintain patency of the tube.)
- Awareness of typical problems with feeding (e.g., vomiting, abdominal distension, diarrhea)
- Awareness of amount of oral intake allowed
- Adherence to feeding schedule to prevent overfeeding or dumping syndrome symptoms
- Type of equipment used by student
- Latex allergy alert (see Chapter 5)
- Universal precautions (Anticipating the tasks to be done, the risk involved, and the personal protective equipment needed will enhance protection of both the caregiver and student.)

PROCEDURE FOR JEJUNOSTOMY FEEDING— CONTINUOUS FEEDING BY PUMP

PROCEDURE

1. Wash hands.

2. Assemble equipment:

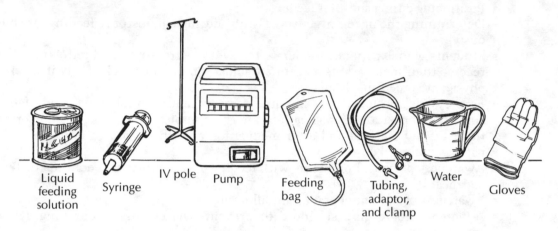

Liquid feeding solution — Syringe — IV pole — Pump — Feeding bag — Tubing, adaptor, and clamp — Water — Gloves

- Liquid feeding solution/formula at room temperature
- 10-ml or -cc syringe
- Feeding pump (optional)
- IV stand (optional)
- Clamp or cap for end of tube
- Water (if prescribed)
- Feeding bag
- Safety pins
- Gloves (optional)

3. Explain the procedure to the student at his or her level of understanding. Encourage the student to participate as much as possible.

4. Position student.

5. Wash hands. Put on gloves.
6. Pour feeding/fluids into feeding bag and run feeding through bag and tubing to the tip. Clamp.

7. Hang bag on pole at height required to achieve prescribed flow. Place tubing into feeding pump mechanism and set for proper flow rate.

8. Insert tip of feeding bag tubing into jejunostomy tube and tape securely. Unclamp J-tube.

POINTS TO REMEMBER

Anticipating the tasks to be done, the risk involved, and the personal protective equipment needed will enhance protection of both the caregiver and student.

Identify size and type of J-tube. Some students get cramps if the feeding solution is too cold.

Used to flush tubing after feeding.

Used to secure J-tube to clothing.

By encouraging the student to assist in the procedure, the caregiver helps the student achieve maximum self-care skills.

Student may be sitting or lying on right side with head elevated at a 30-degree angle. When positioning the student, make sure clamp is not pressing on skin. Tubing may be pinned to shirt. Remember to unpin J-tube before proceeding with feeding.

If medication is prescribed, administer before or after feeding according to student-specific guidelines and flush tubing well before starting feeding.
School activities may continue during feeding provided the student is sedentary.

Do not apply undue traction on jejunostomy tubing.

9. Vent G-tube or skin-level feeding device if indicated during feeding.

May need syringe or drainage bag for venting.

10. Set flow rate on pump.

Check pump periodically for proper infusion rate.

11. Add more fluid to bag before it is completely empty.

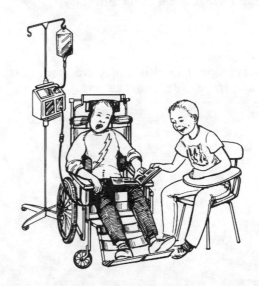

12. If feeding is completed during school time, then clamp feeding bag tubing and clamp J-tube.

Be alert to any changes in the student's tolerance of the feeding. Nausea/vomiting, cramping, pale skin color, sweating, irritability, or diarrhea may indicate that the feeding is being given too quickly or formula is too cold.

13. Disconnect feeding bag from J-tube.
14. Unclamp J-tube and flush with water using a syringe.

Amount of water used for flush may vary according to student-specific recommendations. This clears the tubing of any feeding fluid.

15. Clamp and cap J-tube.
16. Apply dressing, if needed, using universal precautions (see Chapter 5).
17. Make sure tubing is secure and tucked inside clothing. Tubing may be pinned to shirt.

Remember to unpin tube before removing shirt. The feeding may be disconnected while the student is being transported to and from the school program.

18. Wash feeding bag, tubing, and syringe in tap water and store in a clean area.

Most open formula is good for 48 hours. The exceptions are some elemental formulas that are good for only 24 hours. Open formula should be stored in clean plastic containers (not the original can), labeled correctly, in the refrigerator. Formula should be discarded after 48 hours.

19. Remove gloves.
20. Wash hands.
21. Refer to student-specific guidelines regarding activity after feeding.
22. Document feeding/medication and feeding tolerance on log sheet.

Report to family any change in the student's usual pattern.

Possible Problems that Require Immediate Attention

Observation	Reason/Action
Color changes/breathing difficulty	*Some students may have increased upper airway secretions with feedings and may need suctioning. Stop feeding and follow student-specific instructions for suctioning.*
Sweaty skin, pale skin color, increased heart rate, irritability, diarrhea	*Signs of dumping syndrome. This can occur when caloric intake and/or volume of feeding are increased. If this is a new occurrence, stop the feeding until symptoms subside. Notify family of these symptoms. Follow student-specific guidelines.*
Nausea and/or cramping	*Check rate of feeding—rate may need to be decreased.*
	Check temperature of feeding—feeding may be too cold: Stop feeding, let feeding get to room temperature, then administer. If problem continues, notify school nurse, doctor, and family.
Vomiting	*Jejunostomy tube may be dislodged from jejunum. Stop feeding; notify school nurse, doctor, and family.*
	The jejunostomy tube may not be in the proper position. If all of the above have been checked, stop feeding; call school nurse, doctor, and family.
	May need to vent G-tube if it was clamped during jejunal feeding.
May see jejunal feeding contents in G-tube drainage	*J-tube may be dislodged from jejunum. Stop feeding, notify school nurse, doctor, and family.*
Blocked jejunostomy tubing	*May be due to inadequate flushing or very thick fluid. Squeeze or roll tubing with fingers, moving slowly down toward student's stomach. Try a 3-cc syringe filled with warm water held high to facilitate movement of fluid. If blockage remains, do not apply force. Contact school nurse and family.*
Bleeding/drainage	*Make sure tubing is not being pulled. Check the J-tube site for leakage.*
J-tube falls out	*In some students, whose tracts may close quickly, the J-tube may need to be reinserted within 1–2 hours.*
	Cover the site with dry dressing or large bandage. Notify the family.

General Information Sheet

Students with Jejunostomy Tubes

Dear (teacher, lunch aide, bus driver):

_____ [Student's name] has a condition that requires a jejunostomy tube (J-tube). This is a simple and safe way of giving food, medicines, and fluids directly into the intestine because the student is unable to use his or her stomach.

The jejunostomy is a surgical opening into the jejunum (part of the small intestine). A flexible rubber tube (i.e., J-tube) is put into the surgical opening. It is held in place on the outside at all times. The tube is clamped or capped between feedings to prevent leakage. The J-tube usually does not cause the student discomfort and is covered by clothing.

The student may receive feedings or medication through the J-tube as needed during the schoolday in the classroom, the lunchroom, or the health office. Unless he or she has a condition that otherwise would interfere with participation in physical education or other activities, there is no reason why he or she cannot participate fully. Special consideration may be needed, however, for field trips or other activities during which the student may not be able to receive a regularly scheduled feeding.

The following staff members have been trained to deal with any problems that may arise with this student:

_____

_____

_____

For more information about J-tubes or the student's needs, consult the school nurse or family.

Suggested Readings

Faller, N., & Lawrence, K.G. (1993). Comparing low-profile gastrostomy. *Nursing 93, 23*(12), 46–48.

Gauderer, M.W., Olsen, M.M., Stellato, T.A., & Dokler, M.L. (1988). Feeding gastrostomy button: Experience and recommendations. *Journal of Pediatric Surgery, 23*(1), 24–28.

Huddleston, K.C., & Ferraro, A.R. (1991). Preparing families of children with gastrostomies. *Pediatric Nursing, 17*(2), 153–158.

Huth, M.M., & O'Brien, M.E. (1987). The gastrostomy feeding button. *Pediatric Nursing, 13*(4), 24.

Langer, J.C. (1995). What is the role of the pediatric surgeon in the care of children with motility disorders? *The Messenger: A Newsletter Produced by the American Pseudo-Obstruction and Hirschsprung's Disease Society, Inc., 7*(2), 8–9.

Medical Innovations Corporation. (1987). *Surgical placement and nursing guide: MIC gastro-enteric tube*. Milpitas, CA: Author.

Medical Innovations Corporation. (1994). *MIC transgastric jejunal feeding tube patient care guidelines*. Milpitas, CA: Author.

Monturo, C.A. (1990). Enteral access device selection. *Nutrition in Clinical Practice, 5*(5), 207–213.

Neal, J., & Slayton, D. (1992). Neonatal and pediatric PEG tubes. *The American Journal of Maternal/Child Nursing, 17*(4), 184–191.

Shike, M., Wallach, C., Gerdes, H., & Hermann-Zaidins, M. (1989). Skin-level gastrostomies and jejunostomies for long-term enteral feeding. *Journal of Parenteral and Enteral Nutrition, 13*(6), 648–650.

Steele, N.F. (1991). The button: Replacement gastrostomy device. *Journal of Pediatric Nursing, 6*(6), 421–424.

Stellato, T.A., & Gauderer, M.W.L. (1989). Jejunostomy button as a new method for long term jejunostomy feeding. *Surgery, Gynecology, and Obstetrics, 168*(6), 552–554.

INTRAVENOUS LINES

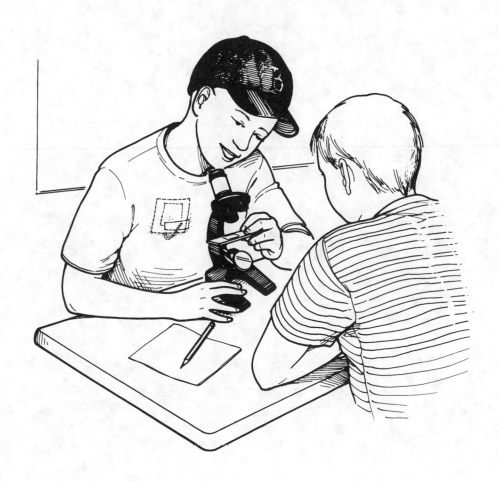

CIRCULATORY SYSTEM

STRUCTURE AND FUNCTION

The circulatory system delivers oxygen and nutrients to different organs of the body and transports carbon dioxide and waste products to the lungs and kidneys for elimination.

The *heart* is a four-chambered pump that is physiologically divided into two sides. The atria are the small collection chambers that collect blood from the veins. The ventricles are the larger, more muscular chambers that pump blood through the arteries.

The right side of the heart collects blood returning from the body via the large veins (i.e., the vena cavae) in the right atrium. The blood then enters the right ventricle through a valve and is pumped to the lungs through the pulmonary artery, where it loses carbon dioxide and gains oxygen.

The oxygenated blood from the lungs enters the left atrium through the pulmonary veins. It then crosses a valve into the left ventricle, which pumps the blood out to the body through the aorta.

The *arteries* are blood vessels with muscular walls that take the blood from the heart to organs in the body. The largest artery, the aorta, is closest to the heart. As the arteries get farther away from the heart, they become smaller with less muscle in their walls.

The *capillaries* are tiny channels, one–blood-cell wide, that connect arteries to veins. These vessels are where the exchange of oxygen and nutrients with carbon dioxide and waste products occurs in every organ.

The *veins* are thin blood vessels that take blood away from the organs toward the heart. Some veins in arms and legs have one-way valves that keep the blood from pooling in the hands and feet. As the veins get closer to the heart, they become larger. Central veins are those inside the abdominal or chest cavities.

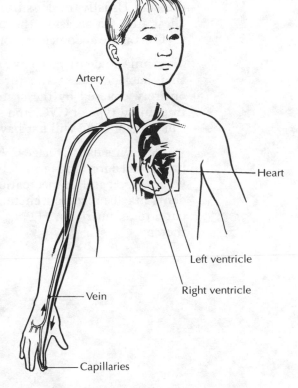

Artery

Heart

Left ventricle

Right ventricle

Vein

Capillaries

CENTRAL VENOUS CATHETER

PURPOSE

A central venous catheter (CVC) is a long-term intravenous line that is inserted surgically into a deep, large vein in the neck or the chest, usually near the heart. The middle portion of the catheter has a Dacron cuff that anchors the catheter under the skin. This cuff also helps to prevent bacteria from traveling up the catheter. The clamp or cap on the end of the tubing prevents blood loss and air entry into the vein. CVCs do not cause any discomfort if they are properly secured.

The exit site (i.e., where the catheter comes out of skin) requires meticulous cleaning and always is covered with a sterile dressing. Usually the dressing is on the upper chest area. On occasion, the exit site for the CVC is on the abdomen or groin.

Some students may have a type of CVC that has an access site (or port) that is entirely covered by the skin. This is the implanted type of CVC, and students with this type of CVC will not have an exit site.

Students usually have CVCs when they have a need for long-term delivery of intravenous food and/or medication. These students may be receiving chemotherapy, total parenteral nutrition (TPN), or antibiotic therapy.

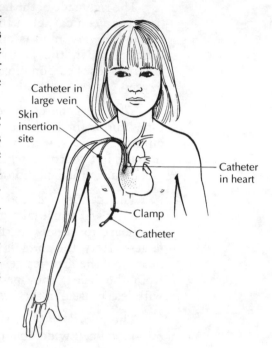

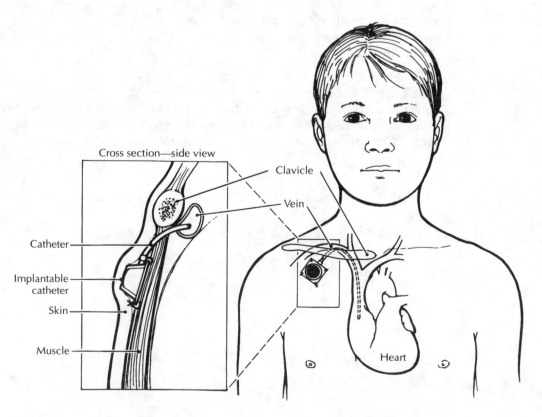

SUGGESTED SETTINGS

As with all medical conditions, every effort should be made to protect the student's privacy. Procedures such as dressing reinforcements or changes should be carried out in a private area of the health office. Because CVCs usually are covered by clothing, students with CVCs should be able to participate in school activities. However, participation in physical education activities should be decided on an individual basis and approved by the student's physician.

SUGGESTED PERSONNEL AND TRAINING

A health assessment must be completed by the school nurse. State nurse practice regulations must be consulted for guidance on delegating health care procedures.

Dressing changes should be performed by a registered nurse with proven competency-based training in appropriate techniques and problem management. Any school personnel who have regular contact with a student who has a CVC must receive general training that covers the student's specific health care needs, potential problems, and how to implement the established emergency plan.

The basic skills checklist on pages 335–336 can be used as a foundation for competency-based training in appropriate techniques. It outlines specific procedures step by step. Once the procedures have been mastered, the completed checklist serves as documentation of training.

THE INDIVIDUALIZED HEALTH CARE PLAN: ISSUES FOR SPECIAL CONSIDERATION

Each student's IHCP must be tailored to the individual's needs. The following section covers the procedure for CVC dressing change as well as possible problems and emergencies that may arise. It is essential to review it before writing the IHCP.

A sample IHCP is included in Chapter 6. It may be copied and used to develop a plan for each student. For a student with a CVC, the following items should receive particular attention:

- The student's underlying condition and potential problems associated with the condition or treatment (e.g., chemotherapy)
- The need for an additional sterile dressing kit with a spare clamp and heparin readily available at all times
- Notification about CVC to school staff who have regular contact with the student
- Reports of any fever to the family or primary physician
- Proper hand washing before and after handling CVC or dressing
- Whether dressings should be changed under sterile conditions
- Determination of when and under what conditions the tubing or the dressing should be handled
- Steps to be taken if a complication occurs (e.g., saline flush, use of heparin)
- Prescribed dosage for heparin flush
- Latex allergy alert (see Chapter 5)
- Universal precautions (Anticipating the tasks to be done, the risk involved, and the personal protective equipment needed will enhance protection of both the caregiver and student.)

Procedure for CVC Dressing Change

Intravenous Lines

PROCEDURE

1. Wash hands.

2. Assemble equipment (i.e., catheter dressing kit):

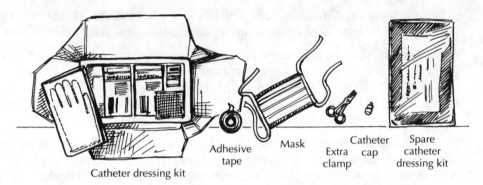

Catheter dressing kit   Adhesive tape   Mask   Extra clamp   Catheter cap   Spare catheter dressing kit

- Mask
- Sterile gloves
- Alcohol swabsticks
- Povidone iodine swabsticks or student-specific cleansing supplies
- Povidone ointment or student-specific antibacterial ointment
- Sterile gauze
- Transparent occlusive dressing
- Adhesive tape

Also needed:
- Extra clamp
- Catheter cap
- Spare catheter dressing kit
- 3-cc syringe for normal saline

3. Explain the procedure to the student according to his or her level of understanding.
4. Put on the mask.
5. Wash hands.

6. Assist the student in removing clothing to uncover the dressing.
7. Position the student.

8. Open the catheter dressing kit on a clean work surface.

9. Remove wet or soiled dressing from the catheter exit site.

POINTS TO REMEMBER

Anticipating the tasks to be done, the risk involved, and the personal protective equipment needed will enhance protection of both the caregiver and student.

Dressing change should be performed in a private area of the health office.

Identify the size and type of central venous catheter.

Different dressing kits may be used that do not contain all of these components. Those items not included in the kit should be supplied separately.

By encouraging the student to assist in the procedure, the caregiver helps the student achieve maximum self-care skills.

Because putting on a mask involves touching the hair, a second hand washing is necessary.

The student may be sitting or lying flat. Have the student turn the head to the side while the catheter is exposed. Avoid having the student breathe on the catheter site.

*Although not all CVC dressing changes are done using sterile procedures, students receiving TPN **do** have sterile dressing changes.*

Discard the dressing in the appropriately marked biomedical waste container.

10. Inspect the skin around the catheter for redness, swelling, or fluid drainage.

11. Put on sterile gloves.

12. Clean the skin with an alcohol swabstick, starting at the center next to the catheter and working outward in widening circles. Repeat the cleaning process two more times, for a total of three cleansings.

This may be a sign of infection. If any of these symptoms are evident, notify the physician and the family.

Start at the exit site.
Be sure to minimize movement of the catheter. This will help decrease skin trauma, thereby decreasing risk for infection. Allow the alcohol solution to dry for approximately 30 seconds.

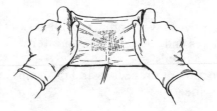

13. Repeat Step 12 using povidone iodine swabsticks. Allow the povidone iodine to dry for about 30 seconds before proceeding.

14. Gently pat the skin dry with sterile gauze.

15. Apply a small dab of antibacterial ointment to the catheter exit site.

16. Lay the gauze over the ointment on the catheter exit site.

17. Using a layer of transparent dressing or other type of dressing indicated in physician's order, cover the gauze and secure the dressing to the skin.

Iodophor solutions require at least 30 seconds to maximize antibacterial and antifungal action.

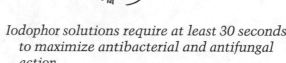

18. Using tape, secure the catheter at a second point to reduce strain on the catheter:
    • Place the first piece of tape as shown.
    • Place a second piece of tape over the first, sealing it along the catheter.
    • Secure the catheter with the free end of tape.

This may be done in a manner other than that illustrated.

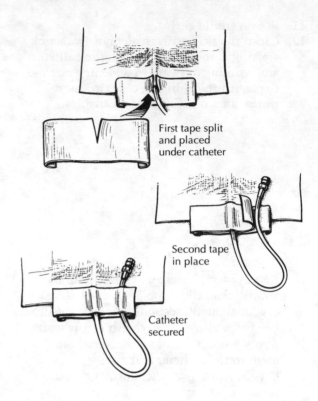

First tape split and placed under catheter

Second tape in place

Catheter secured

19. Remove gloves and mask. Dispose of gloves and supplies appropriately.
20. Wash hands.
21. Document procedure and problems on the log sheet.

22. Write date and time of dressing change on dressing.

Report to the family any changes in the student's usual pattern of tolerating the procedure as well as any unusual drainage.

Possible Problems that Require Immediate Attention

Equipment Needed for Emergencies

Points to Remember

Anticipating the tasks to be done, the risk involved, and the personal protective equipment needed will enhance protection of both the caregiver and the student.

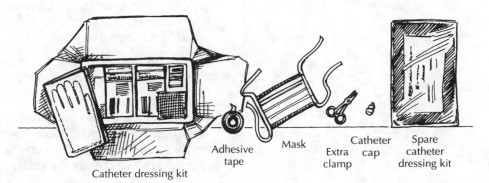

Catheter dressing kit · Adhesive tape · Mask · Extra clamp · Catheter cap · Spare catheter dressing kit

- Smooth-edged clamp
- Sterile gauze
- Adhesive tape
- Sterile gloves (optional)
- Alcohol swabs
- Betadine swabs
- Dressing kit
- Mask
- Heparinized syringe
- Normal saline (sterile)

Observations

Blood in the tubing or bleeding from the end of the tubing

Development of a fever, redness at the CVC site, drainage, increased fatigue, irritability, or headache

Reason/Action

Whenever blood is present, gloves should be worn. Most students will have their CVCs capped while they are in school. If blood is noted in the line or coming from the end of the line, **check to see if the clamp is open.** *If so, close the clamp. Transfer the student to the health office. The catheter may need to be flushed with saline and instilled with heparin if doing so is indicated in the student's IHCP. Notify the family.*

If the clamp has broken or is not functioning properly, the tubing should be firmly pinched closed or clamped and the physician and family contacted immediately. **Activate the emergency plan.**

The family and/or physician should be called at once. These are indications of infection.

CVC is pulled or falls out

Stay calm. Reassure the student. *Whoever is at the site first should cover the CVC exit site with sterile gauze, if immediately available, or clean dressing.*

Inspect the exterior of the dressing. If the dressing is intact and the tape still holds the looped catheter, it is probable that no significant trauma to the student or the line has occurred. The family and the physician should be notified anyway.

If the tape or dressing has been disrupted, they should be taken off and the exit site inspected.

If the catheter has fallen out, apply firm pressure to the exit site (bleeding should be minimal). Notify the physician and family immediately. **Activate the emergency plan.**

Catheter tubing is broken

Clamp the catheter above the break. Notify the school nurse, who will wrap the broken end with a sterile gauze. Notify the family and physician immediately. **Be prepared to initiate the emergency plan.**

The catheter usually can be repaired by the physician at the hospital.

Student complains of chest pain or difficulty in breathing

Have the student lie on his or her left side until the line is clamped. This helps to prevent an air bubble from entering the heart.

Once the tubing is securely clamped and not leaking, transport the student via wheelchair to the school nurse's office. **Do not let the student walk.**

Initiate the emergency plan. The student should be transported as soon as possible to the appropriate hospital emergency room. If the school nurse is not available, pinch the tubing with a clamp or fingers and call the emergency medical team. Notify the family and physician immediately.

General Information Sheet

Students with Central Venous Catheters

Dear (teacher, lunch aide, bus driver):

_____ [Student's name] has a condition that requires a central venous catheter (CVC). This is a plastic tube, like an IV, that has been placed by a surgeon into a large vein close to the heart. A student may have a CVC if he or she is unable to digest food or requires special medications. The tubing usually comes out of the skin on the chest. The exit site is covered by a bandage to protect it and to keep the tubing clean. The CVC does not cause any discomfort if it is secured properly. If the student has an implantable catheter, the tubing will not be visible.

Some students will have the tubing connected to an intravenous fluid solution, but most will have the CVC capped or clamped while they are in school or in transport. In most cases, routine CVC care will be carried out at home or in the health room, unless an emergency occurs.

Most students with CVCs are able to participate in school activities. Participation in physical education and any restrictions must be determined by the physician and the family. Students with CVCs should avoid having the exit site bumped or the tubing pulled.

The CVC is covered by a bandage as well as the student's clothing. No one should touch the tubing or dressing unless a complication occurs. All staff who have contact with students with CVCs should be familiar with the emergency plan and how to initiate it.

The following staff members have been trained to deal with any problems that may arise with this student:

_____

_____

_____

For more information about CVCs, consult the school nurse or the family.

Heparin Lock/
Intermittent Intravenous Device

PURPOSE

A heparin lock is a method of maintaining intravenous (IV) access when a student requires intermittent medication or fluids. An adaptor plug containing heparinized saline is inserted into the hub of the IV catheter. (Heparin prevents blood from clotting in the catheter.) The heparinized saline is replaced regularly by injecting a prescribed dose into the plug. This allows the student increased mobility. These IV catheters are used for short-term courses of medication/fluids.

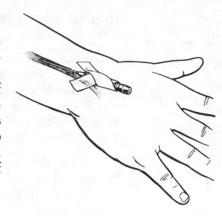

SUGGESTED SETTINGS

Procedures such as dressing reinforcements, changes, and heparin flushes should be performed in the health room. The student's activity may be limited to prevent dislodging the IV catheter.

SUGGESTED PERSONNEL AND TRAINING

A health care assessment needs to be completed by the school nurse. State nurse practice regulations must be consulted for guidance on delegating health care procedures.

A registered nurse with proven competency-based training in appropriate techniques and problem management should administer heparin flushes and provide IV catheter care. Any school personnel with regular contact with a student with a heparin lock or IV catheter must receive general training that covers the student's specific health care needs, potential problems, and how to implement the established emergency plan.

The basic skills checklist on pages 337–338 can be used as a foundation for competency-based training in appropriate techniques. It outlines specific procedures step by step. Once the procedures have been mastered, the completed checklist serves as documentation of training.

THE INDIVIDUALIZED HEALTH CARE PLAN: ISSUES FOR SPECIAL CONSIDERATION

Each student's IHCP should be tailored to the individual's needs. The following section covers the procedures for heparin lock flushes and possible problems and emergencies that may arise. It is essential to review it before writing the IHCP.

A sample plan is included in Chapter 6. It may be copied and used to develop a plan for each student. For a student with a heparin lock, the following items should receive particular attention:

- Protection of the IV site from bumping or other trauma
- Signs of IV site infiltration and infection
- Safe storage and disposal of intravenous supplies
- Medication and heparin/saline flush requirements
- Latex allergy alert (see Chapter 5)
- Universal precautions (Anticipating the tasks to be done, the risk involved, and the personal protective equipment needed will enhance protection of both the caregiver and student.)

PROCEDURE FOR THE ADMINISTRATION OF A HEPARIN FLUSH

PROCEDURE	POINTS TO REMEMBER

PROCEDURE

1. Wash hands.

2. Assemble equipment:

Anticipating the tasks to be done, the risk involved, and the personal protective equipment needed will enhance protection of both the caregiver and the student.

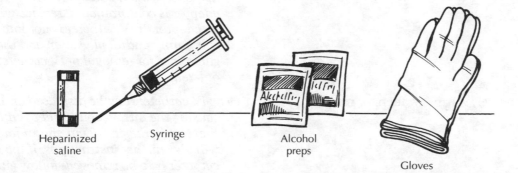

Heparinized saline   Syringe   Alcohol preps   Gloves

Intravenous Lines

- IV catheter with male adapter (in place)
- Saline or heparinized saline (see student-specific guidelines for dosage)

- 3-ml syringe with a 21- to 23-gauge needle
- Two alcohol swabs
- Gloves
- Adhesive tape

Identify size and type of IV device.
Heparinized saline is available in single-dose vials with 10 units of heparin per cc of saline. Vial should be labeled for intravenous use.

3. Position the student and explain the procedure to the student according to his or her level of understanding.
4. Wash hands. Put on gloves.

By encouraging the student to assist in the procedure, the caregiver encourages him or her to achieve maximum self-care skills.

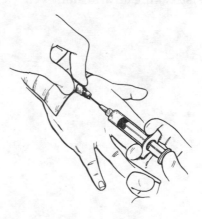

5. Cleanse top of heparinized saline container with alcohol swab.

6. Draw prescribed dosage of heparinized saline into syringe.

7. Cleanse catheter hub with alcohol swab.
8. Slowly inject prescribed dosage of saline or heparinized saline.
9. Remove syringe and needle and dispose of properly.
10. Reinforce dressing, if needed.
11. Remove gloves and wash hands.
12. Document the dosage, time, and condition of IV site on log sheet.

If student complains of pain with injection, inspect IV site. It may be infiltrated.

Report to the family any change in the student's usual pattern of tolerance of procedure.

Possible Problems that Require Immediate Attention

Observation	Reason/Action
IV dressing is wet; there is leakage of blood or fluid	*Male adaptor may be dislodged. IV catheter may be dislodged or IV site is infiltrated.*
	Carefully remove dressing. If IV catheter is intact, apply new dressing. If adaptor is not contaminated, reconnect adaptor to catheter (if disconnected) and apply new dressing. If adaptor is contaminated, replace with a sterile adaptor. If IV catheter is not intact, consult family and/or physician and then follow guidelines for removal of IV catheter if ordered.
IV site is tender, warm, swollen, or red	*The IV catheter may be displaced or dislodged, causing the intravenous fluid to enter the tissue. Notify the physician and/or family, who will give further instructions. If the IV catheter is to be removed, follow guidelines for removal.*
Pain with injection of heparin	*IV catheter may be infiltrated.*
Difficulty injecting saline or heparinized saline into catheter	*Needle may not be in hub properly. Catheter may be clotted. IV site may be infiltrated.*
	Make sure needle is in hub properly. Gently press on plunger; if no results, stop injecting.
	Inspect IV site; if unable to flush or if IV site is infiltrated, notify physician and/or family. If the IV is to be removed, follow guidelines for removal.
Redness/streaking up arm along vein	*May be phlebitis (infection of vein). Notify family and/or physician. Remove IV catheter if ordered.*

Procedure for Removal of IV Catheter

PROCEDURE

1. Wash hands.
2. Assemble equipment:
   - Gloves
   - Sterile gauze
   - Bandage
3. Wash hands. Put on gloves.

4. Open sterile gauze and bandage.
5. Remove dressing, being careful to secure catheter with one hand while removing tape with the other.
6. Hold the hub or end of the catheter; slowly remove from vein.
7. Apply pressure to the IV site.

8. Apply bandage.
9. Dispose of catheter in appropriate receptacle.
10. Remove gloves. Wash hands.
11. Document procedure and condition of site.

POINTS TO REMEMBER

Anticipating the tasks to be done, the risk involved, and the personal protective equipment needed will enhance protection of both the caregiver and student.

Explain procedure to student and have student participate as much as possible.

Hold pressure for at least 5 minutes or more until bleeding stops.

Report to family any change in the student's usual pattern.

General Information Sheet

Students with Heparin Locks

Dear (teacher, lunch aide, bus driver):

_____ [Student's name] has a condition that requires an intravenous (IV) catheter or heparin lock. The IV catheter is a tiny plastic tube placed in a vein in the student's arm or hand. This is a way of giving the student medication or fluids. When the student is not receiving continuous intravenous fluids or medications, a special plug (i.e., heparin lock) is inserted into the end of the intravenous catheter to allow increased mobility while keeping the tube usable. The IV catheter is inserted into the student's vein by a physician or nurse and held in place by tape.

The student can receive medications at home, school, or the hospital. The student's activities may be limited so as not to dislodge the tube.

The following staff members have been trained to deal with any problems that may arise with this student:

_____

_____

_____

For more information about intravenous lines or heparin locks or the needs of this student, consult the school nurse or family.

Suggested Readings

Danek, G.D., & Noris, E.M. (1992). Pediatric IV catheters: Efficacy of saline flush. *Pediatric Nursing, 18*(2), 111–113.

Dragone, M.A. (1996). Cancer. In P. Jackson & J. Vessey (Eds.), *Primary care of the child with a chronic condition* (2nd ed., pp. 193–231). St Louis, MO: Mosby-Yearbook.

Dufour, D.F. (1990). Information for teachers of children with central venous catheters. *Journal of Pediatric Oncology Nursing, 7*(1), 37–38.

Kandt, K.A. (1991). An implantable venous access device for children. *The American Journal of Maternal/Child Nursing, 16*(2), 88–91.

Kleiber, C., Hanrahan, K., Fagan, C.L., & Zittergruen, M.A. (1993). Heparin vs. saline for peripheral IV locks in children. *Pediatric Nursing, 19*(4), 376, 405–409.

Langer, J.C. (1995). What is the role of the pediatric surgeon in the care of children with motility disorders? *The Messenger: A Newsletter Produced by the American Pseudo-obstruction and Hirschsprung's Disease Society, Inc., 7*(2), 8–9.

Marcoux, C., Fisher, S., & Wong, D. (1990). Central venous access devices in children. *Pediatric Nursing, 16*(2), 123–133.

McMullen, A., Fioravanti, I.D., Pollack, V., Rideout, K., & Sciera, M. (1993). Heparinized saline or normal saline as a flush solution in intermittent intravenous lines in infants and children? *The American Journal of Maternal/Child Nursing, 18*(2), 78–85.

Pollack, V.P. (1996). Inflammatory bowel disease. In P. Jackson & J. Vessey (Eds.), *Primary care of the child with a chronic condition* (2nd ed., pp. 507–529). St. Louis, MO: Mosby-Yearbook.

Rountree, D. (1991). The PIC catheter: A different approach. *American Journal of Nursing, 91*(8), 22–26.

Ryder, M.A. (1993). Peripherally inserted central venous catheters. *Nursing Clinics of North America, 28*(4), 937–971.

Viall, C.D. (1990). Your complete guide to central venous catheters. *Nursing 90, 20*(2), 34–41.

Wickham, R.S. (1990). Advances in venous access devices and nursing management strategies. *Nursing Clinics of North America, 25*(2), 345–361.

Young, R.J., & Murray, N.D. (1990). Pediatric home IV nutritional therapy. *Journal of Home Health Care Practice, 2*(4), 35–45.

DIALYSIS

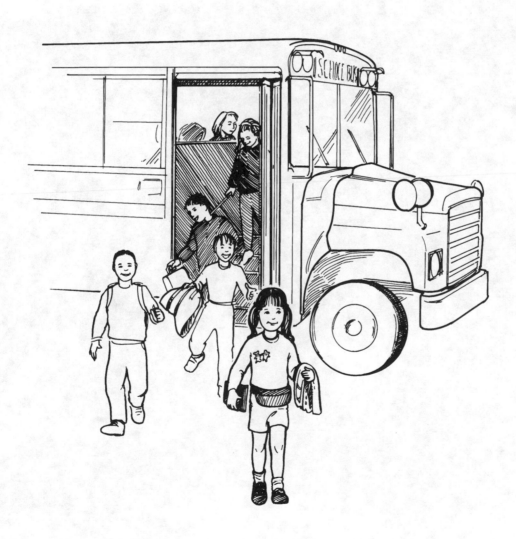

URINARY SYSTEM

STRUCTURE AND FUNCTION

The urinary system filters water and waste material from the blood and removes it from the body as urine.

The *kidneys* are two fist-size organs, one on each side of the spine at the back of the upper abdomen, that regulate the amount of water in the body. Ninety percent of the water that the kidneys remove from the blood is recycled back into the blood after waste is filtered out. The kidneys also regulate blood pressure, growth, calcium absorption, and red blood cell production.

The *blood vessels* include renal arteries that carry blood from the main artery to the kidneys, where waste is filtered out, and the renal veins that take cleansed blood away from the kidneys.

Ureters are narrow tubes that carry the urine from the kidneys to the bladder.

The *bladder* is a reservoir for storing the urine until it is ready to be discharged from the body.

The *urethra* is a tube leading from the bladder to the outside opening of the body through which urine is discharged, and the *meatus* is the external opening where urine comes out. In girls, it is between the labia, just above the vagina; and in boys, it is at the tip of the penis.

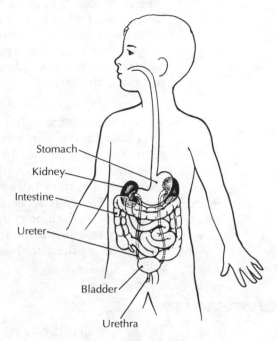

Stomach
Kidney
Intestine
Ureter
Bladder
Urethra

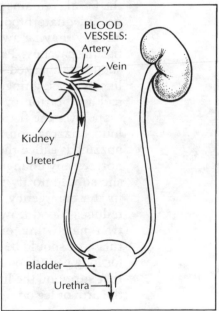

BLOOD VESSELS:
Artery
Vein
Kidney
Ureter
Bladder
Urethra

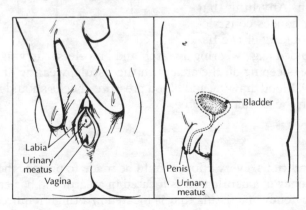

Labia
Urinary meatus
Vagina
Bladder
Penis
Urinary meatus

HEMODIALYSIS

PURPOSE

When a student's kidneys do not function properly (i.e., renal failure), that student may have problems with too much fluid and salt, high blood pressure, and the buildup of toxic waste products. There are two methods of treating the student with renal failure: dialysis and kidney transplantation. *Dialysis* is a therapy that uses a filter to get rid of body waste products and excess fluid. There are two types of dialysis: hemodialysis and peritoneal dialysis.

Usually, a student on hemodialysis is treated for 3 hours at a time, three times a week. During hemodialysis, the student's blood is circulated outside the body through a filter called a *dialyzer*, which allows small molecules and water to pass through a semi-permeable membrane. To perform hemodialysis, an access to the student's blood is needed. The most frequently created access is the arteriovenous fistula. A fistula is created when an artery and a vein are surgically joined, so that arterial blood flows through the vein. The vein becomes enlarged and thick, and large needles can be inserted and removed with each hemodialysis treatment. The most common location for a fistula is in the wrist, but it also can be located in the upper arm or thigh. Hemodialysis is performed in the home or hospital or dialysis unit by specially trained nurses and physicians.

FISTULA CARE

The goal of fistula care is to ensure that the fistula remains patent (i.e., open) and has adequate blood flow. The student already may be aware of how to check fistula patency. Patency of the fistula should be checked several times a day by lightly placing fingers over the fistula to feel a vibration or by placing a stethoscope over the fistula and listening for a loud buzzing sound. The vibration or buzzing is called the *bruit*. If the student notices any changes in the bruit, he or she should notify the people identified in the emergency plan. Anything that reduces blood flow or causes constriction, narrowing, or blocking of the fis-

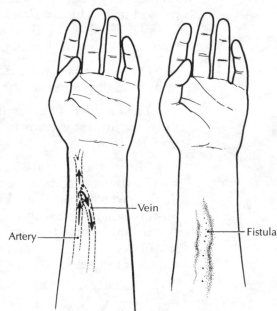

tula area should be avoided (e.g., wearing a watch and bracelets, carrying heavy objects for long periods of time, sleeping on the area with the fistula, wearing dressings or tape that surround the limb). Blood drawing and blood pressure checks should *not* be done on the arm or leg on which the fistula is located.

SUGGESTED SETTINGS

As with all medical conditions, every effort should be made to protect the student's privacy. Checking the patency of a fistula that is located in an arm can be performed in any setting. Checking the patency of a fistula that is located in a thigh requires a private setting, such as the health room.

SUGGESTED PERSONNEL AND TRAINING

A health assessment must be completed by the school nurse. State nurse practice regulations should be consulted for guidance on delegating health care procedures.

The student with an arteriovenous fistula is able to participate in school activities. Participation in physical education and classes in which sharp equipment is used by the student should be decided on an individual basis and specific activities should be approved by the student's physician. Fistula care should be done by a registered nurse with proven competency-based training in appropriate techniques and problem management. Any school personnel who have regular contact with a student who has a fistula must receive general training that covers the student's specific health care needs, potential problems, and how to implement the established emergency plan.

THE INDIVIDUALIZED HEALTH CARE PLAN: ISSUES FOR SPECIAL CONSIDERATION

Each student's IHCP must be tailored to the individual's needs. The following section covers the possible problems and emergencies that may arise for a student with a fistula. It is essential to review it before writing the IHCP.

A sample plan is included in Chapter 6. It may be copied and used to develop a plan for each student. For a student with a fistula, the following should receive particular attention:

- The student's underlying condition and potential problems associated with the condition or treatment
- School staff who have regular contact with the student should be aware that the student has a fistula and be familiar with the baseline appearance of the fistula and vibration of the bruit
- Report fever and/or pain in the fistula to the family or physician
- Report loss of bruit or bulging of the fistula to the family and physician
- Medication requirements (Some students will require additional support and supervision.)
- Student-specific diet restrictions, most significantly foods with high potassium content (Some students will require additional support and supervision.)
- Activity restrictions
- Susceptibility to infections, especially chicken pox
- Latex allergy alert (see Chapter 5)
- Universal precautions (Anticipating the tasks to be done, the risk involved, and the personal protective equipment needed will enhance protection of both the caregiver and student.)

School personnel (e.g., teachers, principals) should consider the following issues when working with a student needing hemodialysis:

- Consider using tape recorders and computers if fistula placement affects student's ability to write.
- Reduce amount of written homework.
- Be aware of frequent hospitalizations.
- Be aware of dialysis schedule.
- Schedule subjects flexibly during dialysis time.
- Prepare textbooks, workbooks, and worksheets for hospital tutor.
- Give credit for tutorial attendance.
- Monitor student performance in class and with hospital tutor.
- Arrange time for make-up work and tests.
- Assign home tutor when illness prevents student from attending school.
- Evaluate performance and review work after long absence.
- Make outlines and teacher's notes available to student.
- Modify amount of work expected by use of teacher–student contracts to attain realistic educational goals.
- Be aware of fatigue.
- Avoid after-school tutorial sessions.
- Provide access to school elevator in the event of fatigue or bone disease.

Possible Problems for the Student Requiring Hemodialysis

Observation	Reason/Action
Oozing or bleeding from a previous needle site	*The formed scab from the last needle puncture has come off. Put on gloves and apply direct pressure to the oozing site using a folded 2" × 2" gauze. Bleeding should stop within 10 minutes. Apply only enough pressure to stop the oozing of blood yet still feel the bruit. Once bleeding has stopped, apply a small Band-Aid.*
Trauma to the fistula	*If the student gets a cut into the fistula, the blood will pump out in a spurting fashion. Put on gloves and apply pressure with sterile gauze (if available) directly to the bleeding site. If bleeding cannot be controlled, apply a tourniquet above the fistula and **activate the emergency plan.** Arterial blood has been rerouted to the vein and the student could lose a large quantity of blood in a very short period of time.*
No bruit (i.e., vibrations, buzzing sound) when fistula is palpated or listened to with a stethoscope	*If fingers are used to palpate the bruit and nothing is felt, use a stethoscope to listen for a bruit. Have the student lie down. Check the student's blood pressure. If blood pressure is low or bruit still cannot be felt, call the dialysis unit or the family.*

Dialysis

Possible Problems that Require Immediate Attention for Any Student with Renal Failure

Observation

Student complains of chest pain, numbness in face or limbs, and generalized weakness

Reason/Action

Most students on dialysis have dietary restrictions on potassium-high foods. A high level of potassium in the blood is an **emergency.** *A high level of potassium in the blood interferes with the heart muscle's pumping action, causing irregular heartbeat, and may lead to cardiac arrest.*

Activate the emergency plan.

Call the family and physician.

Student complains of shortness of breath

The student may have or may be developing fluid in the lungs. Have the student sit and rest for 3 minutes. Check vital signs and document. If difficult breathing continues or increases, activate the emergency plan and notify the family. Have the student remain in a sitting position, leaning forward over a table or chair to facilitate ease of respiration while waiting for the ambulance.

Student complains of sudden onset of localized pain, usually felt while moving or walking

Students with renal failure often have severe bone disease and may experience broken bones with even a minor injury. Some students' bones may become very brittle due to ineffective calcium absorption.

Document location of pain and assess need for immobilizing area of pain. Activate the emergency plan and notify the family.

Dialysis

General Information Sheet

Students with Hemodialysis Fistulas

Dear (teacher, lunch aide, bus driver):

_____ [Student's name] has a condition in which the kidneys do not function properly. This student requires a hemodialysis fistula, which is a surgical joining of an artery and a vein in his or her arm or thigh. The fistula is used to remove waste products from the blood during hemodialysis. This student's fistula is located _____ .

The fistula may be covered by the student's clothing. If the fistula is on an arm, no pressure or tight-fitting objects (e.g., watches, bracelets) should be put on the arm with the fistula. The student should avoid bumping the area around the fistula. Routine care of the fistula will be carried out at home or in the health room, unless an emergency occurs.

The student with a hemodialysis fistula is able to participate in school activities. Participation in physical education activities and classes in which sharp equipment is used by the student should be decided on an individual basis, and specific activities should be approved by the student's physician.

All staff who have contact with the student who has a fistula should be familiar with the emergency plan and how to initiate it.

The following staff members have been trained to deal with any problems that may arise with this student:

_____

_____

_____

For more information about a hemodialysis fistula or the student's needs, consult the school nurse or the family.

PERITONEAL DIALYSIS

PURPOSE

When a student's kidneys do not function properly (i.e., renal failure), that student may have problems with too much fluid and salt, high blood pressure, and the buildup of toxic waste products. There are two methods of treating the student with renal failure: dialysis and kidney transplantation. *Dialysis* is a therapy that uses a filter to get rid of body waste products and excess fluid. There are two types of dialysis: hemodialysis and peritoneal dialysis.

Peritoneal dialysis is the procedure in which dialysis occurs using the abdominal lining as the filter for waste products. There are two forms of peritoneal dialysis:

1. *Continuous Ambulatory Peritoneal Dialysis (CAPD)* is carried out continuously throughout each 24-hour period. A solution called dialysate is instilled by gravity through a catheter into the abdominal space and drained out, by gravity, at regular intervals (i.e., usually four to six times a day).

2. *Continuous Cycling Peritoneal Dialysis (CCPD)* is done over a 12-hour period, usually at night. A machine is set to instill and drain the dialysate at timed intervals (i.e., usually six cycles in a 12-hour period). Depending on the student's comfort, the peritoneal cavity may or may not be left full of dialysate during the 12 hours that he or she is not undergoing CCPD.

A peritoneal dialysis catheter is placed surgically in the abdomen. It is tunneled under the skin and has one or two cuffs attached. The cuffs help to keep the catheter in place and to stop bacteria from traveling along the catheter from the skin into the abdominal cavity. The end of the catheter that shows outside the body has either a cover or a length of tubing with a rolled-up empty dialysate bag attached. The bag is tucked into the student's clothing or in a carrying pouch.

The catheter always must be protected and covered by clothing to prevent tugging or pulling. If the catheter is tugged or pulled, a break in the system or skin tearing could occur.

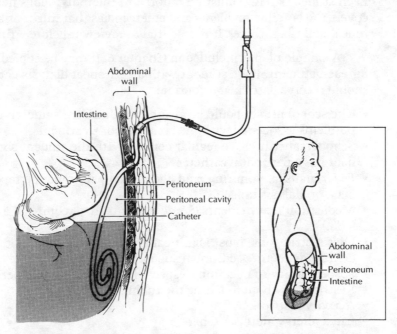

The exit site (i.e., where the catheter comes out through the skin of the abdomen) usually is covered by a small 2" × 2" gauze and held in place with nonabrasive tape after antibiotic ointment or spray has been applied directly to the exit site.

There are two main complications of peritoneal dialysis: infection and abdominal membrane failure. Repeated peritoneal infections can lead to peritoneal membrane failure, and, eventually, peritoneal dialysis will no longer be a treatment option for the student.

SUGGESTED SETTINGS

As with all medical conditions, every effort should be made to protect the student's privacy. Procedures such as dialysate exchange or dressing change must be carried out in the health room or another clean, private room free from interruptions. The student can participate in school activities, but participation in swimming and physical education activities must be decided on an individual basis and approved by the student's physician.

SUGGESTED PERSONNEL AND TRAINING

A health assessment must be completed by the school nurse. State nurse practice regulations should be consulted for guidance on delegating health care procedures.

Any school personnel who have regular contact with a student with a peritoneal dialysis catheter must receive general training that covers the student's specific health care needs, potential problems, and how to implement the established emergency plan.

Because the technique for performing peritoneal dialysis must be adhered to rigidly, only personnel with competency-based training should perform this procedure. The training in this technique usually takes place in the dialysis unit responsible for the student's care. Those chosen for training are selected by the caregivers and the family. Changing the dressing at the exit site can be performed by a registered nurse using a sterile technique. The goal is to keep the skin around the catheter site clean and dry. Skin breakdown can eventually lead to peritonitis (i.e., abdominal infection).

THE INDIVIDUALIZED HEALTH CARE PLAN: ISSUES FOR SPECIAL CONSIDERATION

Each student's IHCP must be tailored to the individual's needs. The following section covers the possible problems and emergencies that might arise for a student with a peritoneal dialysis catheter. It is essential to review it before writing the IHCP.

A sample plan is included in Chapter 6. It may be copied and used to develop a plan for each student. For a student with a peritoneal dialysis catheter, the following items should receive particular attention:

- The school nurse should be aware of the student's underlying condition and potential problems associated with the condition or treatment
- School staff who have regular contact with the student should be aware that the student has a peritoneal catheter
- Fever, nausea, vomiting, and abdominal pain must be reported to the family, physician, or dialysis unit
- Medication requirements (Some students may require additional support and supervision.)
- Diet restrictions, most significantly foods with high potassium content (Some students may require additional support and supervision.)
- Susceptibility to infections, especially chicken pox and peritonitis
- Restrictions about touching the tubing or the dressing
- Activity restrictions
- Latex allergy alert (see Chapter 5)
- Universal precautions (Anticipating the tasks to be done, the risk involved, and the personal protective equipment needed will enhance protection of both the caregiver and student.)

Dialysis

Possible Problems for the Student Requiring Peritoneal Dialysis that Require Immediate Attention

Observation	**Reason/Action**
Exit site dressing falls off	*Using sterile technique, apply sterile 2" × 2" split gauze around the catheter where it exits skin. Cover catheter and gauze with a second gauze. Secure with nonabrasive tape and notify family.*
Catheter is pulled or tugged	*Check catheter for any leaks or breaks in the tubing. Using aseptic technique, take dressing off, and check exit site for any indication of trauma or tears in the skin. If any leaking or trauma has occurred, notify family or dialysis unit immediately. Cover affected areas with sterile dressing.*
Cover on the end of the catheter comes off	*Cover the catheter end with sterile gauze. Make sure roller clamp has remained tight and dialysate is not leaking. If clamp is open, close it. Notify family.*
Tubing has become disconnected	*If the catheter and the tubing have disconnected, cover open end of catheter with a sterile dressing. Stop the flow of dialysate from the catheter by bending the catheter. Tape the folded, bent catheter to stop dialysate flow. Call family or dialysis unit immediately.*
Student complains of abdominal pain, fever, nausea, vomiting	*Have student rest. Take vital signs.*
	Call family or dialysis unit immediately. (Abdominal infection, or peritonitis, can happen within a few hours.)
	This is a potential emergency. Be prepared to activate the emergency plan.

Dialysis

Possible Problems that Require Attention
for Any Student with Renal Failure

Observation	Reason/Action
Student complains of chest pain, numbness in face or limbs, and generalized weakness	*Most students on dialysis have dietary restrictions on potassium-high foods. A high level of potassium in the blood is an* **emergency.** *A high level of potassium in the blood interferes with the heart muscle's pumping action, causing irregular heartbeat, and may lead to cardiac arrest.*
	Activate the emergency plan.
	Call the family or physician.
Student complains of shortness of breath	*The student may have or may be developing fluid in the lungs. Have the student sit and rest for 3 minutes. Check vital signs and document. If difficult breathing continues or increases, activate the emergency plan and notify the family. Have the student remain in a sitting position, leaning forward over a table or chair to facilitate ease of respiration while waiting for the ambulance.*
Student complains of sudden onset of localized pain, usually felt while moving or walking	*Students with renal failure often have severe bone disease and may experience broken bones with even a minor injury. Some students' bones may become very brittle.*
	Document location of pain and assess need for immobilizing area of pain.
	Activate the emergency plan and notify the family.

General Information Sheet

Students with Peritoneal Dialysis Catheters

Dear (teacher, lunch aide, bus driver):

_____ [Student's name] has a condition in which the kidneys do not function properly. He or she requires a peritoneal dialysis catheter. This is plastic tube that has been placed surgically into the student's abdomen to help remove waste products from the body.

The student will have a catheter closed with a cover or connected to a special fluid solution bag. The tubing and fluid bag are covered by the student's clothing. No one should touch the catheter or bag unless a problem occurs. Routine care of the dialysis catheter tubing will be carried out at home or in the health room, unless an emergency occurs.

Most students with peritoneal dialysis catheters are able to participate in school activities. Participation in swimming and physical education activities must be decided on an individual basis by the student's physician. Students with peritoneal dialysis catheters should avoid significant blunt trauma to their abdomen or situations in which the tubing might be pulled.

All staff who have contact with the student with a peritoneal dialysis catheter should be familiar with the emergency plan and how to initiate it.

The following staff members have been trained to deal with any problems that may arise with this student:

_____

_____

_____

For more information about peritoneal dialysis catheters or the student's needs, consult the school nurse or family.

Suggested Readings

Graham-Macaluso, M.M. (1991). Complications of peritoneal dialysis: Nursing care plans to document teaching. *American Nephrology Nurses' Association (ANNA) Journal, 18*(5), 479–483.

Taylor, J.H. (1996). Chronic renal failure. In P. Jackson & J. Vessey (Eds.), *Primary care of the child with a chronic condition* (2nd ed., pp. 689–716). St Louis, MO: Mosby-Yearbook.

Dialysis

Clean Intermittent Catheterization

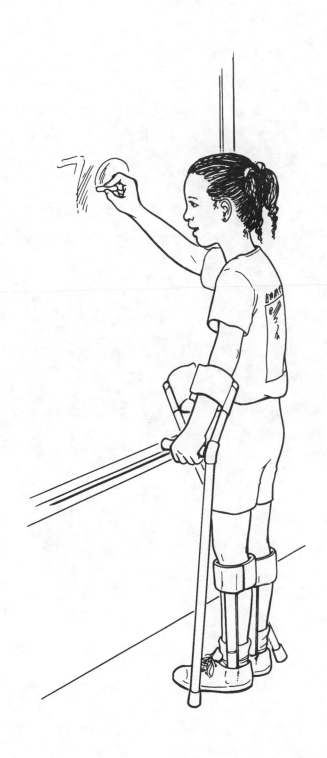

URINARY SYSTEM

STRUCTURE AND FUNCTION

The urinary system filters water and waste material from the blood and removes it from the body as urine.

The *kidneys* are two fist-size organs, one on each side of the spine at the back of the upper abdomen, that regulate the amount of water in the body. Ninety percent of the water that the kidneys remove from the blood is recycled back into the blood after waste is filtered out. The kidneys also regulate blood pressure, growth, calcium absorption, and red blood cell production.

The *blood vessels* include renal arteries that carry blood from the main artery to the kidneys, where waste is filtered out, and the renal veins that take cleansed blood away from the kidneys.

Ureters are narrow tubes that carry the urine from the kidneys to the bladder.

The *bladder* is a reservoir for storing the urine until it is ready to be discharged from the body.

The *urethra* is a tube leading from the bladder to the outside opening of the body through which urine is discharged, and the *meatus* is the external opening where urine comes out. In girls, it is between the labia, just above the vagina; and in boys, it is at the tip of the penis.

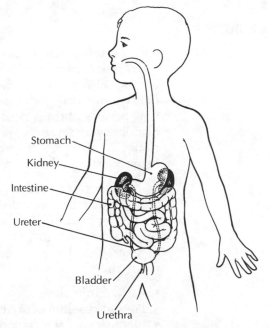

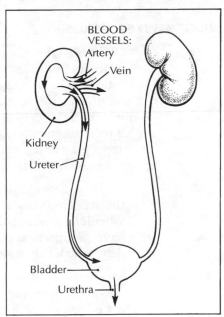

CLEAN INTERMITTENT CATHETERIZATION

PURPOSE

Clean intermittent catheterization (CIC) is a generally clean procedure used to empty the bladder. Infrequently, the procedure may require sterile technique depending on student-specific needs. CIC helps prevent urinary tract infections in students who have difficulty emptying their bladders. When the bladder remains filled with stagnant urine for long periods of time, rapid bacterial growth and infection may result. Catheterizing the bladder every few hours eliminates urine before bacteria can multiply to cause an infection. CIC also prevents wetting caused by overflow incontinence, a condition in which urine overflows the bladder and dribbles out the urethra.

CIC is often used when the nerves that stimulate the bladder do not function properly. For instance, a condition called *neurogenic bladder* is associated with myelodysplasia (i.e., spina bifida) and other conditions in which the nerves from the spinal cord to the bladder are damaged (e.g., spinal injuries resulting from accidents). Because of nerve damage, the bladder is completely or partially unable to empty, which can lead to the following:

- Risk of infection
- Possible backup of urine to the kidney resulting in kidney damage
- Incontinence (i.e., lack of control of urine leading to wetting)

SUGGESTED SETTINGS

CIC can be done in regular bathroom facilities in the home, school, or hospital. CIC also may be done in the nurse's office or any other facility where the student is ensured privacy. If recommended sites are not private, appropriate accommodations (e.g., screens, doors) should be made.

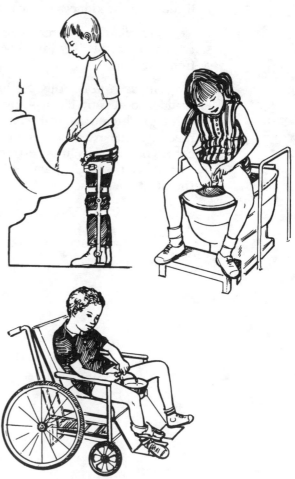

If toilet facilities are used by the student, those facilities must be wheelchair accessible and should have railings or supports for the student who needs assistance.

Some students may need to lie down while being catheterized—a cot or bed in the health room would be appropriate.

SUGGESTED PERSONNEL AND TRAINING

A health assessment must be completed by the school nurse. State nurse practice regulations should be consulted for guidance on delegating health care procedures.

An adult with proven competency-based training in appropriate techniques and problem management can do this procedure safely and effectively. All students should be encouraged to learn the procedure and do it themselves, if able. It is important to recognize that if a student does self-catheterization, he or she may still need some supervision. School personnel who have regular contact with the student who requires CIC should receive general training that covers the student's specific health care needs, potential problems, and how to implement the established emergency plan.

The basic skills checklist on pages 339–342 can be used as a foundation for competency-based training in appropriate techniques. It outlines specific procedures step by step. Once the procedures have been mastered, the completed checklist serves as documentation of training.

THE INDIVIDUALIZED HEALTH CARE PLAN: ISSUES FOR SPECIAL CONSIDERATION

Each student's IHCP must be tailored to the individual's needs. The following section covers the procedure for CIC and possible problems and emergencies that may arise. It is essential to review it before writing the IHCP.

A sample plan is included in Chapter 6. It may be copied and used to develop a plan for each student. For a student who requires catheterization, the following items should receive particular attention:

- Medications that would affect urine color, amount, and odor
- Flexible timing of catheterization to accommodate classroom schedule, field trips, and other school events
- Fostering independence in performing the procedure, depending on the student's developmental ability
- An extra set of clothing in the educational setting
- Individual baseline status, including urine color, amount, and pattern of continence
- Position of student during catheterization
- Student's history of urinary tract infections
- Student's ability to self-catheterize (The student who is capable of self-care should have ready access to his or her equipment and a clean, private bathroom with a sink.)
- Student's need of assistance with clothing and leg braces
- Whether procedure is to use clean or sterile technique
- Latex allergy alert (see Chapter 5)
- Universal precautions (Anticipating the tasks to be done, the risk involved, and the personal protective equipment needed will enhance protection of both the caregiver and student.)

CIC

PROCEDURE FOR
CLEAN INTERMITTENT CATHETERIZATION—MALE

PROCEDURE

1. Wash hands.

2. Assemble equipment:

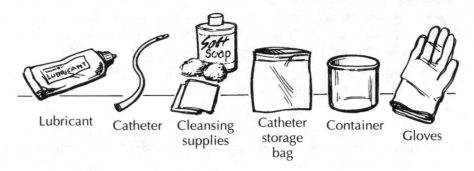

Lubricant   Catheter   Cleansing supplies   Catheter storage bag   Container   Gloves

- Water-soluble lubricant (e.g., K-Y jelly, Lubrifax, Surgel)
- Catheter (e.g., plastic, polyvinylchloride, metal)
- Wet wipes or cotton balls (nonsterile) plus mild soap and water or student-specific cleansing supplies
- Storage receptacle for catheter
- Container for urine or toilet
- Gloves (if person other than student does procedure)

3. Explain the procedure to the student at his level of understanding. Have him do as much of the procedure as he is capable of, with supervision as needed.
4. Position the student.

5. Wash hands and put on gloves.
6. Show the student, depending on his age, the location of the urethral opening.
7. Lubricate the tip of the catheter with a water-soluble lubricant and place on clean surface.

POINTS TO REMEMBER

Anticipating the tasks to be done, the risk involved, and the personal protective equipment needed will enhance protection of both the caregiver and student.

If the student does the procedure unassisted, gloves are not needed.

By encouraging the student to assist in the procedure, the caregiver helps him achieve maximum self-care skills.

The student may be catheterized lying down, standing, or sitting. If able, he may stand at the toilet. If unable to sit or stand, he may lie on his back. This procedure requires a receptacle to catch the flow of urine from the catheter.

CIC

8. Cleanse the penis in the following manner:
   a. Hold the penis below the glans at a 45- to 90-degree angle from the abdomen depending on position of student or student-specific guidelines.
   b. If the student is not circumcised, retract the foreskin.

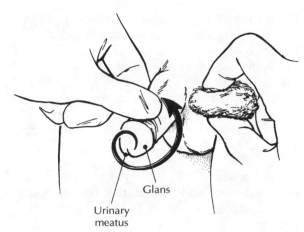

Glans

Urinary
meatus

Always start at the meatus and wash toward the base of the penis. This helps remove bacteria from the area.

   c. Wash the glans with soapy cotton balls or student-specific cleansing supplies. Begin at the urethral opening, and, in a circular manner, wash away from the meatus. Repeat twice for a total of three washings. Use a clean cotton ball each time you wash the penis.
9. Locate the urethral opening. Hold the penis at a 45- to 90-degree angle from the abdomen, depending on position of student or student-specific guidelines. Insert catheter gently into the urethral opening. Some resistance may be met at the bladder sphincter. Use gentle but firm pressure until the sphincter relaxes. Encouraging the child to relax (i.e., breathe deeply) may also be helpful.
10. Insert the catheter until there is a good flow of urine. When the flow stops, insert catheter slightly more and then withdraw a little to make sure all urine is drained. Rotate the catheter so that catheter openings have reached all areas of the bladder.

Do not force catheter. If you feel unusual resistance, notify the family. *Make sure the other end of the catheter is either in a receptacle or over the toilet to catch urine.*

It is also helpful to have the student bear down a couple of times while the catheter is in place. If trained to do so, apply external manual pressure to encourage the urine flow until the flow stops. This must be done with the catheter in place.

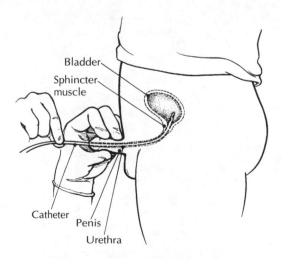

Bladder
Sphincter
muscle

Catheter
Penis
Urethra

11. When bladder is emptied, pinch catheter and withdraw. (If using metal catheter, put finger over end.)

This prevents urine still in the catheter from flowing back into the bladder during withdrawl.

12. If the student is not circumcised, pull the foreskin over the glans when finished.
13. Remove gloves and wash hands.
14. Assist student in dressing.
15. Put on gloves.
16. Measure and record the urine volume if ordered. Dispose of urine, clean equipment, and store in appropriate container.

Examples of storage receptacles include a sealed plastic bag, a urine specimen container, and a pencil case. The used catheter(s) should be sent home with student to be cleaned.

17. Wash hands.
18. Document on log sheet that the procedure was done.

Report to the family any change (e.g., cloudy urine, mucus, blood, foul odor, color changes, unusual wetting between catheterizations; these may be signs of infection).

CIC

Procedure for
Clean Intermittent Catheterization—Female

PROCEDURE

1. Wash hands.

2. Assemble equipment:

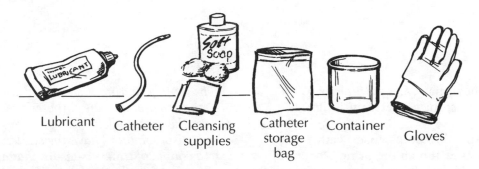

Lubricant   Catheter   Cleansing   Catheter   Container   Gloves
supplies   storage
bag

- Water-soluble lubricant (K-Y jelly, Lubri-fax, Surgel)
- Catheter (e.g., plastic, polyvinylchloride, metal)
- Wet wipes or cotton balls (nonsterile) plus mild soap and water or student-specific cleansing supplies
- Storage receptacle for catheter
- Container for urine or toilet
- Gloves (if person other than student does procedure)
- Mirror (if student normally uses)

3. Explain the procedure to the student at her level of understanding. Have her do as much of the procedure as she is capable of, with supervision as needed.
4. Position the student.

5. Wash hands and put on gloves.
6. Use a mirror to show the student, depending on her age, the location of the urethral opening.

POINTS TO REMEMBER

Anticipating the tasks to be done, the risk involved, and the personal protective equipment needed will enhance protection of both the caregiver and student.

If the student does the procedure unassisted, gloves are not needed.

By encouraging the student to assist in the procedure, the caregiver helps her achieve maximum self-care skills.

The student may be catheterized lying down or sitting. If able, she may sit on the toilet with legs straddled. A student unable to sit may lie on her back. This procedure requires a receptacle to catch the flow of urine from the catheter.

CIC

7. Lubricate the tip of the catheter with a water-soluble lubricant. Place on clean surface.

8. Separate the labia (i.e., vaginal lips) and hold open with fingers. Cleanse in a direction from the top of the labia toward the rectum. Wash three times: once down each side and once down the middle. Use a clean cotton ball each time.

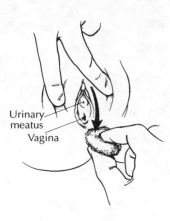

Urinary meatus
Vagina

9. Locate the urinary meatus (opening). Gently insert the catheter until there is urine.
10. When urine flow stops, insert catheter slightly more. If no more urine is obtained, withdraw it slightly and rotate catheter so that catheter openings have reached all areas of the bladder.

The female urethra is short and straight. Keep the other end of the catheter over the toilet or the receptacle.

It is also helpful to have the student bear down a couple of times to ensure that all urine has been drained completely. If trained to do so, apply manual external pressure until the urine stops flowing. This must be done with the catheter in place.

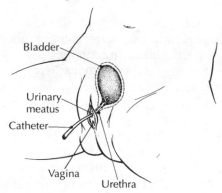

Bladder

Urinary meatus
Catheter

Vagina   Urethra

11. When bladder is completely empty, pinch catheter and withdraw. (If using metal catheter, put finger over end.)
12. Remove gloves and wash hands.
13. Assist student in dressing.
14. Put on gloves.
15. Measure and record the urine volume if ordered. Dispose of urine, clean equipment, and store in appropriate container.

16. Wash hands.
17. Document on log sheet that the procedure was done.

This prevents urine still in catheter from flowing back into the bladder during withdrawal.

Examples of storage receptacles include a sealed plastic bag, a urine specimen container, a pencil case, and a cosmetic bag. The used catheter(s) should be sent home with student to be cleaned.

Report to the family any change (e.g., cloudy urine, mucus, blood, foul odor, color changes, unusual wetting between catheterizations; these may be signs of infection).

Possible Problems that Require Immediate Attention

Observations	Reason/Action
Bleeding from urethra	*This may be due to trauma to the urethra or urinary tract infection. Discontinue catheterization. Contact family and physician.*
Inability to pass catheter	*This may be due to increased sphincter tone caused by anxiety or spasm. Encouraging the child to relax (i.e., breathe deeply) may be helpful.*
	In boys: Reposition the penis and use gentle but firm pressure until the sphincter relaxes. Sometimes it helps to have boys flex at hips to decrease reflex resistance of bladder sphincter.
	In girls: Check catheter placement. The catheter may be in the vagina. If catheter is in the vagina, do not reinsert; use a clean catheter.
	If unsuccessful, notify family or physician for further instructions.
No urine as a result of catheterization	*This may be due to improper placement of catheter or the bladder may be empty. Check position of catheter.*
Cloudy urine, mucus, blood, foul odor, color changes, or unusual wetting between catheterizations	*This may be due to a urinary tract infection. Always report to family any changes in the student's usual pattern or tolerance of procedure.*

CIC

General Information Sheet

Students Who Use Clean Intermittent Catheterization

Dear (teacher, lunch aide, bus driver):

_____ [Student's name] has a condition that requires clean intermittent catheterization (CIC). CIC is a simple and safe procedure that helps the student empty his or her bladder because the bladder is unable to empty on its own. This helps to prevent wetness or urinary infections.

The student or another person empties the bladder by putting a clean, small tube (i.e., catheter) into the bladder and letting the urine drain out. This should be done in a clean, private space, preferably in the bathroom or in the health room. Most students need to do this every 4–6 hours during the day.

Unless the student has a condition that otherwise would interfere with his or her participation in physical education or other school activities, there is no reason why he or she cannot participate fully. Special consideration may need to be given to the timing of catheterization, based on the student's schedule, for field trips or other activities during which the student may not have access to a bathroom. This procedure should be done in a private place.

The following staff members have been trained to deal with any problems that may arise with this student:

_____

_____

_____

For more information about this procedure or the student's needs, consult the school nurse or the family.

Suggested Readings

Bloom, D.A., McGuire, E.J., & Lapides, J. (1994). A brief history of urethral catheterization. *The Journal of Urology, 151*(2), 317–325.

Brown, J.P. (1990). A practical approach to teaching self-catheterization to children with myelomeningocele. *Journal of Enterostomal Therapy, 17*(2), 54–56.

Brown, J.P., & Reichenbach, M.B. (1989). Screening children with myelodysplasia for readiness to learn self-catheterization. *Rehabilitation Nursing, 14*(6), 334–337.

Farley, J.A., & Dunleavy, M.J. (1996). Myelodysplasia. In P. Jackson & J. Vessey (Eds.), *Primary care of the child with a chronic condition* (2nd ed., pp. 580–597). St. Louis, MO: Mosby-Yearbook.

Segal, E.S., Deatrick, J.A., & Hagelgans, N.A. (1995). The determinants of successful self-catheterization programs in children with myelomeningoceles. *Journal of Pediatric Nursing, 10*(2), 82–88.

Smith, K.A. (1990). Bowel and bladder management of the child with myelomeningocele in the school setting. *Journal of Pediatric Health Care, 4*(4), 175–180.

CIC

OSTOMY CARE

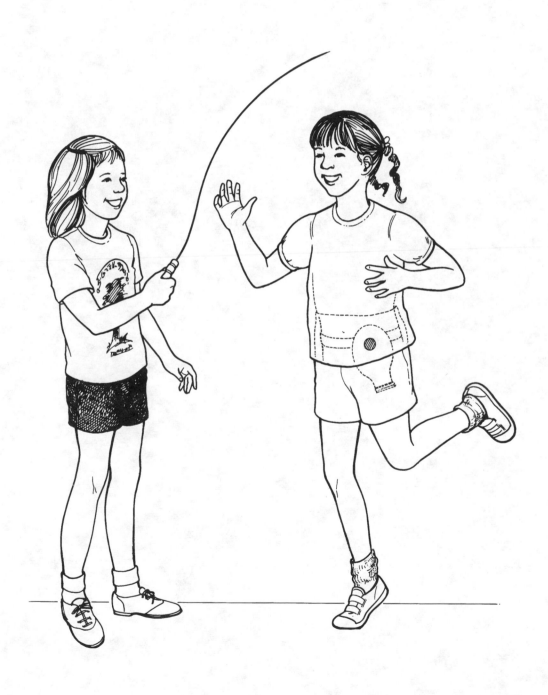

GASTROINTESTINAL SYSTEM

STRUCTURE AND FUNCTION

The gastrointestinal system breaks down food into basic nutrients that can feed the cells of the body. Functionally, the gastrointestinal tract is divided into two parts: upper and lower.

The upper gastrointestinal tract is where digestion and absorption of most of the nutrients occur. The mouth, throat, esophagus, stomach, and small intestine are components of this part of the digestive tract.

The *mouth* is where processing of food starts. Chewing is important because digestion is more effective with smaller particles. The food is swallowed and passes through the throat, then through the esophagus.

The *esophagus* is a straight tube approximately 10 inches in length in an adult. It extends from the base of the throat behind the trachea to the stomach.

The *stomach* is a curved, pouch-like organ that is located under the diaphragm in the upper left portion of the abdomen. The stomach partially digests food and regulates passage of food into the intestine.

The *small intestine* is approximately 12 feet long in an adult. The duodenum, jejunum, and ileum are parts of the small intestine. Food passes from the stomach through the small intestine, where most digestion and absorption of nutrients take place.

The lower gastrointestinal tract consists of the *large intestine*, where water is reabsorbed and undigested food is consolidated into fecal waste.

The large intestine extends from the end of the small intestine to the *rectum*. The *anus* is the opening to the outside of the body.

Digestion takes place in two ways:

- *Mechanical*: Chewing and stomach contractions break down food.
- *Chemical*: Food is broken down by digestive acids and enzymes.

The digested food is absorbed through the lining of the intestine and then enters the bloodstream, where it is carried to the cells and tissues throughout the body.

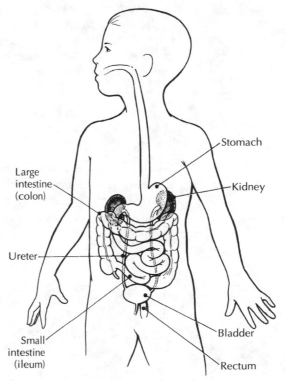

Ostomies for Elimination

An ostomy for elimination is a surgically created opening into the intestine or urinary tract to permit the elimination of stool or urine. The ostomy may be temporary or permanent.

An ostomy may be necessary when there is inadequate function caused by the following:

- Obstruction (blockage)
- Inflammatory bowel disease
- Infection
- Birth defects
- Accident or injury
- Abnormal motility
- Cancer

A *stoma* is the opening of the ostomy on the skin. A piece of intestine or urinary tract is brought out to the surface of the abdomen and folded back onto itself, then stitched in place on the skin. A stoma is shiny, wet, and dark pink in color, similar to the inside lining of the mouth. The shape is usually round or oval and the size may vary. Stomas are rich in blood supply and may bleed slightly if irritated or rubbed. Because the stoma itself does not have nerve endings, irritation of the stoma does not cause discomfort. However, the skin surrounding the stoma does have nerve endings and may be sensitive to manipulation of the stoma or contact with the stoma discharge.

Students usually wear a pouch over the stoma to collect urine or stool. The location of the stoma in the urinary or intestinal tract determines the type, amount, and consistency of the drainage. These factors determine how quickly the pouch fills and how frequently it needs to be emptied. Other students may have a continent (i.e., self-containing) ostomy that does not require a pouch but requires periodic drainage by passing a tube (i.e., catheter) into it.

Ostomies can be located on different parts of the abdomen depending on which part of the intestine or urinary tract is affected. Common types of ostomies include the following:

- Colostomy—a surgically created opening in the large intestine
- Ileostomy—a surgically created opening in the small intestine
- Urostomy—a surgically created opening into any part of the urinary tract (Types of urostomies include conduit, ureterostomy, or vesicostomy.)

COLOSTOMY

PURPOSE

A colostomy is a surgical opening in the large intestine that is used to drain stool when part of the colon does not function properly as a result of the following:

- Obstruction (blockage)
- Inflammation or infection
- Birth defects
- Accident or injury
- Abnormal motility

The end of the remaining part of the colon is brought out to the surface of the abdomen and stitched in place after it has been folded back onto itself to create the stoma. Depending on the reason for the colostomy, the anatomical location of the stoma may vary.

Some students have two stomas from either a loop colostomy or a double-barrel colostomy. In these cases, the last part of the colon may not function, or only part of the colon may have been removed. One of the stomas will function as the colostomy, where the stool comes out. The other opening, which is closer to the rectum, is a *mucus fistula*. No stool comes out of this stoma, only mucus, which the colon normally makes. Some students who have colostomies like this occasionally may pass mucus from their rectum when they sit on the toilet. The ostomy is covered by a pouch that collects the stool.

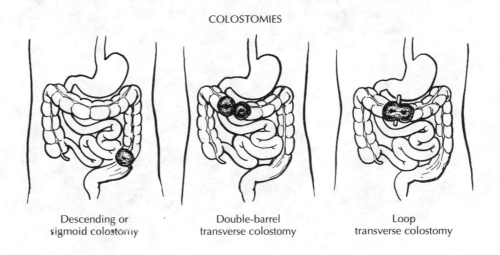

COLOSTOMIES

| Descending or sigmoid colostomy | Double-barrel transverse colostomy | Loop transverse colostomy |

STOMA CARE

The goal of stoma care is to keep the skin and stoma clean and healthy. Good skin care is essential because discharge from the ostomy can be irritating to the skin around the stoma. A properly fitting barrier should be applied around the stoma to protect the skin from any leakage.

SUGGESTED SETTINGS

The student or caregiver empties the pouch in a private place (e.g., bathroom, health office), and stoma care is done when needed. The pouch should be emptied when it is one third to one half full or when a leak occurs. A student should be able to participate in all school activities, including physical education.

SUGGESTED PERSONNEL AND TRAINING

A health assessment must be completed by the school nurse. State nurse practice regulations should be consulted for guidance on delegating health care procedures.

Stoma care can be done by the student, school nurse, or other adult with proven competency-based training in appropriate techniques and problem management. School personnel who have regular contact with a student with a colostomy should receive general training that covers the student's specific health care needs, potential problems, and how to implement the established emergency plan.

THE INDIVIDUALIZED HEALTH CARE PLAN: ISSUES FOR SPECIAL CONSIDERATION

Each student's individualized health care plan must be tailored to individual needs. The following section covers the procedure for colostomy care and possible problems and emergencies that may arise. It is essential that this section be reviewed before writing the health care plan.

A sample health care plan is included in Chapter 6. It may be copied and used to develop a plan for each student. For a student with a colostomy, the following items should receive particular attention:

- Student's ability for self-care (The student capable of self-care should have ready access to his or her equipment and a private bathroom with a sink.)
- Student's change of clothing in school
- Baseline status of the colostomy (e.g., stool consistency, frequency, stoma care)
- Latex allergy alert (see Chapter 5)
- Universal precautions (Anticipating the tasks to be done, the risk involved, and the personal protective equipment needed will enhance protection of both the caregiver and student.)

Ostomy Care

PROCEDURE FOR CHANGING A COLOSTOMY POUCH

PROCEDURE

1. Wash hands.

2. Assemble equipment:

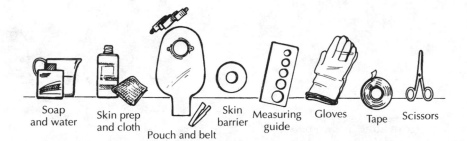

Soap and water   Skin prep and cloth   Pouch and belt   Skin barrier   Measuring guide   Gloves   Tape   Scissors

- Water
- Skin cleanser solution
- Soft cloth or gauze
- Clean pouch and belt, if needed

- Skin barrier
- Measuring guide, if needed
- Disposable gloves, if pouch is to be changed by someone other than student
- Tape, if needed
- Scissors, if specified
- Protective powder and paste, if used

3. Explain procedure at the student's level of understanding.

4. Wash hands and put on gloves.

5. Empty contents of pouch student is wearing.

6. Carefully remove the used pouch and skin barrier by pushing the skin away from the bag, instead of pulling the bag off the skin.

7. Wash the stoma area using clean cloth or gauze. **Do not scrub.** Cover the stoma with gauze, then clean the skin around the stoma.

POINTS TO REMEMBER

Anticipating the tasks to be done, the risk involved, and the personal protective equipment needed will enhance protection of both the caregiver and student.

Each student should have a complete setup at school with a spare pouch and clip/pouch closure.

By encouraging the student to assist in the procedure, the caregiver helps the student achieve maximum self-care skills.

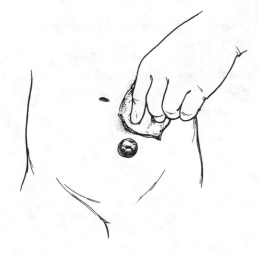

Ostomy Care

8. Inspect skin for redness, rash, bleeding, or blistering.

9. Pat stoma and skin dry. Apply protective powder around stoma. Brush excess powder off skin.

10. If a skin barrier is used that requires fitting, measure stoma per student-specific guidelines. Place skin barrier on skin around stoma.

If there is skin irritation, check student-specific guidelines. Do not put medication, ointment, or adhesive on the damaged skin. Report skin irritation to school nurse and/or family. A small amount of pinpoint bleeding may normally occur.

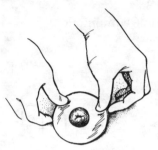

11. Peel off backing from adhesive on pouch and apply paste to pouch, if needed. Securely apply pouch closure to bottom of pouch.

12. Remove used gauze and discard in appropriate receptacle.

13. Center the new pouch directly over the stoma.

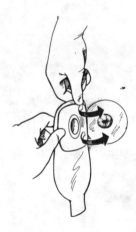

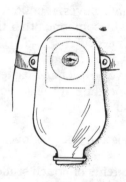

14. Firmly press the pouch to the skin barrier so there are no wrinkles and no leaks.

15. Dispose of used pouch in appropriate receptacle.

16. Remove gloves and wash hands.

17. Document on log sheet that the procedure was done.

If indicated, open the pouch to allow in a small amount of air. Then seal the drain. If a belt is used to fasten pouch, attach to pouch.

Rever to universal precautions.
Report to family any change in stool pattern, skin irritation, or tolerance of the procedure.

Ostomy Care

Possible Problems When Changing a Colostomy Pouch

Observations	Reason/Action
Odor	*A properly cared for colostomy should not have a persistent odor when the pouch is closed. If there is an odor, check for a leak around the stoma or in the pouch itself.*
Leakage	*Check to see if pouch is too full or has a leak. Other causes include inadequate or improper stoma care, improper pouch size for stoma, or a change in stool pattern (e.g., diarrhea).*
Bleeding from stoma	*The stoma is irritated very easily. This may happen if it is rubbed too roughly during cleaning or nicked with a fingernail. Usually the bleeding stops quickly. If it does not, apply gentle pressure and notify the family. If a large area of the stoma appears to be bleeding, notify the family, school nurse, or physician.*
Irritation/skin breakdown around stoma; skin is raw or weeping	*Usually this is due to improper stoma care, such as poor seal of the pouch or inadequate barrier on the skin. If the skin is just red, make sure that skin barrier is applied properly. Also, check that the student is not using any new barrier or adhesive preparation (possible allergic reaction). Contact the family, school nurse, or physician.*
A rash with small red spots	*Student may have a yeast infection. Clean and dry the skin carefully and notify the family.*
Change in stool pattern	*If the student is having either looser stools than before or much fewer, notify the family. This may be due to diet changes or illness.*
Part of intestine showing through stoma	*If the amount of intestinal tissue showing is more than usual, the stoma may be prolapsing (i.e., intestine being pushed out through the opening). The tissue may appear swollen, and the student may experience cramping and vomiting. Contact the school nurse, family, and physician immediately.*

Ostomy Care

General Information Sheet

Students with Colostomies

Dear (teacher, lunch aide, bus driver):

_____ [Student's name] has a condition that requires a colostomy. This is an opening on the surface of the abdomen into the large intestine, which allows the body to eliminate feces because the student is unable to do so. The opening, or stoma, is covered by a pouch that serves as a container for waste until it can be emptied. The student or another person empties the pouch and cleans the stoma in the bathroom when needed.

Unless the student has a condition that otherwise interferes with his or her participation in physical education or other activities, there is no reason why he or she cannot participate fully. It is very difficult for a stoma to be injured. It can be bumped, leaned on, or slept on without problems. The pouch is firmly attached and should not come off under normal circumstances. The student should be allowed easy access to private bathroom facilities.

The following staff members have been trained to deal with any problems that may arise with this student:

_____

_____

_____

For more information about colostomies or the student's needs, consult the school nurse or the family.

Ileostomy

PURPOSE

An ileostomy is a surgical opening in the small intestine that is used to drain feces if the colon has been removed or is unable to be used due to disease, injury, or blockage. The end of the ileum is brought out to the surface of the abdomen and is stitched in place after it has been folded back onto itself to create the stoma.

The stoma may seem to protrude like a nipple, unlike the flatter stoma in a colostomy. This is because the fecal matter from ileostomies is very irritating to the surrounding skin, and the nipple helps to direct drainage into the ostomy bag. Because food is not completely digested without the colon, discharge from the ileostomy stoma is usually pasty but may be watery. Discharge will be fairly constant with more after meals and a little less during the night. Foods that are difficult to digest, such as tomato skins and corn, will be passed from the ileostomy looking very much the same as when eaten. Students with ileostomies must be careful about what they eat so the ileostomy does not become blocked.

Another type of ileostomy, now used for some students, is the *continent ileostomy*. In this type of ileostomy, a surgeon makes an internal pouch from the end of the ileum under the skin. A valve is also made from the end of the intestine, which keeps most gas and the stool inside the pouch until it is emptied. The internal pouch is emptied four to six times a day by putting a tube (i.e., catheter) through the stoma to open the valve and drain the contents. Students with a continent ileostomy will still have a stoma, but their stoma care is usually simpler than is that needed for the other type of ileostomy.

STOMA CARE

The goal of stoma care is to keep the skin and stoma clean and healthy. Good skin care is essential, because discharge from the ostomy can be irritating to the skin around the stoma. A properly fitting barrier should be applied around the stoma to protect the skin from any leakage.

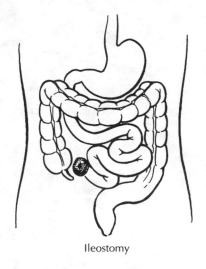

Ileostomy

SUGGESTED SETTINGS

The student or caregiver empties the pouch in a private place, such as a bathroom or the health room, and does stoma care when needed. The pouch should be emptied before it is full or if a leak occurs. The student should be able to participate in all school activities, including physical education.

SUGGESTED PERSONNEL AND TRAINING

A health assessment must be completed by the school nurse. State nurse practice regulations should be consulted for guidance on delegating health care procedures.

Stoma care can be done by the student, school nurse, or other adult with proven competency-based training in appropriate techniques and problem management. School personnel who have regular contact with a student with an ileostomy should receive general training that covers the student's specific health care needs, potential problems, and how to implement the established emergency plan.

THE INDIVIDUALIZED HEALTH CARE PLAN: ISSUES FOR SPECIAL CONSIDERATION

Each student's individualized health care plan must be tailored to the individual's needs. The following section covers the procedure for ileostomy care, as well as possible problems and emergencies that may arise. It is essential that these guidelines be reviewed before writing the IHCP.

A sample plan is included in Chapter 6. It may be copied and used to develop a plan for each student. For a student with an ileostomy, the following items should receive particular attention:

- Student's ability for self-care (The student capable of self-care should have ready access to his or her equipment and a private bathroom with a sink.)
- Some students with ileostomies may require a modified diet
- Baseline status of the ileostomy (e.g., stool consistency, frequency)
- Access to change of clothes
- Latex allergy alert (see Chapter 5)
- Universal precautions (Anticipating the tasks to be done, the risk involved, and the personal protective equipment needed will enhance protection of both the caregiver and student.)

PROCEDURE FOR CHANGING AN ILEOSTOMY POUCH

PROCEDURE

1. Wash hands.

2. Assemble equipment:

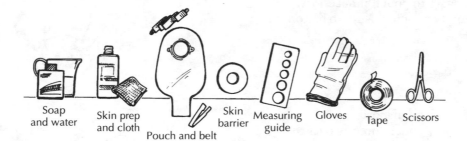

Soap and water • Skin prep and cloth • Pouch and belt • Skin barrier • Measuring guide • Gloves • Tape • Scissors

- Water
- Skin cleanser solution
- Soft cloth or gauze
- Clean pouch and belt, if needed

- Skin barrier
- Measuring guide, if needed
- Disposable gloves, if pouch is to be changed by someone other than student
- Tape, if needed
- Scissors, if specified
- Protective powder and paste, if used

3. Explain procedure at the student's level of understanding.

4. Wash hands and put on gloves.

5. Empty contents of used pouch into toilet.
6. Carefully remove the used pouch and skin barrier by pushing the skin away from the pouch, instead of pulling the pouch off the skin.
7. Wash the stoma with soap and water using clean cloth or gauze. Cover the stoma with gauze or cloth and clean the skin around the stoma.

POINTS TO REMEMBER

Anticipating the tasks to be done, the risk involved, and the personal protective equipment needed will enhance protection of both the caregiver and student.

Each student should have a complete set-up at school with a spare pouch.

By encouraging the student to assist in the procedure, the caregiver helps the student achieve maximum self-care skills.
Not necessary if student is doing procedure unassisted.

If a skin barrier that requires fitting is used, measure stoma.

Do not scrub the stoma or the skin.

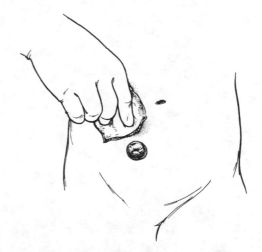

8. Inspect the skin for redness, rash, or blistering.

9. Pat skin dry. Apply protective powder around stoma. Brush excess powder off skin.
10. Place skin barrier on skin around stoma.
11. Peel off backing from adhesive on pouch, and apply paste to pouch if necessary. Securely apply pouch closure to bottom of pouch.

If there is skin irritation, check student-specific guidelines. Do not put medication, ointment, or adhesive on the damaged skin. Report skin irritation to school nurse and/or family.

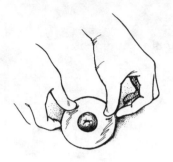

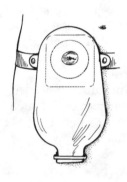

12. Remove gauze and dispose.
13. Center the new pouch directly over the stoma.

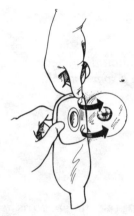

14. Firmly press the pouch to the skin barrier so there are no leaks or wrinkles.
15. Dispose of used pouch in appropriate receptacle.
16. Remove gloves and wash hands.
17. Document on log sheet that procedure was completed and note any significant changes.

If indicated, open the pouch to allow in a small amount of air. Then seal drain.
Refer to universal precautions.

Report to the family any change in stool pattern or tolerance of the procedure.

Possible Problems When Changing an Ileostomy Pouch

Observations	**Reason/Action**
Odor	*A properly cared for ileostomy should not have a persistent odor. If there is an odor, check for an improperly cleaned pouch or belt or a leak around the stoma or in the pouch itself.*
Leakage	*Check to see if the pouch is too full or has a leak. Other causes include inadequate or improper care, wrong pouch size for stoma, or change in amount of fecal drainage.*
Bleeding from stoma	*The stoma is irritated very easily. This may happen if it is rubbed too hard during cleaning or nicked with a fingernail. Usually the bleeding stops quickly. If it does not, apply gentle pressure and notify the family. If a large area of the stoma appears to be bleeding, notify the family, school nurse, or physician.*
Irritation/skin breakdown around stoma; skin is raw or weeping	*Usually this is caused by improper stoma care or an inadequate barrier on the skin. Fecal discharge from ileostomies is very irritating to the skin because of the presence of digestive juices in the fluid. Therefore, it is very important to have a proper seal and skin barrier. Also, check that the student is not using any new preparation that might be causing an allergic reaction. Contact the family, school nurse, or physician.*
Rash with small red spots	*Student may have a yeast infection. Clean and dry the skin carefully and notify the family.*
Change in stool pattern	*If the student either has more watery stools than usual or has not had any discharge from the ileostomy, notify the family. This may be due to diet changes or illness.*
Part of intestine showing through stoma	*If the amount of intestinal tissue showing is more than usual, the stoma may be prolapsing (i.e., intestine being pushed out through the opening). The tissue may appear swollen, and the student may experience cramping and vomiting. Contact the school nurse, family, and physician immediately.*

Ostomy Care

General Information Sheet

Students with Ileostomies

Dear (teacher, lunch aide, bus driver):

_____ [Student's name] has a condition that requires an ileostomy. This is an opening on the surface of the abdomen into the small intestine, which allows the body to eliminate stool because the student is unable to do so. The opening, or stoma, is covered by a pouch that serves as a container for waste until it can be emptied. The student or another person empties the pouch and cleans the stoma, when needed, in the bathroom.

Unless the student has a condition that otherwise would interfere with his or her participation in physical education or other activities, there is no reason that he or she cannot participate fully. It is very difficult for a stoma to be injured. It can be bumped, leaned on, or slept on without problems. The pouch is firmly attached and should not come off under normal circumstances. The student should be allowed easy access to private bathroom facilities.

The following staff members have been trained to deal with any problems that may arise with this student:

_____

_____

_____

For more information about ileostomies or the student's needs, consult the school nurse or family.

Ostomy Care

Urostomy

URINARY SYSTEM—STRUCTURE AND FUNCTION

The urinary system filters water and waste material from the blood and removes it from the body as urine.

The *kidneys* are two fist-size organs, one on each side of the spine at the back of the upper abdomen, that regulate the amount of water in the body. Ninety percent of the water that the kidneys remove from the blood is recycled back into the blood after waste is filtered out. The kidneys also regulate blood pressure, growth, calcium absorption, and red blood cell production.

The *blood vessels* include renal arteries that carry blood from the main artery to the kidneys, where waste is filtered out, and the renal veins that take cleansed blood away from the kidneys.

Ureters are narrow tubes that carry the urine from the kidneys to the bladder.

The *bladder* is a reservoir for storing the urine until it is ready to be discharged from the body.

The *urethra* is a tube leading from the bladder to the outside opening of the body through which urine is discharged, and the *meatus* is the external opening where urine comes out. In girls, it is between the labia, just above the vagina; and in boys, it is at the tip of the penis.

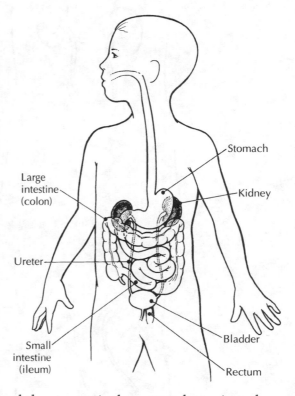

PURPOSE

A urostomy, or urinary diversion, is an artificial site for urine to come out of the body. A urostomy is made by a surgeon when the bladder has been removed or bypassed. Like other types of ostomies, the stoma for the urostomy is on the abdomen, and the urine drains into a pouch or bag or may be eliminated by catheterizing the stoma.

The following are different types of urinary diversions (see illustrations on next page):

- *Urostomy or conduit:* The ureters are attached surgically to a piece of the intestine and then brought out to the surface of the abdomen to form a stoma. The appearance is like an ileostomy, but stool does not drain out. Some urostomies have a continence mechanism. The stoma for the continent urostomy (see illustration on next page) is much smaller than an ostomy that continually drains urine. It is necessary to catheterize the continent stoma at least four to five times per day.
- *Ureterostomy:* One or both of the ureters are brought directly out to the surface of the abdomen. Sometimes the ureterostomy stomas will be pale pink or look as if they are covered by skin. Because the bladder has been bypassed, the ureterostomy continuously drains urine into the pouch.
- *Vesicostomy:* A vesicostomy (see illustration on next page) is an opening from the bladder directly to the surface of the skin. Some vesicostomies are called "continent" if the surgeon has made a pouch out of the bladder under the skin to hold the urine inside it until it is drained with a catheter. Continent vesicostomies also have a

stoma. The more usual types of vesicostomy allow the urine to drain continuously into a pouch or dressing covering the stoma. Most vesicostomies are used as temporary means of draining urine.

UROSTOMIES

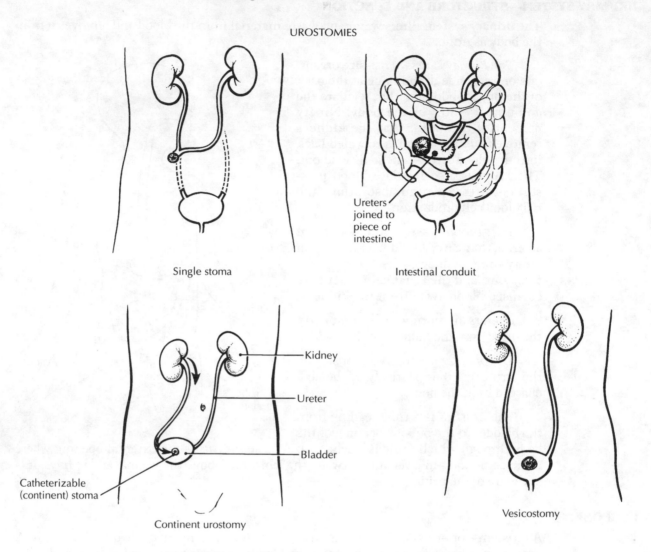

Single stoma

Ureters joined to piece of intestine

Intestinal conduit

Kidney

Ureter

Bladder

Catheterizable (continent) stoma

Continent urostomy

Vesicostomy

STOMA CARE

The goal of stoma care is to keep the skin and stoma clean and healthy. Good skin care is essential as discharge from the ostomy can be irritating to the skin around the stoma. A properly fitting barrier should be applied around the stoma to protect the skin from any leakage.

A small adhesive bandage may be worn over a continent stoma. Some children prefer to wear nothing over the stoma.

SUGGESTED SETTINGS

Stoma care and catheterization should be done in a private place, such as a bathroom or the health room. The pouch should be emptied before it is full or if a leak occurs. Some students may want to have an extra change of clothes at school. The student should be able to participate in all school activities, including physical education.

SUGGESTED PERSONNEL AND TRAINING

A health assessment must be completed by the school nurse. State nurse practice regulations should be consulted for guidance on delegating health care procedures.

Stoma care and catheterization of the continent stoma can be done by the student or by the school nurse or other adult with proven competency-based training in appropriate techniques and problem management. Any school personnel who have regular contact with a student with a urostomy must receive general training that covers the student's specific health care needs, potential problems, and how to implement the established emergency plan.

The basic skills checklist on pages 347–350 can be used as a foundation for competency-based training in appropriate techniques. It outlines specific procedures step by step. Once the procedures have been mastered, the completed checklist serves as documentation of training.

THE INDIVIDUALIZED HEALTH CARE PLAN: ISSUES FOR SPECIAL CONSIDERATION

Each student's individualized health care plan should be tailored to the individual's needs. The following section covers the procedure for urostomy care as well as potential problems that may arise. It is essential that these guidelines be reviewed before writing the IHCP.

A sample plan is included in Chapter 6. It may be copied and used to develop a plan for each student. For a student with a urostomy, the following items should receive particular attention:

- Student's ability for self-care (The student should have ready access to his or her equipment and private bathroom facilities with a sink. Each student should have enough equipment at school for at least 1 week.)
- Urostomies should not have an odor (An odor may indicate infection or a leak.)
- Access to a change of clothing in school
- Student's baseline status (e.g., urine volume, urine color)
- Latex allergy alert (see Chapter 5)
- Universal precautions (Anticipating the tasks to be done, the risk involved, and the personal protective equipment needed will enhance protection of both the caregiver and student.)

PROCEDURE FOR CHANGING A UROSTOMY POUCH

PROCEDURE

1. Wash hands.

2. Assemble equipment:

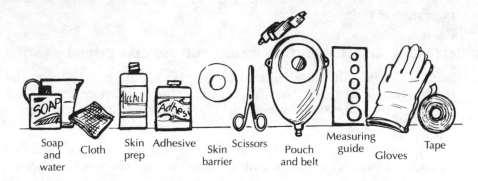

Soap and water | Cloth | Skin prep | Adhesive | Skin barrier | Scissors | Pouch and belt | Measuring guide | Gloves | Tape

- Soap and water
- Soft cloth or gauze
- Skin preparation
- Clean pouch and belt, if needed

- Disposable gloves, if pouch is to be changed by someone other than student
- Skin barrier
- Measuring guide
- Scissors, if specified
- Tape, if needed
- Adhesive
- Container to store used pouch
- Disinfectant solution for cleaning pouch

3. Explain procedure at the student's level of understanding.

4. Position the student.
5. Wash hands and put on gloves.
6. Empty contents of used pouch into toilet.
7. Carefully remove the used pouch and skin barrier by pushing the skin away from the pouch, instead of pulling the pouch off the skin.

POINTS TO REMEMBER

Anticipating the tasks to be done, the risk involved, and the personal protective equipment needed will enhance protection of both the caregiver and student.

Each student should have a complete setup at school with a spare pouch.
For ureterostomies, the pouch should have an antireflux valve to prevent urine from going back into the stoma.

By encouraging the student to assist in the procedure, the caregiver helps the student achieve maximum self-care skills.

If a skin barrier is used that requires fitting, measure stoma per student-specific guidelines.

8. Wash the stoma area using a clean cloth or gauze.

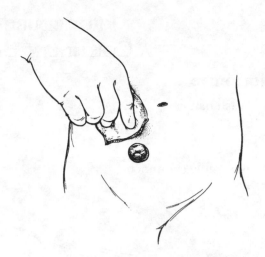

9. Cover the stoma with gauze or cloth and clean the skin around the stoma. **Do not scrub the stoma or the skin**.
10. Inspect skin for redness, rash, or blistering.

If there is skin irritation, check student-specific guidelines. Do not put medication, ointment, or adhesive on the damaged skin. Report skin irritation to school nurse and family.

11. Pat skin dry.

12. Place skin barrier on skin around stoma per student-specific guidelines.
13. Peel off backing of adhesive on the pouch or apply adhesive to pouch.
14. Remove gauze and dispose.
15. Remove gloves.
16. Center the new pouch directly over the stoma.

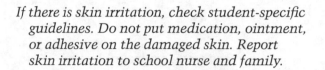

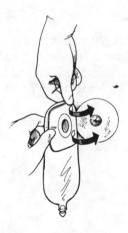

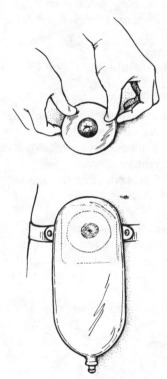

17. Firmly press the pouch to the skin barrier so there are no wrinkles or leaks. Attach belt if used.
18. Dispose of used pouch in appropriate receptacle.
19. Wash hands.
20. Document on log sheet that the procedure was completed.

If indicated, open the pouch to allow in a small amount of air. Then seal bottom if the pouch has a bottom drain.

Report to family any change in urine pattern.

Ostomy Care

PROCEDURE FOR CATHETERIZING A CONTINENT UROSTOMY/VESICOSTOMY

PROCEDURE

1. Wash hands.

2. Assemble equipment:

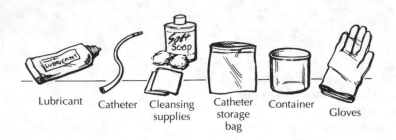

Lubricant   Catheter   Cleansing supplies   Catheter storage bag   Container   Gloves

- Soap and water or alcohol-free towelette
- Disposable gloves, if stoma is to be catheterized by someone other than student
- Catheter
- Water-soluble lubricant
- Catheter storage bag
- Container to collect and dispose of urine if unable to perform procedure while student sits on toilet
- Small adhesive bandage or stoma covering

3. Explain procedure at the student's level of understanding.

4. Position the student.
5. Wash hands and put on gloves.
6. Lubricate catheter tip with lubricant.

7. Wash the stoma using cleansing supplies.

POINTS TO REMEMBER

Anticipating the tasks to be done, the risk involved, and the personal protective equipment needed will enhance protection of both the caregiver and student.

Each student should have enough equipment at school for at least 1 week.

By encouraging the student to assist in the procedure, the caregiver helps the student achieve maximum self-care skills.
Student may be lying down or sitting.

It is important to lubricate the catheter to ensure easy passage and prevent tissue trauma.

8. Insert the catheter into the stoma until a flow of urine is passed.

Insert the catheter approximately ½–1 inch further.

Make sure the other end of the catheter is in either a receptacle to catch urine or over the toilet.

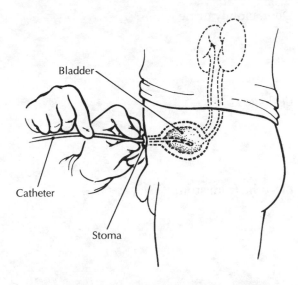

Bladder

Catheter

Stoma

9. Leave the catheter in the stoma until the flow of urine stops.

The flow of urine may be stopped by a mucus plug. The catheter should be removed and rinsed, lubricated, and reinserted. Sometimes the continent urostomy will need to be gently irrigated if there is presence of persistent mucus. A physician's order is needed for urostomy irrigation.

10. Slowly pinch the catheter and remove it from the stoma.
11. Remove gloves and wash hands.
12. Reapply adhesive bandage or stoma covering to stoma.
13. Put on gloves.
14. Measure and record urine volume if ordered. Dispose of urine.
15. Wash hands. Document on log sheet that the procedure was done.

Clean equipment and store in home container.

Report to the family any change (e.g., cloudy urine, mucus, blood, foul odor, color changes, unusual wetting between catheterizations).

Possible Problems that Require Immediate Attention

Observations	Reason/Action
Odor, cloudy urine	*Fresh urine should not have an odor. If there is an odor, check for a leak around the stoma or in the pouch itself.* **Urinary tract infections may cause the urine to have a strong smell.**
Leakage	*Check to see if the pouch is too full or has a leak. Other causes include inadequate or improper stoma care (e.g., inadequate adhesive) or incorrect pouch size for stoma. The continent stoma may be too full.*
Bleeding from stoma	*The stoma is irritated very easily. This may happen if it is rubbed too hard during cleaning or nicked with a fingernail. Usually the bleeding stops quickly. If it does not, apply gentle pressure and notify the family. If a large area of the stoma appears to be bleeding, notify the family or the physician.*
Irritation/skin breakdown around stoma; skin is raw or weeping	*Usually this is due to improper stoma care or to inadequate barrier on the skin. Also, check that the student is not using any preparation that might be causing an allergic reaction. Contact the family or physician.*
A rash with small red spots	*Student may have a yeast infection. Clean and dry the skin carefully and notify the family.*
Decrease or change in the flow of urine	*This may occur if the ureterostomy has narrowed. Notify the family of any change in urine flow.*

General Information Sheet

Students with Urostomies

Dear (teacher, lunch aide, bus driver):

_____ [Student's name] has a condition that requires a urostomy. This is an opening on the surface of the abdomen, which allows the urine to come out of the body when the student is unable to pass urine in the usual way. Depending on the student's condition, the opening will be in one of a number of parts of the urinary system. The opening, or stoma, is covered by a plastic pouch that serves as a container for waste until it can be emptied. The student or another person empties the pouch and cleans the stoma, when needed, in the bathroom. Some students catheterize their stomas.

Unless the student has a condition that otherwise interferes with his or her participation in physical education or other activities, there is no reason why he or she cannot participate fully. It is very difficult for a stoma to be injured. The pouch is firmly attached and should not come off under normal circumstances. The student should be allowed easy access to private bathroom facilities.

The following staff members have been trained to deal with any problems that may arise with this student:

_____

_____

_____

For more information about urostomies or the student's needs, consult the school nurse or the family.

Suggested Readings

Erwin-Troth, P. (1988). Teaching ostomy care to the pediatric client: A developmental approach. *Journal of Enterostomal Therapy, 15*(3), 126–130.

Langer, J.C. (1995). What is the role of the pediatric surgeon in the care of children with motility disorders? *The Messenger: A newsletter produced by the American Pseudo-obstruction and Hirschsprung's Disease Society, 7*(2), 8–9.

Motta, G.J. (1987). Life span changes: Implications for ostomy care. *Nursing Clinics of North America, 22*(2), 333–339.

Mullen, B.D., & McGinn, K.A. (1992). *The ostomy book.* Palo Alto, CA: Bull Publishing Co.

Perrone, P.V. (1996). Inflammatory bowel disease. In P. Jackson & J. Vessey (Eds.), *Primary care of the child with a chronic condition* (2nd ed., pp. 507–529). St. Louis, MO: Mosby-Yearbook.

Reilly, N.J. (1994). Advances in quality of life after cystectomy: Urinary diversions. *Innovations in Urological Nursing: Urological Diversions, 5*(2).

Rodriguez, D.B. (1982). Teaching the preschooler with two ostomies. *Journal of Enterostomal Therapy, 9*(1), 18–19.

RESPIRATORY CARE

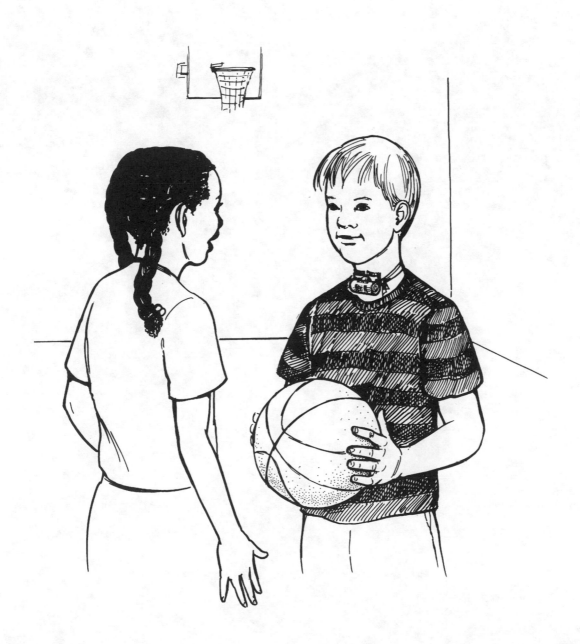

RESPIRATORY SYSTEM

STRUCTURE AND FUNCTION

The primary function of the respiratory system is the exchange of gases in the air with gases dissolved in the blood. Oxygen from the air is transferred to the blood, and carbon dioxide from the blood is removed to the air. Effective and efficient transfer of gases depends on all of the parts of the respiratory system. Chronic or acute disease of any of these parts may impair gas exchange. There are several parts to the respiratory system.

In the *upper airway*, air enters the lungs through the nose and mouth to reach the *pharynx* (i.e., back of the throat) and passes through the *larynx* (i.e., voice box) and into the *trachea* (i.e., windpipe).

As air enters the nose, hairs in the nostrils filter out the larger dust particles. Air then passes through the nose, where a large area of moist mucus membrane adds moisture and warms the air to body temperature. Air then passes through the larynx and down into the trachea. This passage of air through the larynx during inhalation (i.e., breathing in) and exhalation (i.e., breathing out) is necessary for normal speech production. *Mucus* comes from the tissues that line both the upper and lower airways. If mucus is not warmed and humidified, it can dry and thicken or harden, causing a blockage in the airway.

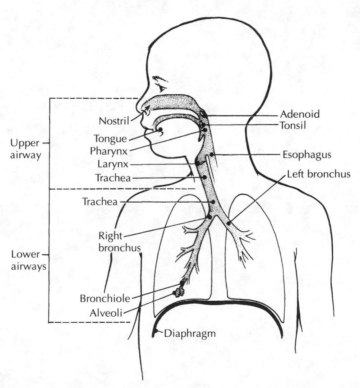

In the *lower airways*, the trachea divides into the two main *bronchi*. Each bronchus then subdivides into smaller bronchi, which in turn divide. This division into smaller and smaller airways continues many times. Finally, the *bronchioles* (i.e., small bronchi) end in the *alveoli*, where the exchange of oxygen and carbon dioxide takes place. The bronchi are lined with mucus and are covered with *cilia* (i.e., tiny hairs) that help remove particles of dust. All but the smallest airways also are surrounded by smooth muscle and can tighten and narrow if irritated (e.g., as in asthma).

Gas exchange takes place in the alveolus. The alveolus is only one cell thick. It is in contact with the blood so gas can diffuse from the blood to the alveolus or from the alveolus to the blood.

The *diaphragm* and *intercostal muscles* are the main muscles for normal breathing. The diaphragm is located below the lungs and is attached to the lower ribs and the spine. When it contracts, it pulls down, and air enters the respiratory system. The intercostal muscles connect nearby ribs and help to expand the lungs so air can enter the respiratory system.

The *heart* pumps blood to the lungs and to the body. If there is heart disease or disease of the *blood vessels* in the lungs, gas exchange may not be adequate, and the patient may require extra oxygen (see pp. 259–270).

DISORDERS AFFECTING THE RESPIRATORY SYSTEM

Diseases may affect any of the parts of the respiratory system and lead to ineffective gas exchange. Disorders that may chronically impair the respiratory system can be divided into several major categories. A student may be affected by one or more of these disorders. It is helpful, however, to think in terms of the major systems affected. Ongoing support of the respiratory system ranges from supplemental oxygen to full mechanical ventilation through a tracheostomy tube. How much support a person needs is a function of the major system involved and the severity of the disease. The following are some examples:

1. Disorders that affect the stimulus to breathe
    - Brain damage from trauma, drowning, suffocation, or difficulties at birth
    - Certain progressive neurological diseases

2. Disorders that affect the strength of the respiratory muscles
    - Progressive degenerative muscle diseases such as muscular dystrophy or spinal cord injuries

3. Disorders that affect the upper airway
    - Structural abnormalities of the oral or nasal cavity (e.g., cleft palate, choanal atresia [blocked nasal passages])
    - Abnormal development of the facial bones or muscles
    - Disorders affecting the normal coordination of the swallowing mechanism and the mechanisms that protect the airway from food or liquid
    - Conditions such as muscular dystrophy, brain damage, or progressive neurological diseases, which interfere with normal function of the esophagus
    - Abnormalities of the larynx, trachea, or bronchi, such as stenoses (narrowing), blockage (by tumor or swelling), or abnormally floppy airways

4. Disorders affecting the lower airways
    - Swelling, scarring, and other structural blockages in the trachea
    - Cystic fibrosis, which causes increased amounts of thick mucus in the lungs and airway
    - Asthma, which may also necessitate chronic oxygen use

5. Disorders of the alveoli
    - Pneumonia
    - Bronchopulmonary dysplasia
    - Pulmonary toxicity from cancer chemotherapy

Supplemental Oxygen Use

PURPOSE

Oxygen provides for body functions, relieves shortness of breath, and reduces the workload of the heart. Oxygen use is indicated for physical conditions in which a student is unable to get enough oxygen into the body or needs more oxygen, such as chronic lung conditions (e.g., bronchopulmonary dysplasia [BPD], cystic fibrosis [CF], heart problems).

SUGGESTED SETTINGS

When in contact with a student using oxygen, the following warning is in effect:

WARNING:

- **THERE SHOULD BE NO SMOKING, OPEN FLAME, OR HEAT SOURCE CLOSE TO THE OXYGEN; THESE MAY INCREASE THE RISK OF FIRE.**
- **EQUIPMENT AND OXYGEN SUPPLY MUST BE CHECKED AT LEAST DAILY, OR MORE OFTEN, DEPENDING ON THE EQUIPMENT.**

SUGGESTED PERSONNEL AND TRAINING

A health assessment must be completed by the school nurse. State nurse practice regulations should be consulted for guidance on delegating health care procedures.

The school nurse or other adult with proven competency-based training in appropriate techniques and problem management may administer oxygen through a nasal cannula or mask. Use of a tracheostomy collar may require a registered nurse or respiratory therapist with training, depending on the care needs of the student with a tracheostomy. Any school personnel who have regular contact with a student who requires oxygen must receive general training that covers the student's specific health care needs and potential problems and must understand how to implement the established emergency plan.

The basic skills checklists on pages 351–354 can be used as a foundation for competency-based training in appropriate techniques. Specific procedures for oxygen use are outlined step by step. Once the procedures have been mastered, the completed checklists serve as documentation of training.

THE INDIVIDUALIZED HEALTH CARE PLAN: ISSUES FOR SPECIAL CONSIDERATION

Each student's individualized health care plan (IHCP) must be tailored to the individual's needs. The following section covers the procedure for oxygen use and possible problems and emergencies that may arise. It is essential that this section be reviewed before writing the IHCP.

A sample plan is included in Chapter 6. It may be copied and used to develop a plan for each student. For a student who requires oxygen, the following items should receive particular attention:

- Student's underlying condition and possible problems associated with the condition or treatment
- Oxygen safety precautions including posting of "oxygen in use" warnings
- Spare oxygen supply and safe storage when not in use
- Adaptation of classroom for necessary equipment, storage, and transport (e.g., length of tubing, oxygen source)
- Signs and symptoms shown by the student when not receiving adequate oxygen (e.g., cyanosis, agitation, distress)
- Student's baseline status, including color, respiratory rate, pulse, and blood pressure
- Student's ability to request oxygen or assistance
- Percentage and/or liter flow of oxygen prescribed (for daily use and emergencies)
- Access to oxygen supply throughout school building (i.e., portable or stationary)

- Latex allergy alert (see Chapter 5)
- Universal precautions (Anticipating the tasks to be done, the risk involved, and the personal protective equipment needed will enhance protection of both the caregiver and student)

OXYGEN SAFETY PRECAUTIONS

- Do not smoke or allow open flames near oxygen. Store oxygen away from heaters, radiators, and hot sun.

- Never permit oil, grease, or highly flammable material to come into contact with oxygen cylinders, liquid oxygen, valves, regulators, or fittings. Do not lubricate with oil or other flammable substances, and do not handle equipment with greasy hands or rags.

- Never put anything over an oxygen gas tank.

- Know the name of the home oxygen supply company contact person. Have the telephone number posted in an obvious place and on the emergency plan.

- Return any defective equipment to the authorized company for replacement.

- Have spare oxygen readily accessible based on the student's needs. This should be stored safely in a secure place.

- Keep extra tubing and tank equipment (e.g., wrenches) in an easily accessible place.

- Protect dry regulator from becoming dislodged. A hissing noise may indicate a leak in system.

- Be sure that the tank (when using oxygen gas) is securely placed in its stand and cannot fall or be knocked over.

- Be careful that the oxygen tubing does not become kinked, blocked, punctured, or disconnected.

- Use only the flowmeter setting prescribed by the student's physician.

- Notify the fire department that oxygen is in use in the school.

- Secure the oxygen tank or liquid system for transport in an upright position. Make sure the gauge and valve stem are protected from damage.

EQUIPMENT

OXYGEN SOURCES

Oxygen gas Pure oxygen gas is stored under pressure in a metal tank or cylinder. Tanks come in different sizes, ranging from small (portable) to large (stationary). The tank size used by the student depends on the amount of oxygen flow needed. The amount of oxygen available in the tank is indicated by the pressure gauge on the tank.

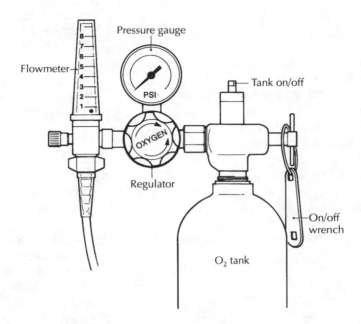

Oxygen concentrator This is an electronically powered machine that removes nitrogen from room air and concentrates the remaining oxygen for delivery to the student. This type of system delivers a lower concentration of oxygen at low liter flows. An oxygen concentrator requires an electrical outlet and is not portable. Some units may contain a back-up battery in the event of a power failure. Each unit has an air filter that requires periodic cleaning.

Additional equipment for oxygen concentrator systems includes the following:

- Humidification source
- Oxygen tubing, mask, cannula, or tracheostomy collar
- Emergency oxygen tank for power failure

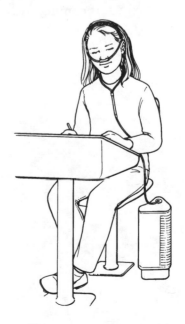

Oxygen liquid Oxygen liquid systems utilize a thermal storage container that keeps the pure oxygen as a liquid at –300° Fahrenheit. A smaller portable container (i.e., thermos) usually is used to deliver the oxygen to the student. Depending on the prescribed liter flow for the student, the thermos may require refilling from the larger storage tank.

Additional equipment for both gas and liquid systems includes the following:

- Tank stand or carrier
- Regulator with pressure gauge and flowmeter
- Wrench for gas tank valve
- Humidification source
- Oxygen tubing, mask, cannula, or tracheostomy collar

Respiratory Care

Procedure for Using a Nasal Cannula

A nasal cannula is used to deliver a low-to-moderate concentration of oxygen. It can be used as long as nasal passages are open; a deviated septum, swelling of the passage, mucus, or polyps may interfere with adequate oxygen intake. A nasal cannula is easy to use. Eating, talking, and coughing are possible.

PROCEDURE

1. Wash hands.

2. Assemble equipment
   - Oxygen source and backup
   - Cannula and tubing (plus extra connecting tubing)
   - Humidity source, if needed
   - Adaptor for connect tubing
   - Scissors
3. Explain procedure at the student's level of understanding.

4. Wash hands.
5. Attach cannula tubing to oxygen source securely.

6. Set liter flow on the flowmeter as prescribed by the physician. **Never change this setting without first contacting the physician**. Turn on the oxygen source.

7. Check cannula prongs to make sure that oxygen is coming out.

POINTS TO REMEMBER

Anticipating the tasks to be done, the risk involved, and the personal protective equipment needed will enhance protection of both the caregiver and student.

Extra connecting tubing may be used to increase mobility.

Scissors are used to cut adaptor to size.
By encouraging the student to assist in the procedure, the caregiver is helping the student to achieve maximum self-care skills.

Make sure a proper adaptor is available for the oxygen source. Check that tank has enough oxygen. Attach humidifier, if ordered. Check that all pieces are secured tightly to prevent leaks.
A highly visible information card stating oxygen liter flow must be attached to the regulator. A too-high oxygen flow may irritate the nose. Oxygen liter flow can be ordered as a set liter flow rate (e.g., 3 liters per minute) or as a range (e.g., 3–5 liters per minute) based on student's needs. For emergencies, see page 269.
Hold them up to your hand or check to feel for flow coming out. If no flow is felt, check oxygen supply, connections, flow rate, and tubing for obstruction.

8. Insert prongs into student's nose. **Make sure both prongs are in the nostrils.**

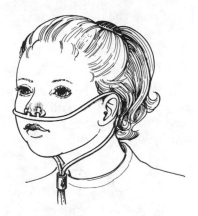

9. Wash hands.
10. Document procedure and problems on student's log sheet.

Gently insert prongs into the student's nostrils (one in each side). Loop the tubing over each ear then under the chin; secure by sliding the clasp up under the chin. Make sure that it is comfortable for the student. If the student is not comfortable, the cannula tubing may be secured behind the head rather than under the chin.

Report to family any changes in student's pattern.

PROCEDURE FOR USING AN OXYGEN MASK

An oxygen mask can deliver higher or lower concentration of oxygen than the nasal cannula and is useful when nasal passages are blocked.

PROCEDURE

1. Wash hands.

2. Assemble equipment:
   • Oxygen source and backup
   • Appropriate size mask and tubing (plus a spare)
   • Extra connecting tubing plus adaptor
   • Humidity source, if needed

3. Explain procedure at the student's level of understanding.

4. Set oxygen flow on flowmeter to the rate prescribed by the physician. **Do not change setting without first contacting the physician.** Turn on the oxygen source.

5. Check that oxygen flow is coming out of the mask.

6. Place the mask over the student's nose and mouth.

7. Wash hands.
8. Document procedure and problems on student's log sheet.

POINTS TO REMEMBER

Anticipating the tasks to be done, the risk involved, and the personal protective equipment needed will enhance protection of both the caregiver and student.

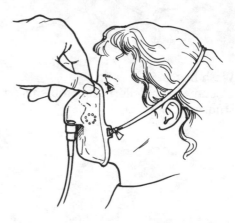

By encouraging the student to assist in the procedure, the caregiver helps the student achieve maximum self-care skills.

Excessive flow rates may cause irritation to the skin. A highly visible information card stating oxygen liter flow must be attached to the regulator. Oxygen liter flow can be ordered as a set liter flow rate (e.g., 3 liters per minute) or as a range (e.g., 3–5 liters per minute) based on student's needs. For emergencies, see page 269.

Hold mask up to your cheek to feel gas flow. If no flow is felt, check oxygen supply, connections, flow rate, and tubing for obstruction.

Tighten the elastic band over the student's head and pinch mask over the bridge of the nose for a good fit. Make sure that the student is comfortable with the mask and that the mask does not touch the eyes.

Report to family any changes in student's usual pattern.

PROCEDURE FOR USING A TRACHEOSTOMY COLLAR

The tracheostomy collar is one means of delivering oxygen or humidified air to the tracheostomy. The tracheostomy collar may be used with a humidifying device and tubing to prevent dry and/or thick secretions from plugging the tracheostomy and to administer oxygen to the student.

PROCEDURE

1. Wash hands.

2. Assemble equipment:
   - Extra nebulizer/humidifier
   - Heating device, if indicated
   - Wide bore tubing
   - Tracheostomy collar
   - Oxygen tubing
   - Nipple adaptor
   - Oxygen source, if needed

POINTS TO REMEMBER

Anticipating the tasks to be done, the risk involved, and the personal protective equipment needed will enhance protection of both the caregiver and student.

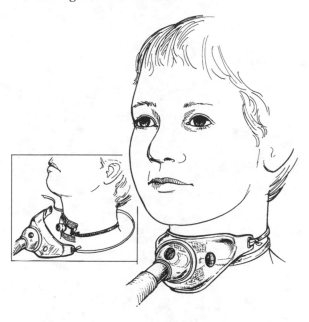

3. Explain procedure at the student's level of understanding.

4. Set up humidification device.

5. Dial percent of oxygen as ordered.

6. Connect to compressed air/oxygen source. Turn on oxygen source. **Do not change setting without first contacting the physician.**

7. Connect to heater and/or humidifier if required.

8. Place one end of wide bore tubing on the collar and the other on the humidifier or heater.

By encouraging the student to assist in the procedure, the caregiver helps the student achieve maximum self-care skills.

There are several types of humidification devices. Check student-specific guidelines and set up according to specific instructions.

Some students may require only compressed air.

A highly visible information card stating oxygen liter flow must be attached to the regulator. Oxygen liter flow can be ordered as a set liter flow rate (e.g., 3 liters per minute) or as a range (e.g., 3–5 liters per minute) based on student's needs. For emergencies, see page 269.

Some students may use cool mist. With prolonged humidification, moisture collection in the tubing can block the flow of air/oxygen and may require periodic removal.

9. With compressed air/oxygen source on, look at mist at the end of tubing. You should see a fine mist when held up to the light.

If this is not present, check that all connections are on securely and compressed air/oxygen is flowing. Turn on higher flow, then return to flow ordered to see if mist is present.

10. Place collar on student's neck over tracheostomy tube in the midline.

Adjust tracheostomy collar so that it is snug but not uncomfortable for student.

11. Wash hands.

12. Document procedure and problems on student's log sheet.

Report to family any change in student's usual pattern.

Respiratory Care

Possible Problems that Require Immediate Attention for Students Requiring Oxygen

Observations

The student shows any of the following signs of respiratory distress:
- Shortness of breath or rapid breathing rate
- Agitation
- Blueness or pallor of the lips, nails, or earlobes
- Pulling in of the muscles at the neck or chest
- Confusion, dizziness, or headache
- Rapid or pounding pulse

Reason/Action

Stay calm and reassure student.

Check student:
- *Position student to open airway. Make sure mouth, nose, or tracheostomy tube is not obstructed by food or mucus.*
- *Check tracheostomy tube placement.*
- *Make sure collar is not out of position or obstructing tracheostomy tube.*

Check equipment (check oxygen flow—if flow is weak or inadequate):
- *Make sure tank is not empty or defective. If so, replace with back-up tank.*
- *Make sure valve, regulator, and flowmeters are on proper settings.*
- *Make sure tubing is not blocked or kinked.*
- *Check all connections from oxygen source to student.*
- *Make sure tubing, mask, cannula, and collar are not blocked.*
- *Make sure humidifier bottle is properly attached.*
- *Make sure tubing is not obstructed by water collecting in it from condensed mist. Empty water from tubing frequently when using mist.*

May indicate the need for increased oxygen flow. Prior to school entry, obtain physician order for emergency oxygen use (percent and flow rate).

The equipment and oxygen flow are adequate, but the student continues to show signs of respiratory distress, becomes unconscious, or has a respiratory arrest.

Initiate emergency procedure and notify family. Begin cardiopulmonary resuscitation if needed.

A Possible Problem that Does Not Require Immediate Attention

Observation

Redness, dryness, or bleeding of the skin

Reason/Action

May be due to irritation from the device or from insufficient humidity.

Notify family to discuss problem with physician.

Never use powders or petroleum products on the student's face.

General Information Sheet

Students Who Use Supplemental Oxygen

Dear (teacher, lunch aide, bus driver):

_____ [Student's name] has a condition that requires the use of additional oxygen. When used appropriately, this is a safe method that allows the student to be normally active. Oxygen is kept in a small tank or thermos and goes everywhere the student does. The oxygen is given to the student through a mask or small plastic tubing close to the student's nose. Students with tracheostomies receive oxygen through a collar that fits over the tube. Some students need oxygen continuously, while others may need it only intermittently.

Depending on the student's condition, she or he may be able to participate in many school activities with some modifications, which are determined by the school staff, the family, physician, and school nurse. **There should be no smoking or open flames in the room in which oxygen is being used. The oxygen tanks should not come into contact with oil, grease, greasy hands, or rags.**

It is recommended that you participate in cardiopulmonary resuscitation training. It is also important to learn how to recognize the warning signs of breathing problems.

The following staff members have been trained to deal with any problems that may arise with this student:

_____

_____

_____

For more information about oxygen use or the student's needs, consult the school nurse or the family.

Respiratory Care

TRACHEOSTOMY

PURPOSE

A tracheostomy is a surgical opening in the neck into the trachea (windpipe), which allows air to go in and out of the lungs. The opening in the neck is called a stoma. A metal or plastic tube, called a tracheostomy tube, may be inserted through the stoma into the trachea; some students may not need a tracheostomy tube. There are various types of tracheostomy tubes that are held in place with a tie around the neck.

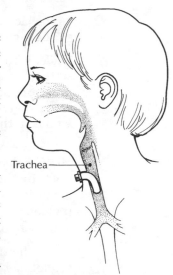

Trachea

Some students will have a tracheostomy because of an injury or condition that requires bypassing the normal breathing passages. Others require a tracheostomy because of neurological, muscular, or other conditions that make it difficult for them to breathe effectively or to clear secretions or mucus out of their breathing passages without assistance. A tracheostomy allows long-term access to a ventilator or respirator (i.e., breathing machine) and an easy way to clear the trachea of mucus. Many students with tracheostomies are able to speak. Most are able to eat and drink by mouth but may need dietary modifications.

SUGGESTED SETTINGS

Students with tracheostomies, in most cases, can attend classes in general classrooms. Some may need to be accompanied by a trained caregiver at all times in the educational setting or during transport. Many students with tracheostomies participate in school activities with modifications that should be determined by the family, physician, school nurse, and school staff. **All staff in contact with students with tracheostomies should have specialized cardiopulmonary resuscitation training. They should be able to recognize signs of breathing difficulty and should know how to activate the emergency plan for their setting.**

Students with tracheostomies should avoid areas with a lot of dust or other airborne particles, such as chalk dust. Such areas should be avoided because the air the student breathes enters the lungs directly without being filtered, humidified, and warmed by the nose and mouth.

Regular tracheostomy care prescribed to maintain the student's health and function should be done at home. If additional regular care is required, however, it should be done in a private, clean area, such as the health room. In an emergency, care should be given wherever the student is. Therefore, it is imperative that a complete set of equipment for tracheostomy care, including all items in the go-bag (p. 355) and suction machine be with the student at all times.

SUGGESTED PERSONNEL AND TRAINING

A health assessment must be completed by the school nurse. State nurse practice regulations should be consulted for guidance on delegating health care procedures.

Tracheal care for students who require care in school, such as suctioning, saline instillation, use of a tracheostomy collar, or other daily care, should be provided by a registered nurse or licensed respiratory therapist unless state medical and nursing practice standards specify otherwise. These caregivers should have proven, competency-based training in appropriate techniques and problem management. **All staff in contact with students with tracheostomies should have specialized cardiopulmonary resuscitation training. They should be able to recognize signs of breathing difficulty and should know how to activate the emergency plan for their setting.**

There are different service delivery models available for tracheostomy care that involve nonmedical personnel. The recommendations herein are conservative and are based on the following issues:

- The lack of standardization in nursing and medical practice
- The highly technical nature and potential risk to the student

Under some circumstances, after a student with a tracheostomy has been in the school setting for a period of time and it is clear that the student's medical condition is stable, it may be appropriate for the health care team and the family to consider using a nonmedical caregiver who has received appropriate training and supervision by a school nurse who is in the building at all times.

Some students need less frequent care or require no routine tracheostomy care at all. The decision regarding the placement of the caregiver for such a student must be made by the family, physician, and school nurse and be based on the student's medical condition, tracheal care needs, and adaptation to school. Other considerations should include the varied locations of the student in the school, the school nurse-to-pupil ratio, and a school nurse being in the building at all times.

If the trained caregiver and back-up personnel are unable to be available on a given school day, the student should not attend school. However, an optional arrangement could be made between the school and the family so someone from the family would be available to attend school to function as the caregiver for the student.

Any school personnel who have regular contact with a student with a tracheostomy must receive general training that covers the student's specific health care needs, potential problems, and how to implement the established emergency plan.

The basic skills checklists on pages 356–358 can be used as a foundation for competency-based training in appropriate techniques and problem management. They outline specific procedures step by step. Once the procedures have been mastered, the completed checklists serve as a documentation of training.

THE INDIVIDUALIZED HEALTH CARE PLAN: ISSUES FOR SPECIAL CONSIDERATION

Each student's individualized health care plan (IHCP) must be tailored to the individual's needs. The following sections cover the procedures for tracheostomy care and possible problems and emergencies that may arise. It is essential that these sections be reviewed before writing the IHCP.

A sample plan is included in Chapter 6. It may be copied and used to develop a plan for each student. For a student who requires tracheal care, the following items should receive particular attention:

- Student's underlying condition and possible problems associated with the condition or treatment
- Student's baseline status (e.g., color, respiratory rate, pulse, blood pressure, secretions)
- Student's care requirements (e.g., suctioning)
- Student's ability to request assistance
- Student's proneness to emergencies
- Signs and symptoms of respiratory distress shown by this student
- Type of tracheostomy tube used (e.g., inner cannula, cuffed)
- Accessibility to equipment and back-up equipment
- An alternate means of warming and moisturizing the air may be necessary at times to prevent the mucus from becoming too thick
- Student's need for additional fluids
- Student's speech may be affected—alternative means of communication may be necessary (i.e., American Sign Language, Passey-Muir valve, communication board)
- Personnel and equipment needed for transportation (e.g., travel bag)
- Availability of caregivers

- Staffing needs to provide care for the student (one to one)
- Means of communication (e.g., walkie-talkies, intercoms, telephones) among different areas of the school
- Latex allergy alert (see Chapter 5)
- Universal precautions (Anticipating the tasks to be done, the risk involved, and the personal protective equipment needed will enhance protection of both the caregiver and student.)

Do not use powders; aerosols (i.e., room deodorizers); small particles, such as sand, glitter, lint, chalk dust, and animal hair; small pieces of food and water; or glue or chemicals with strong fumes near a student with a tracheostomy. Students who may have accidental contact with any of these potential hazards should have some kind of protective covering for the tracheostomy.

Required Equipment for Tracheostomy Care

REQUIRED EQUIPMENT

POINTS TO REMEMBER

Anticipating the tasks to be done, the risk involved, and the personal protective equipment needed will enhance protection of both the caregiver and student.

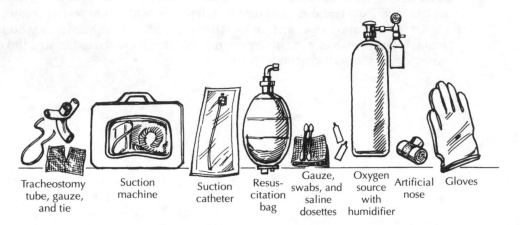

Tracheostomy tube, gauze, and tie | Suction machine | Suction catheter | Resuscitation bag | Gauze, swabs, and saline dosettes | Oxygen source with humidifier | Artificial nose | Gloves

- Spare tracheostomy tube and obturator with gauze pads and ties or Velcro collar
- Scissors
- Suction machine
- Equipment for suctioning (e.g., suction catheters)
- Sterile or clean gauze, cotton-tip swabs, if required
- Pipe cleaners
- Saline dosettes if prescribed
- Manual resuscitator with adaptor

- One half hydrogen peroxide and one half normal saline or one half distilled water
- Device to deliver humidity, if prescribed
- Device to deliver oxygen, if prescribed
- Device, such as an artificial nose, for protecting tracheostomy from dry or cold air and dust or other particles

- Sterile or disposable gloves, per student-specific guidelines
- Manual suction device
- Syringe to inflate or deflate tracheostomy cuff

Not all tracheostomy tubes require obturator use.

This equipment must accompany the student at all times, *including transport and classroom activities. A backpack or other carrying device could serve as a travel bag. This equipment should be checked daily.*

It is encouraged that a manual resuscitation bag with adaptor be obtained if the student does not have one at home to bring to school.

The artificial nose must be changed if it appears to be saturated with moisture or secretions. ***Do not rinse.*** *Discard if saturated.*
Refer to universal precautions in Chapter 5.

Back-up suction if battery fails.

Respiratory Care

Possible Problems that Require Immediate Attention for Students with Tracheostomies

Observations

DO NOT LEAVE STUDENT ALONE.
The student shows any of the following signs of respiratory distress:
- Coughing
- Color changes
- Wheezing or noisy breathing
- Agitation
- Retraction

Tracheostomy tube is dislodged

Suction catheter will not pass or there is no air movement from tracheostomy

Aspiration of foreign material (e.g., food, sand) into tracheostomy

Reason/Action

This may be due to a plugged tracheostomy tube from mucus, aspiration of foreign matter, accidental decannulation, or dislodged tracheostomy tube.

Reassure student. Check air movement from tracheostomy. Check placement of tracheostomy tube. It tracheostomy tube is in place, suction.

Reposition tracheostomy tube, if possible. If unable to reposition tube, insert new (spare) tracheostomy tube. Check air movement. Give breaths with resuscitation bag, if indicated. Administer oxygen if prescribed in emergency plan, and initiate emergency plan and begin cardiopulmonary resuscitation if necessary. Notify family and physician.

Change inner cannula if present or replace tracheostomy tube. Check air movement. Give breaths with resuscitation bag, if necessary. Give oxygen, if prescribed in emergency plan, and initiate emergency plan and begin cardiopulmonary resuscitation if necessary. Notify family and physician.

Suction first. Do not give breath with resuscitation bag. This may force aspirate into lungs.
Give breaths with resuscitation bag after initial suctioning.

Check air movement.

If tracheostomy tube remains blocked by foreign material, change tracheostomy tube. Check air movement.

Add saline and give breaths with resuscitation bag. Repeat suctioning. Repeat above steps until aspirated secretions are clear or gone.

Give breaths with resuscitation bag if indicated.

Administer oxygen if prescribed in emergency plan.

Bronchospasm (wheezing) may also occur. The student may require medication.

Respiratory distress or arrest can occur with any aspiration. Be prepared to initiate emergency plan. Begin cardiopulmonary resuscitation after suctioning, if needed. Notify family and physician.

Potential Problems that
Do Not Require Immediate Attention

Observations	*Reason/Action*
Increased secretions or thicker than usual mucus	*May require more frequent suctioning. These changes, or yellow or green mucus, may indicate infection. This should be documented in the daily log, and the family should be informed. Thicker mucus also may be a sign of insufficient humidity.*
Fever	*May be a sign of respiratory infection. Notify family.*
Redness or crusting at the stoma	*May be due to a tracheal infection. The site should be thoroughly cleaned and the problem documented in the daily log and reported to the family.*
Bleeding or pain at stoma site	*May be due to infection or trauma. Notify family.*
Bloody secretions from tracheostomy	*May be due to infection or trauma from vigorous suctioning. Notify family.*

Respiratory Care

General Information Sheet

Students with Tracheostomies

Dear (teacher, lunch aide, bus driver):

_____ [Student's name] has a condition that requires a tracheostomy. This is an opening in the neck into the windpipe, which allows the student to breathe if he or she is unable to breathe well through the nose or mouth. The opening, or stoma, may have a metal or a plastic tracheostomy tube inside to keep it open and to allow air to pass in and out of the windpipe and lungs. The tube is secured by trach ties that are tied around the student's neck. The student's tracheostomy tube may be covered with a device that provides humidity or oxygen. Some people have nothing covering the opening of the tube.

Most students with tracheostomies are able to eat and drink by mouth. If the student cannot eat or drink, his or her physician will give you specific instructions. Many students are able to speak normally. If the student's condition prevents him or her from speaking, other means of communication will be used. Not all students who have tracheostomies require routine tracheostomy care in school. Many students can manage their care, but some who require regular tracheostomy care such as suctioning, a procedure to remove mucus from the tracheostomy tube, will have a trained caregiver with them.

Most students with tracheostomies are able to participate in school activities. A team including the student's family and educational and health personnel will help develop a specific health care plan. Classroom issues will be addressed in the care plan, such as the accommodation of health care during the school day with minimal interference, the avoidance of activities (e.g., swimming) that could affect the function of the tracheostomy, and avoidance of infectious exposure such as colds.

The following staff members have been trained to deal with any problems that may arise with this student:

_____

_____

_____

It is recommended that you participate in cardiopulmonary resuscitation training and request specialized training for people with tracheostomies.

For more information about this procedure or the student's needs, consult the school nurse or family.

TRACHEAL SUCTIONING

PURPOSE

Tracheal suctioning is a means of clearing the airway of secretions or mucus. This is accomplished by using a vacuum-type device through the tracheostomy. Tracheal suctioning is performed when a person cannot adequately clear secretions on his or her own. Indications for suctioning include the following:

- Noisy, rattling breathing sounds
- Secretions (i.e., mucus) visible and filling opening of tracheostomy
- Signs of respiratory distress (e.g., difficulty breathing, agitation, paleness, excessive coughing, cyanosis [blueness], nasal flaring, retracting)
- No air moving through tracheostomy (listen for sounds)
- Before eating or drinking if congested
- After respiratory treatments (e.g., inhalation therapy, assisted breathing with a self-inflating manual resuscitator), chest percussion, and drainage

Depending on the student's age, he or she may be able to request suctioning when needed or assist with the procedure.

SUGGESTED SETTINGS FOR NONEMERGENCY SUCTIONING

Designate a clean area outside the classroom, if possible, for suctioning. Suctioning can be a noisy procedure and may be distracting and disruptive to the rest of the class.

If an electrically powered suction machine is used, the setting must have an accessible, working, grounded electric outlet.

SUGGESTED PERSONNEL AND TRAINING

A health assessment must be completed by the school nurse. State nurse practice regulations should be consulted for guidance on delegating health care procedures.

Tracheal suctioning should be performed by a registered nurse or a licensed respiratory therapist with proven competency-based training in appropriate techniques and problem management, unless state medical and nursing practice standards specify otherwise. **All staff in contact with students with tracheostomies should have specialized cardiopulmonary resuscitation training. They should be able to recognize signs of breathing difficulty and should know how to activate the emergency plan for their setting.**

If the trained caregiver and back-up personnel are unable to be available on a given school day, the student should not attend school. However, an optional arrangement may be made between the school and the family so someone from the family would be available to attend school to function as the caregiver for the student.

Any school personnel who have regular contact with a student who requires tracheal suctioning must receive general training that covers the student's specific health care needs, potential problems, and how to implement the established emergency plan.

The basic skills checklist on pages 358–359 can be used as a foundation for competency-based training in appropriate techniques. It outlines procedures step by step. Once the procedures have been mastered, the completed checklist serves as documentation of training.

THE INDIVIDUALIZED HEALTH CARE PLAN: ISSUES FOR SPECIAL CONSIDERATION

Each student's individualized health care plan (IHCP) must be tailored to the individual's needs. The following section covers the procedure for tracheal suctioning and possible problems and emergencies that may arise. It is essential that this section be reviewed before writing the IHCP.

A sample plan is included in Chapter 6. It may be copied and used to develop a plan for each student. For a student who requires tracheal suctioning, the following items should receive particular attention:

- Student's underlying condition and possible problems associated with the condition or treatment
- Student's baseline status (e.g., color, respiratory rate, pulse, color and consistency of secretions, usual frequency of suctioning, usual indications for suctioning)
- Student's ability to request suctioning or do it independently
- Availability and use of back-up manual suctioning equipment
- Accessibility of equipment
- Signs and symptoms of respiratory distress shown by the student (e.g., cyanosis, agitation)
- Need for saline instillation
- Need for breaths with a manual resuscitation bag
- Length of tracheostomy tube measured to determine depth of suctioning
- Latex allergy alert (see Chapter 5)
- Universal precautions (Anticipating the tasks to be done, the risk involved, and the personal protective equipment needed will enhance protection of both the caregiver and student.)

Respiratory Care

PROCEDURE FOR TRACHEAL SUCTIONING

PROCEDURE

All equipment for suctioning must be assembled and ready for immediate use at all times and checked daily by the trained caregiver. If the equipment is not present or not functional, the student should not attend school.

1. Wash hands.

2. Assemble the equipment and materials on a small, clean work surface:

POINTS TO REMEMBER

Anticipating the tasks to be done, the risk involved, and the personal protective equipment needed will enhance protection of both the caregiver and student.

A disposable, waterproof underpad may be used.

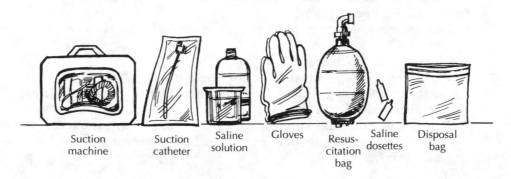

| Suction machine | Suction catheter | Saline solution | Gloves | Resus-citation bag | Saline dosettes | Disposal bag |

- Suctioning machine and manual backup

*All students **must** have a means of suctioning (e.g., a portable suction machine or manual device) that can accompany them during all school activities as well as transport. A manual means of suctioning also must be available as a backup at all times for those students who use suction machines.*

- Suction catheter of prescribed size

To determine how deep to insert the catheter, it is essential to know the length of the tracheostomy tube. This information is written on the package or may be obtained from the family or primary caregiver.

- Sterile saline or sterile water to clear catheter
- Container for saline or water
- Disposable gloves
- Self-inflating manual resuscitation bag with tracheostomy adaptor
- Saline dosettes (for instillation) if indicated
- Plastic bag for disposal of materials
- Syringe to inflate and deflate cuff, if used

Refer to universal precautions in Chapter 5.

3. Position student as recommended/ordered.

When at school, most students are suctioned while seated upright.

4. Explain procedure at student's level of understanding.

By encouraging the student to assist in the procedure, the caregiver helps the student achieve maximum self-care skills.

5. Wash hands.
6. Turn on suction machine and check for function.

7. Encourage student to cough to expel secretions.

Coughing may eliminate need for suctioning.

8. Open suction catheter or kit.

Peel paper back without touching the inside of the package to maintain sterility.

9. Open saline dosette if instillation is ordered.
10. Fill container with sterile saline or sterile water.

This will be used to moisten the catheter and to clear out secretions in the catheter.

11. Put on gloves.

The dominant hand should remain "clean." It should not touch anything but the catheter. The nondominant hand should be used to turn on switches or touch other objects.

12. Holding the end of the suction catheter in dominant hand, attach it to the suction machine tubing (held in other hand).

Leave the other end of catheter in its covering.

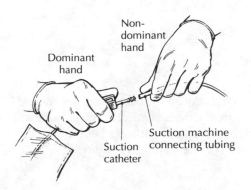

13. Turn on machine to appropriate vacuum setting (if machine has vacuum setting) for student.

This should be ordered by physician.

14. Encourage student to cough and to take a deep breath if possible. If prescribed, manually ventilate with resuscitation bag.

Coughing helps to bring secretions up toward the tracheostomy. By taking a deep breath (or manually ventilating), the student will get more oxygen into his or her lungs. This will also help to loosen secretions.

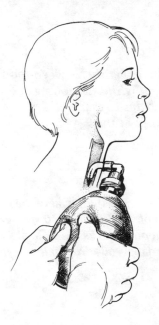

15. Hold suction catheter 2–3 inches from tip with dominant hand and insert tip in sterile saline or sterile water.

16. Grasp catheter connection with other hand; cover vent hole with thumb to suction a small amount of saline through catheter.

This tests that suction is functioning.

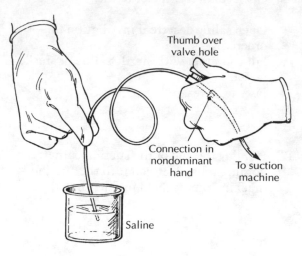

17. With thumb off vent hole, gently and quickly insert catheter into tracheostomy. Do not insert catheter beyond the distal end of the tracheostomy tube.

If the catheter is inserted too deeply, this can cause irritation/injury to the trachea, as well as bronchospasm. Coughing indicates that the suction catheter possibly has passed the end of the tracheostomy tube.

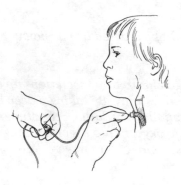

18. Cover vent hole with thumb while withdrawing catheter.

Rotate catheter gently between thumb and index finger while suctioning and withdrawing. This helps to reach all secretions in the tracheostomy tube.

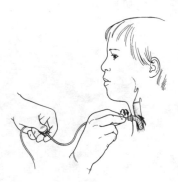

Each insertion and withdrawal of the catheter must be completed within 5–10 seconds. Prolonged suctioning blocks the student's airway and can cause a dangerous drop in the oxygen level.

19. Allow student to breathe or give breaths with resuscitator bag between suctioning passes. Suction saline again through catheter to rinse secretions from catheter and tubing.

The student needs to clear lungs of carbon dioxide and get new oxygen/air into lungs.

20. If prescribed, insert several drops of saline into tracheostomy with nondominant hand. Manually ventilate with resuscitation bag to disperse saline, if ordered.

This helps to loosen and thin out thick or dry secretions.

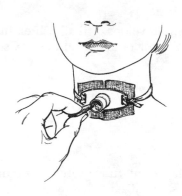

21. If moist, gurgling noises or whistling sounds are heard or if mucus is seen at the tracheostomy opening, repeat suctioning procedure (Steps 14–20).

If appropriate, ask the student if he or she needs repeat suctioning.

22. Suction the nose and then the back of mouth if indicated after completion of tracheal suctioning.

If the nose and mouth are suctioned, the catheter cannot be reused to suction the tracheostomy.

23. For each suctioning session, a new catheter should be used.

Consult family and physician for student-specific use.

24. Disconnect catheter from suction tubing. Wrap catheter around gloved hand. Pull gloves off inside out.
25. Discard used suction catheter in appropriate receptacle. Wash hands.

Refer to universal precautions in Chapter 5.

26. Note color, consistency (e.g., thin, thick), and quantity of secretions.

Report any changes from student's usual pattern to family.

27. Document procedure on student's log sheet.
28. Be sure suction equipment and supplies are restocked and checked daily and are ready for immediate use.

Possible Problems When Suctioning

Observations

The student develops difficulty breathing during suctioning or is not relieved by suctioning

The tracheostomy tube or inner cannula becomes dislodged

Bleeding occurs during suctioning:
- The secretions become blood-tinged and the student is not in respiratory distress

- A large amount of blood is suctioned from the tracheostomy or the student develops respiratory distress while being suctioned

Bronchospasm occurs during suctioning

Reason/Action

Do not leave student alone. Reassure student.

If tracheostomy tube is blocked (suction catheter will not pass), change inner cannula, if present, or replace entire tracheostomy tube.

Give breaths with resuscitation bag.

Give oxygen.

Reposition using gentle pressure. If unable to reposition tube, insert new tube. Be prepared to initiate emergency plan.

Stop suctioning.

Check vacuum pressure setting. Adjust to lower setting, if appropriate. Continue suctioning as necessary to clear the airway. Use the manual resuscitation bag and oxygen if needed.

Initiate the emergency plan and begin cardiopulmonary resuscitation if necessary.

Reassure student.

May be due to excessive suctioning. Allow student to calm him- or herself. If unable to remove catheter, disconnect from suction tubing and hold oxygen near end of suction catheter. When bronchospasm relaxes, remove catheter. If bronchospasm persists, student may require medication. Notify family and physician.

Respiratory Care

General Information Sheet

Students Who Need Suctioning

Dear (teacher, lunch aide, bus driver):

_____ [Student's name] has a condition that requires suctioning. Suctioning helps the student breathe better by clearing secretions/mucus from the airway. Depending on the student's age, he or she may be able to request suctioning when needed or assist in the procedure.

A student needing suctioning will have the necessary equipment at all times.

Most students who need suctioning are able to participate in school activities. A team including the students, parents, and educational and health personnel will help develop a specific health care plan.

The following staff members have been trained to deal with any problems that may arise with this student:

_____

_____

_____

For more information about suctioning or the student's needs, consult the school nurse or family.

Tracheostomy Tube Changes

PURPOSE

Tracheostomy tubes are routinely changed to prevent mucus from building up within the tubing. Mucus may block the tube and prevent air from entering the lungs. The tube also may need to be changed if it is blocked or accidentally dislodged. **In a school setting, this procedure should be done only in an emergency situation.**

SUGGESTED SETTINGS

Routine tracheostomy tube changes are performed in the home. This is ideally done when the student has an empty stomach and when the airway is relatively free of mucus. If a tracheostomy tube plugs (becomes blocked) or comes out, the tube should be changed or reinserted wherever the student is, even if conditions are not ideal.

SUGGESTED PERSONNEL AND TRAINING

A health assessment must be completed by the school nurse. State nurse practice regulations should be consulted for guidance on delegating health care procedures.

Tracheostomy tube changes should be performed by a registered nurse or a respiratory therapist with proven competency-based training in appropriate techniques and problem management, unless state medical and nursing practice standards specify otherwise. **All staff in contact with students with tracheostomies should have specialized cardiopulmonary resuscitation training. They should be able to recognize signs of breathing difficulty and should know how to activate the emergency plan for their setting.**

If the trained caregiver(s) and back-up personnel are unavailable on a given school day, the student should not attend school. However, an optional arrangement may be made between the school and the family so someone from the family would be available to attend school to function as the caregiver for the student.

Any school personnel who have regular contact with a student who requires a possible emergency tracheostomy tube change must receive general training that covers the student's specific health care needs, potential problems, and how to implement the established emergency plan.

The basic skills checklist on pages 361–362 can be used as a foundation for competency-based training in appropriate techniques and problem management. It outlines specific procedures step by step. Once the procedures have been mastered, the completed checklist serves as a documentation of training.

THE INDIVIDUALIZED HEALTH CARE PLAN: ISSUES FOR SPECIAL CONSIDERATION

Each student's individualized health care plan (IHCP) must be tailored to the individual's needs. The following section covers the procedure for tracheostomy tube changes as well as possible problems and emergencies that may arise. It is essential that this section be reviewed before writing the IHCP.

A sample plan is included in Chapter 6. It may be copied and used to develop a plan for each student. For a student who requires tracheostomy tube changes, the following items should receive particular attention:

- Student's need for support during reinsertion
- Student's underlying condition and possible problems associated with the condition or treatment (e.g., tracheal stenosis)
- Student's baseline status (e.g., color, respiratory rate, pulse)
- Type and size of tracheostomy tube (e.g., inner cannula, cuffed)

- Signs and symptoms of respiratory distress (e.g., cyanosis, agitation)
- Student's ability to request assistance
- Student's ability to breathe without a tracheostomy tube
- Difficulty with reinsertion of a dislodged tracheostomy tube
- Latex allergy alert (see Chapter 5)
- Universal precautions (Anticipating the tasks to be done, the risk involved, and the personal protective equipment needed will enhance protection of both the caregiver and student.)

PROCEDURE FOR CHANGING A TRACHEOSTOMY TUBE

PROCEDURE

1. Wash hands.

Anticipating the tasks to be done, the risk involved, and the personal protective equipment needed will enhance protection of both the caregiver and student. Should be done in a clean area with good lighting. Usually two people are needed. If an emergency situation occurs, tracheostomy tube change may be done by one person.

2. Assemble equipment:

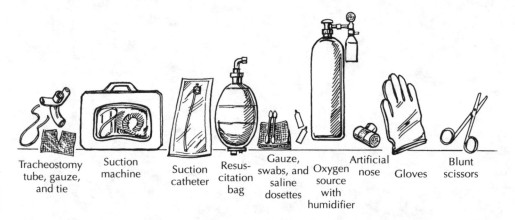

Tracheostomy tube, gauze, and tie • Suction machine • Suction catheter • Resuscitation bag • Gauze, swabs, and saline dosettes • Oxygen source with humidifier • Artificial nose • Gloves • Blunt scissors

- Prescribed type and size of tracheostomy tube for student
- Twill tape or other ties
- Obturator if applicable
- Blunt scissors
- Stethoscope
- Resuscitation bag
- Oxygen, if ordered
- Suctioning device and supplies

Always have a clean tracheostomy tube available and ready for use.

The obturator is used as a guide for insertion.

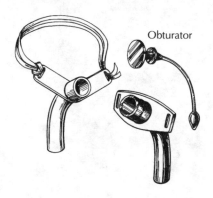

Obturator

- Syringe if cuffed
- Sterile water-soluble lubricant or sterile saline
- One size smaller tracheostomy tube
- Blanket roll, if needed
- Gloves

3. Explain procedure to the student at his or her level of understanding.

4. Position the student as ordered.

5. Wash hands.

Never use Vaseline or oil-based lubricants.

To position student's neck.

By encouraging the student to assist in the procedure, the caregiver helps the student achieve maximum self-care skills.

Have small children and infants lie on their backs with a blanket roll under the shoulders.

6. Open tracheostomy tube package.

7. Put on gloves.

8. Put obturator into clean tracheostomy tube, if applicable.

9. Attach tracheostomy ties to tube.

*Keep tube clean. **Do not** touch curved part of tube.*

10. Lubricate end of tracheostomy tube with water-soluble lubricant or sterile saline.

11. Suction tracheostomy and nose and mouth, if needed.

12. Give two to four breaths with resuscitation bag, if indicated.

Some students may have a Velcro holder or other means of securing tracheostomy tube around neck.

This makes airway as clear as possible.

If oxygen is used, make sure tubing is attached and oxygen is flowing.

13. Have assistant hold old tube in place while cutting the ties.

If tube is being changed by one person, do not cut ties until clean tracheostomy tube is in hand.

14. When the new tube is ready (in hand), have assistant remove old tube.

15. If the tube does not have an obturator, insert the clean (new) tube at a right angle to the stoma, rotating it downward as it is inserted. If an obturator is present, insert tube straight into stoma. Hold in place until secured.

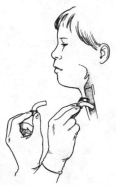

16. If an obturator is used, immediately remove it after the tube is inserted. Insert inner cannula at this time. Hold in place until secured.

17. Listen and feel for air movement through tracheostomy tube.

18. Secure tube in place with ties or holder.

Hold the tracheostomy tube in place at all times. A person is unable to breathe when the obturator is in place in the tracheostomy tube.

Observe the student for signs of distress (e.g., blueness, agitation, shortness of breath).

The tracheostomy ties should be tied in a double knot. The ties should be loose enough to slip one finger between the ties and the neck.

19. While assistant is holding the new tube in place, listen with stethoscope to assess breath sounds. Watch chest rise with breath.

A small amount of bleeding may occur around stoma or be in secretions after a tracheostomy change. If unusual or persistent bleeding is present, notify the family and seek medical attention.

20. Do skin care, if needed (see student-specific guidelines), and reapply gauze around and under tracheostomy tube and ties.

Save metal tracheostomy tube and send home to be sterilized.

21. Give two to four breaths with resuscitation bag and suction if needed.

22. Discard used equipment according to universal precautions guidelines (see Chapter 5).

23. Student may resume previous activities.

24. Remove gloves and wash hands.

25. Document procedure and problems on student's log sheet.

Notify family of any changes in the student's usual pattern.

Possible Problems with Tracheostomy Tube Changes that Require Immediate Attention

Observations

The tracheostomy tube comes out:

- Student is not showing signs of distress

- Student shows signs of respiratory distress

- Tube can be inserted and the student is still having difficulty

The tracheostomy tube cannot be reinserted

It is still possible to insert the tracheostomy tube

If insertion of tracheostomy tube is not possible and the student has respiratory distress and/or respiratory arrest

Reason/Action

Never leave student alone. Call for assistance.
Follow procedure for tracheostomy tube change outlined on pages 288–289.

Attempt to insert tracheostomy tube as outlined in procedure.

- *Reassure the student.*
- *Assess airway and breathing.*
- *Administer oxygen via the tracheostomy.*
- *Suction the tracheostomy.*
- *Use bronchodilators, if ordered.*
- *Use manual resuscitator bag, if indicated.*

If distress persists, initiate emergency plan and begin cardiopulmonary resuscitation.

This may be due to a false passage or bronchospasm:

Never leave student alone. Call for assistance.

- *Reassure the student.*
- *Encourage the student to take a deep breath—be prepared to insert tube if stoma opens.*
- *Administer flow of oxygen directly to the tracheostomy stoma.*
- *Reposition the student.*

- *Attempt to insert the smaller tracheostomy tube or thread a suction catheter through the new tracheostomy tube and attempt to insert catheter through stoma into trachea as a guide for tracheostomy tube.*
- *Slide tracheostomy tube over catheter into stoma and remove catheter without dislodging tracheostomy tube.*

Begin cardiopulmonary resuscitation with mouth-to-mouth breaths, following universal precautions. Cover trach stoma with your thumb if an air leak is present. Initiate the emergency plan.

Aspiration of foreign material (e.g., food, sand)

Suction first. Using the manual resuscitator bag before suctioning may force aspirate into lungs.

Give breaths with resuscitation bag after initial suctioning.

Check air movement.

Add saline and give breaths with resuscitation bag. Repeat suctioning. Repeat above steps until aspirated secretions are clear or gone.

If tracheostomy tube remains blocked by foreign material, change tracheostomy tube. Check air movement.

Give breaths with resuscitation bag if indicated.

Administer oxygen if prescribed in emergency plan.

Bronchospasm (wheezing) also may occur. The student may require medication.

Respiratory distress or arrest can occur with any aspiration. Be prepared to initiate emergency plan. Begin cardiopulmonary resuscitation after suctioning, if needed. Notify family and physician.

Respiratory Care

MANUAL RESUSCITATION BAG

PURPOSE

A manual resuscitator or self-inflating bag is used to deliver breaths manually when a student is unable to breathe on his or her own. This device may be used with a mask to cover the nose and mouth or with a special adaptor for a tracheostomy tube.

Situations in which a manual resuscitator may need to be used include the following:

- Student is having difficulty breathing on his or her own.
- A ventilator malfunctions.
- Routine respiratory care for a student is needed.
- Student stops breathing and needs to be resuscitated.

Students who have tracheostomies or who use ventilators should have manual resuscitation bags with them at all times.

SUGGESTED SETTINGS

In optimal circumstances, manual resuscitation (e.g., ambuing, bagging) should be done in an area designated for health care procedures. In an emergency, it must be done wherever needed.

SUGGESTED PERSONNEL AND TRAINING

A health assessment must be completed by the school nurse. State nurse practice regulations should be consulted for guidance on delegating health care procedures.

Manual resuscitation should be performed by a registered nurse or a respiratory therapist or a delegated adult with proven competency-based training in appropriate techniques and problem management, following state medical and nursing practice standards.

If the trained caregiver and back-up personnel are unavailable on a given school day, the student should not attend school. However, an optional arrangement may be made between the school and the family so that someone from the family would be available to attend school to function as the caregiver for the student.

Any school personnel who have regular contact with a student who may require the use of a manual resuscitator must receive general training that covers the student's special health care needs, potential problems, and how to implement the established emergency plan.

Respiratory Care

Procedure for Using a
Manual Resuscitator with Tracheostomy

PROCEDURE

1. Wash hands.

2. Assemble equipment:
   - Oxygen source with appropriate tubing if needed
   - Manual resuscitator
   - Adaptor for tracheostomy tube
   - Go-bag items

3. Explain the procedure to the student at his or her level of understanding.

4. Check that resuscitator is functioning properly.

5. Position student.

6. Attach resuscitator bag to tracheostomy tube.

7. If the student is able to breathe independently, coordinate the manual breaths with his or her own breaths. Give a breath by squeezing the resuscitation bag as the student begins to inhale (i.e., chest begins to rise).

POINTS TO REMEMBER

Anticipating the tasks to be done, the risk involved, and the personal protective equipment needed will enhance protection of both the caregiver and student.

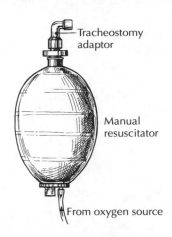

Tracheostomy adaptor

Manual resuscitator

From oxygen source

By encouraging the student to assist in the procedure, the caregiver helps the student achieve maximum self-care skills.

Place adaptor, which is connected to the bag, against a gauze or tissue in hand. Squeeze bag to be sure it is functioning. (If it is functioning, slight resistance will be felt.)

Position may vary; see student-specific guidelines. If oxygen is to be used, make sure tubing is attached and that oxygen is flowing.

Hold tracheostomy tube with one hand to prevent accidental dislodgement while attaching adaptor to it.

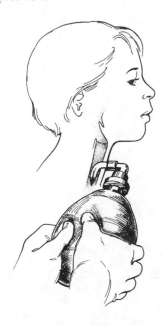

Respiratory Care

If you feel resistance and/or the student looks distressed, be sure you are giving breaths with the student's own effort and that the tube is patent.

8. If the student is unable to breathe on his or her own, squeeze the resuscitation bag at a regular rate to deliver prescribed breaths per minute.

9. Remove resuscitation bag from tracheostomy tube.
10. Wash hands.
11. Document procedure and problems on student's log sheet.

If the student has no breathing rate prescribed, a standard range of breaths per minute is
20–24 for infants
16–20 for children
12–16 for adolescents and adults
Hold tracheostomy tube with one hand to prevent pulling/dislodging it.

Notify the family of any problem.

Respiratory Care

Nose and Mouth Suctioning

PURPOSE

Nasal and/or oral suctioning are performed when the student needs assistance in clearing secretions from the airway. Indications of this include the following:

- Noisy, rattling, or gurgling breathing sounds
- Secretions (e.g., mucus or saliva) pooling in the back of the throat
- Respiratory distress (e.g., difficulty breathing, agitation, paleness, excessive coughing or choking, cyanosis [blueness])

The student may request suctioning and may be able to assist with the procedure.

SUGGESTED SETTINGS

Routine, nonemergency suctioning can be done in a clean, private area outside of the classroom, such as the health room or a corner of the classroom. Suctioning can be a noisy procedure and may be distracting and disruptive to the rest of the class.

If a suction machine that requires electricity is used, the setting must have an accessible electric outlet. All students who require routine suctioning must have a portable suction machine and suctioning equipment to accompany them in transport.

SUGGESTED PERSONNEL AND TRAINING

A health assessment must be completed by the school nurse. State nurse practice regulations should be consulted for guidance on delegating health care procedures.

Nose and mouth suctioning should be performed by a caregiver with proven competency-based training in appropriate techniques and problem management. All school personnel who have regular contact with a student who requires nose and mouth suctioning must receive general training that covers the student's special health care needs, potential problems, and how to implement the established emergency plan.

The basic skills checklist on page 369 can be used as a foundation for competency-based training in appropriate techniques. It outlines specific procedures step by step. Once the procedures have been mastered, the completed checklist serves as a documentation of training.

THE INDIVIDUALIZED HEALTH CARE PLAN: ISSUES FOR SPECIAL CONSIDERATION

Each student's individualized health care plan (IHCP) must be tailored to the individual's needs. The following section covers the procedures for nose and mouth suctioning as well as possible problems and emergencies that may arise. It is essential that this section be reviewed before writing the IHCP.

A sample plan is included in Chapter 6. It may be copied and used to develop a plan for each student. For a student who needs nose and mouth suctioning, the following items should receive particular attention:

- Student's underlying condition and the possible complications arising from the condition or treatment
- Student's baseline status (e.g., color, respiratory rate, pulse, usual amount of secretions, frequency of suctioning)
- Signs and symptoms of respiratory distress (e.g., agitation, cyanosis, noisy breathing)
- Ability of the student to request assistance
- Usual indications for suctioning
- Latex allergy alert (see Chapter 5)
- Universal precautions (Anticipating the tasks to be done, the risk involved, and the personal protective equipment needed will enhance protection of both the caregiver and student.)

Respiratory Care

Procedure for Nose and Mouth Suctioning Using Suction Machine

PROCEDURE

1. Wash hands.

2. Assemble the equipment:

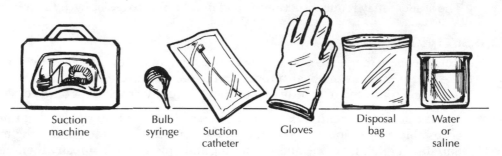

Suction machine   Bulb syringe   Suction catheter   Gloves   Disposal bag   Water or saline

- Suction machine (battery operated or plug-in) and tubing
- Bulb syringe or other manual backup
- Suction catheter of the appropriate size
- Disposable gloves
- Plastic bag for disposal of materials
- Water or saline to clean catheter, with container

3. Position student. Explain the procedure to the student, according to his or her level of understanding. If able, the student should assist.

4. Turn on suction machine to check function.

5. Encourage the student to cough to expel secretions.

6. Open suction catheter or kit without touching the inside of package.

7. Put on gloves.

8. In the dominant hand, hold the catheter and attach appropriate end to the suction machine. Keep the other end of the catheter in the package.

9. Turn on machine with other hand to prescribed suction pressure.

10. Hold suction catheter 2–3 inches from the tip with dominant hand.

POINTS TO REMEMBER

Anticipating the tasks to be done, the risk involved, and the personal protective equipment needed will enhance protection of both the caregiver and student.

All equipment for suctioning must be assembled and ready for immediate use at all times. It must be checked daily by designated personnel.

This cleans and lubricates the catheter.

Position may vary and should be recommended in student-specific guidelines. By encouraging the student to assist in the procedure, the caregiver is helping the student achieve maximum self-care skills.

This may eliminate the need for suctioning or may bring secretions up for easier suctioning.
This keeps catheter clean and reduces risk of transmitting infection.
Dominant hand, which is used to manipulate catheter, should remain clean.

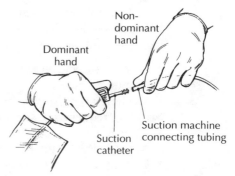

Non-dominant hand

Dominant hand

Suction catheter

Suction machine connecting tubing

Portable machines may not have adjustable pressure settings.

11. Grasp catheter connection with other hand; cover vent hole with thumb to suction a small amount of water through the catheter.

This tests that suction machine is working and lubricates the catheter.

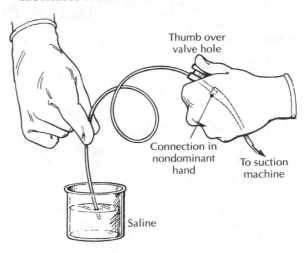
Thumb over valve hole
Connection in nondominant hand
To suction machine
Saline

12. Remove covering from end of suction catheter with nondominant hand while holding catheter in dominant hand.
13. With thumb off vent hole, insert catheter gently into the nose to the prescribed depth suggested in student-specific guidelines.

Always suction the nose first. There are more bacteria in the mouth. Many students may only need to have the anterior part of the nose suctioned. Be gentle; the nose bleeds easily. Make sure catheter tip has been lubricated with saline or water-soluble lubricant.
If the nose secretions are too thick, put a few drops of saline in each nostril.

14. Cover vent hole with nondominant thumb while suctioning and withdrawing catheter. Gently rotate catheter between thumb and index finger while suctioning and withdrawing.
15. Suction up some water to rinse secretions out of catheter.
16. If nasal congestion persists, repeat nasal suction.
17. With thumb off vent hole, insert catheter gently into the mouth.

Rotating the suction catheter diminishes damage to the mucus membrane. If the catheter sticks, remove thumb from vent hole to release suction.

Parts of the mouth to be suctioned include the back of the throat, the cheeks, and under the tongue. Be careful when suctioning the back of the throat, as this may cause the student to gag and vomit.

18. Cover vent hole with nondominant thumb. Gently rotate catheter between thumb and index finger while suctioning and withdrawing.
19. Suction up some water to rinse secretions out of catheter.
20. If gurgling noises persist, repeat mouth suctioning procedure with the same catheter.
21. Discard catheter.
22. Discard gloves in an appropriate receptacle.
23. Wash hands.
24. Note color, consistency, and amount of secretions on daily procedure log sheet.

This helps to minimize trauma to the membranes of the mouth.

If, after suctioning of the mouth, repeat suctioning of the nose is needed, use a clean catheter.

Report to the family any changes from the student's usual pattern.

Procedure for Nose and
Mouth Suctioning with a Bulb Syringe

PROCEDURE

1. Wash hands.

2. Assemble equipment:
   - Bulb syringe
   - Saline
   - Tissues
   - Gloves

3. Wash hands.

4. Explain the procedure to the student, according to his or her level of understanding.

5. Position student.

6. Put on gloves.

7. Squeeze the bulb syringe away from student and place the tip gently into the nose or mouth, where secretions are visible or audible, and let the bulb fill up.

8. Remove the bulb syringe from the nose or mouth.

9. Holding the syringe over a tissue or basin, squeeze the bulb to push out the secretions, then let it fill with air.

10. Repeat Steps 7–9 as needed until nose and mouth are clear.

11. If the nose secretions are too thick, put a few drops of saline in each nostril before suctioning with bulb syringe.

12. Clean bulb syringe in hot soapy water, rinse with fresh water, let dry, and store.

13. Dispose of tissues in appropriate receptacle.

14. Remove gloves.

15. Wash hands.

16. Note color, consistency, and amount of secretions on student's log sheet.

POINTS TO REMEMBER

Anticipating the tasks to be done, the risk involved, and the personal protective equipment needed will enhance protection of both the caregiver and student.

Always suction nose first.

Position varies. See student-specific guidelines.

When suctioning the mouth, suction under the tongue, in the cheeks, and in the back of the throat. Be careful when suctioning the back of the throat, as this may cause the student to gag and vomit.

Report to the family any changes from the student's usual pattern.

Possible Problems with Nose and Mouth Suctioning that Require Immediate Attention

Observations

Student develops a nosebleed during suctioning

Student gags or vomits during suctioning

Reason/Action

Stop suctioning. Gently squeeze bridge of nose with your fingers and hold for 5 minutes. Once bleeding has stopped, do not use that side of the nose to suction until permission is given by the family or physician.

Catheter is probably down too far. Pull back a short distance and complete suctioning. If vomiting occurs, stop suctioning and remove catheter. Position student to keep airway open. Wait until vomiting has stopped. Make sure that the student is able to breathe easily. After vomiting, the student may require repeat suctioning. Be careful that catheter is not down too far.

Respiratory Care

General Information Sheet

Students Who Need Suctioning

Dear (teacher, lunch aide, bus driver):

_____ [Student's name] has a condition that requires suctioning. Suctioning helps the student breathe better by clearing secretions/mucus from the airway. Depending on the student's age, he or she may be able to request suctioning when needed or assist in the procedure.

A student needing suctioning will have the necessary equipment at all times.

Most students who need suctioning are able to participate in school activities. A team including the students, parents, and educational and health personnel will help develop a specific health care plan.

The following staff members have been trained to deal with any problems that may arise with this student:

_____

_____

_____

For more information about suctioning or the student's needs, consult the school nurse or family.

Respiratory Care

Nebulizer Treatments

PURPOSE

Nebulizer treatments deliver medication in mist form directly into the lungs. When air from the compressor (i.e., air pump) is pushed through the tubing and into the medicine chamber (i.e., nebulizer cup), the medicine breaks up into a mist that the student inhales. Small dosages of medication inhaled directly into the lungs cause fewer side effects than the same medication taken in oral form. Medication by nebulizer also reaches the bronchioles more rapidly, and less coordination and breathing effort are required than when using a metered dose inhaler.

Aerosol treatments are beneficial for children who are too young to master the metered dose inhaler and for students with moderate to severe asthma whose lung function is greatly impaired. Nebulizer treatments also are used to deliver antibiotics and other medications.

SUGGESTED SETTINGS

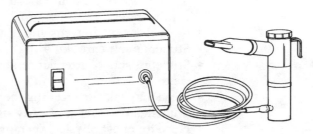

Select an area such as a health room or office for privacy. The air compressor may be moderately noisy. A *nebulizer unit* is attached to the air outlet on the compressor. It consists of the *nebulizer cup*, which holds the medicine, and the *nebulizer*, which produces the mist. A *T adaptor*, placed on the nebulizer, passes air to the mouthpiece and allows exhaled air to pass out.

The *mouthpiece* is placed between the teeth and allows for a tight seal with the lips. A *face mask* or a *tracheostomy mask* can be used instead of a mouthpiece and attaches directly to the nebulizer unit. The *connecting tubing* connects from the end of the nebulizer unit to the air outlet of the compressor.

Note: Nebulizer units vary in design, which affects the size and speed of the mist particles and length of treatment. Some units are more durable and can withstand greater use and cleaning.

A *power-driven air compressor* is available in different models. All have the same basic features: an *air outlet*, to which the nebulizer tubing is connected; and an *air inlet*, which pulls air into the compressor through a *filter*.

The filter needs to be kept clean and should be replaced periodically.

SUGGESTED PERSONNEL AND TRAINING

A health care assessment must be completed by the school nurse. State nurse regulations should be consulted for guidance on delegating health care procedures.

A nebulizer treatment may be administered by the school nurse, family, teacher, student aide, or other person with proven competency-based training in appropriate techniques and problem management. Before deciding on the appropriate person to administer the treatment, information about state regulations and school policy for medication administration in school must be considered. Medication administration protection measures (e.g., use of filters in the exhalation port, tightly fitting mask during treatment), if indicated, also should be followed. The student should be encouraged to assist with the nebulizer treatment as much as possible. Any school personnel who have regular contact with a student who requires a nebulizer treatment should receive general training that covers the student's specific health care needs, potential problems, and how to implement the established emergency plan.

The basic skills checklist on page 372 can be used as a foundation for competency-based training in appropriate techniques. It outlines the procedure step by step. Once the procedures have been mastered, the completed checklist serves as documentation of training.

THE INDIVIDUALIZED HEALTH CARE PLAN: ISSUES FOR SPECIAL CONSIDERATION

Each student's individualized health care plan (IHCP) must be tailored to the individual's needs. The following section covers the procedures for nebulizer treatment and possible problems and emergencies that may arise. It is essential to review it before writing the IHCP.

A sample plan is included in Chapter 6. It may be copied and used to develop a plan for each student. For a student who requires nebulizer treatment, the following items should receive particular attention:

- Need for student to receive nebulizer treatment
- Need for activity modifications
- Knowledge of guidelines and protective measures specific to the medication being administered
- Knowledge of allergens and triggers of wheezing for students with asthma
- Student's self-care skills
- Student's school attendance/absences related to increase in episodes of respiratory distress
- Need for peak flow readings before treatment
- Student's knowledge of early signs of respiratory distress
- Need for chest physical therapy and/or suctioning
- Treatment administration as "regularly scheduled" or "treatment as needed"
- Response to treatment and necessity for repeat treatments (per physician or nurse practitioner's order)
- Latex allergy alert (see Chapter 5)
- Universal precautions (Anticipating the tasks to be done, the risk involved, and the personal protective equipment needed will enhance protection of both the caregiver and student.)

Procedure for Aerosol Treatment by Nebulizer with Air Compressor

PROCEDURE

1. Determine need for treatment based on specific physician's or nurse practitioner's order. The student may ask for treatment.
2. Wash hands.

3. Assemble equipment:

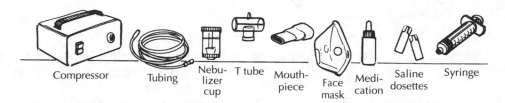

Compressor   Tubing   Nebulizer cup   T tube   Mouthpiece   Face mask   Medication   Saline dosettes   Syringe

- Compressor/gas cylinder
- Connecting tubing
- Nebulizer cup
- Mouthpiece or mask, T adaptor
- Medication
- Diluting solution
- Saline dosettes
- Syringe
- Filter disc/exhalation filter, if needed

4. Place the unit on a firm, flat surface.

5. Attach the end of the nebulizer tubing to the compressor's air outlet. Unscrew the top from the nebulizer cup.
6. Place the prescribed amount of medicine and diluent into the nebulizer cup.
7. Reattach the nebulizer cap tightly.
8. Attach the connecting tubing to the nebulizer cup outlet.
9. Have the student sit in a comfortable position.

10. Turn on power switch.

POINTS TO REMEMBER

Assess student's status: respiratory rate, depth, effort, pulse, restlessness, color, retractions, cough, and wheezing.

Anticipating the tasks to be done, the risk involved, and the personal protective equipment needed will enhance protection of both the caregiver and student.

Some compressors are electrically powered. Others are battery operated.

Some medications do not require diluent solution.

Encourage student to participate in the procedure. Assess student's pulse and respiratory rate.

A fine mist should be visible.

11. Have student place mouthpiece in mouth between teeth and seal lips around mouthpiece or place mask over nose and mouth (or tracheostomy).

If a student is able to use mouthpiece for treatment, he or she should be encouraged to take slow, deep breaths during entire treatment.

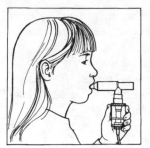 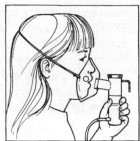

Note: This illustration does not apply to students receiving medications that need a filter in exhalation port or tightly fitting mask during treatment.

12. Have student begin to breathe in through the mouthpiece or mask.

Have student breathe at a normal rate and depth. Observe the expansion of the student's chest.

13. Every 1–2 minutes have student take a deep breath, hold breath briefly, then exhale slowly and resume normal breathing.

Deep breaths ensure that the medicine is being delivered to the lower airways, not just the mouth. A treatment may last 10–15 minutes. Give student time to rest during procedure if needed. If mist stops and medicine can be seen on sides of cup, tap side of cup, and the mist should start again. Allow all medicine to aerosolize.

14. At the end of treatment turn off power switch.
15. Remove mouthpiece or mask.
16. If ordered, have student take several deep breaths, and cough up secretions.
17. Assess student's respiratory status.

If student still is having difficulty breathing or is wheezing, follow student-specific plan.

18. Disassemble equipment.
19. Refer to cleaning instructions.
20. Wash hands.
21. Document treatment.

Report to family any changes in the student's usual pattern of tolerating the procedure.
May be done at home. Cleaning the equipment prevents clogging and malfunction and reduces infection. Student-specific nebulizer cup, tubing, and mouthpiece can be reused after cleaning. Compressors can be used for multiple students.

22. Cleaning and care of equipment: After every use, rinse nebulizer assembly, mouthpiece, and mask under warm running water for 30 seconds. Shake off excess water. Lay on clean cloths to dry. Cover with cloth or paper towel. When parts are dry, store them in a clean plastic bag. Follow manufacturer's instructions regarding replacement of filter. Do not wash tubing. Once or twice a week: Clean nebulizer parts more thoroughly. Soak parts in solution of 1 cup white vinegar and 2 cups warm water for 30 minutes. Rinse thoroughly after soaking. Alternatively, parts may be sterilized by boiling or may be cleaned in dishwasher. See product instructions accompanying the unit.

Problems that Require Immediate Attention for Students Requiring Nebulizer Treatment

Observation	Reason/Action
Tightness in chest Coughing Wheezing Shortness of breath Retractions (i.e., pulling in of rib cage) Cough or wheeze gets worse	*Give nebulizer treatment according to physician's orders. Most inhaled bronchodilator medicines produce an effect within 5–10 minutes.*
Breathing gets increasingly difficult	*Stay calm. Reassure student. Document vital signs.*
Struggling to breathe or hunching over after treatment is finished	*Follow student-specific emergency plan. Notify school nurse, family, and physician.*

Possible Problems that Are Not Emergencies

Student needs to rest or becomes light-headed during treatment	*Too-rapid breathing, as well as some medications, may cause dizziness. Discontinue treatment. Turn off unit. Continue treatment when student is feeling better.*
Student becomes jittery or shaky during bronchodilator treatment	*Some medications may cause increased heart rate. See student-specific guidelines.*

General Information Sheet

Students Who Need Nebulizer Treatments

Dear (teacher, lunch aide, bus driver):

_____ [Student's name] has a condition that requires nebulizer treatments. Nebulizer treatments deliver medication in mist form directly into the lungs. Nebulizer treatments are also used to give antibiotics and other medications.

A student needing nebulizer treatments will have the necessary equipment in school at all times.

Most students who need nebulizer treatments are able to participate in school activities. A team including the students, parents, and educational and health personnel will help develop a specific health care plan.

The following staff members have been trained to deal with any problems that may arise with this student:

_____

_____

_____

For more information about nebulizer treatments or the student's needs, consult the school nurse or family.

Respiratory Care

USE OF MECHANICAL VENTILATORS

This section provides a general overview of basic ventilator terminology, appropriate personnel, and possible problems and emergency management. It is not intended to be used as a comprehensive reference for ventilator management for an individual student. Several such manuals are available. See Suggested Readings on page 315. In addition, it is essential to obtain student-specific information for each student from the appropriate medical providers.

PURPOSE

Mechanical ventilation is used to sustain life when a person is unable to breathe sufficiently on his or her own. Students with conditions such as neurological damage, muscle weakness, and severe pulmonary disease may need ventilator assistance.

The ventilator or respirator is a machine that can be used to provide total respiratory support for a person who is unable to breathe independently. A ventilator also may be used to assist a student who is able to breathe but whose respiratory ability is inadequate. Some students may require a few breaths a minute in addition to their own or positive end expiratory pressure (PEEP) to keep the lungs open. Other students require full respiratory support for a prescribed period of time during the day or night for rest.

Many different types of ventilators are used, depending on the student's size, the student's medical condition, and the preference of the student's physician. The most common basic type of ventilator is a *positive pressure ventilator*. This machine breathes for a person by pushing air or oxygen-rich gas into the lungs, usually through a tracheostomy tube. This type of ventilator can be relatively small and portable.

A *negative pressure ventilator* pulls air into the lungs by pulling the person's chest wall outward as the person lies in a vacuum chamber. There are various negative pressure ventilators, including the iron lung, the *raincoat*, and other portable home devices. Negative pressure ventilators are only recommended for people with specific conditions such as muscular weakness. A tracheostomy tube is not required with negative pressure ventilators.

Portable ventilators are usually mounted on the bottom shelf of a wheelchair. The battery is partitioned away from the ventilator in case battery fluid begins to leak.

SUGGESTED SETTINGS

In many cases, the ventilator must be with the student in school and in the transportation vehicle. All settings always should have available grounded electrical outlets and a back-up power source.

Any student who travels to school with a ventilator must carry with him or her a "go bag" containing a manual resuscitation bag, a spare tracheostomy tube, and suction supplies. See "go-bag" checklist on page 355.

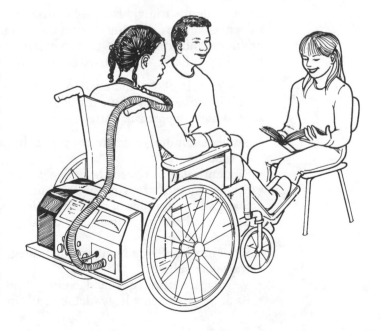

SUGGESTED PERSONNEL AND TRAINING

A health assessment must be completed by the school nurse. State nurse practice regulations should be consulted for guidance on delegating health care procedures.

Care of the student assisted by a ventilator should be performed by a qualified registered nurse or respiratory therapist. Any other health professional caring for a student assisted by a ventilator should have taken a competency-based training program.

Providing educational services to a student assisted by mechanical ventilation is a complex and challenging commitment. There are various health care delivery service models, and some utilize nonmedical personnel to provide ventilator care.

All caregivers should

- Be aware of state nurse practice acts that may specify care delivery and delegation issues
- Be trained in student-specific ventilator procedures due to the technical and unique nature of care
- Be immediately available to the student who is dependent on mechanical ventilation in all school environments, including the classroom and transportation vehicle
- Understand the amount of assistance each student requires from the ventilator
- Know specialized cardiopulmonary resuscitation for students with tracheostomies

If the trained caregiver and back-up personnel are unavailable on a given school day, the student should not attend school. However, an optional arrangement may be made between the school and the family so that someone from the family would attend school to function as the caregiver for the student.

All school personnel who have regular contact with a student who requires mechanical ventilation must receive general training that covers the student's specific health care needs, potential problems, and how to implement the established emergency plan.

The basic skills checklists for ventilator machine and circuit and ventilator alarms—troubleshooting on pages 374–377 can be used as a foundation for ventilator training. Their use alone does not constitute comprehensive competency-based training. Additional training in student-specific techniques, equipment, and health care needs is essential and should be documented.

THE INDIVIDUALIZED HEALTH CARE PLAN: ISSUES FOR SPECIAL CONSIDERATION

Each student's individualized health care plan (IHCP) must be tailored to the individual's needs. The following section reviews information about ventilator use and possible problems and emergencies that may arise. It is essential that this section and a reference for the specific ventilator used be reviewed before writing the IHCP.

A sample plan is included in Chapter 6. It may be copied and used to develop a plan for each student. For a student who requires the use of a ventilator, the following items should receive particular attention:

- Student's underlying condition and the possible problems arising from the condition or treatment
- Student's degree of ventilator dependency
- Student's ability to request assistance
- Signs and symptoms of respiratory distress (e.g., cyanosis, agitation)
- Student's baseline status (e.g., usual ventilator settings, respiratory rate, color, lung sounds, pulse)
- Student's need for a highly skilled caregiver with him or her in the classroom and the transport vehicle
- Ventilator settings checked every 1–2 hours
- Back-up power supply available at all times (e.g., battery, generator)

- Latex allergy alert (see Chapter 5)
- Universal precautions (Anticipating the tasks to be done, the risk involved, and the personal protective equipment needed will enhance protection of both the caregiver and student.)

Procedure for Checking Ventilator Features

PROCEDURE

Standard ventilator features that should be checked at least daily and on arrival at school. Check the following:

1. Power source:
   - Internal battery

   - External battery

   - Accessible, functioning electrical outlets
   - Back-up battery
   - Emergency power supply
2. Oxygen source:

   - Connection to ventilator and spare tubing
   - Adequate supply of oxygen, spare tank, and gauge

3. Humidification source:
   - Passive condensor
   - Heat–moisture exchanger

4. Patient pressure manometer
5. Ventilator circuit:
   Tubing and spare tubing required:
   - Pressure tubing

   Valves:
   - Exhalation valve
   - PEEP valve
   - Other adaptors needed for a particular student plus spares of each

6. Alarms:
   - High and low pressure
   - Volume
   - Power source
7. Other equipment that should be checked daily:
   - Manual resuscitator bag and adaptor or mask
   - Spare tracheostomy tube and supplies
   - Suctioning equipment
   - Saline dosettes

POINTS TO REMEMBER

Must be connected for machine to function.
The internal battery is generally a 12-volt DC battery intended for emergency use only.
The external battery is connected to the ventilator via a cable. If fully charged, it will operate for approximately 10 hours.

The back-up battery is usually kept at home.

An oxygen source may be included, if prescribed for the student.

Oxygen may be supplied in gas or liquid form. Ensure adequate supply of oxygen is available for the day. Identify flow in liters per minute (LPM) and percentage of oxygen.
Any student who has his or her nose and mouth bypassed by a tracheostomy tube needs a humidifier. Always remember to have an adequate amount of water in the humidifier and have it set at a safe temperature. Some students may use a heat–moisture exchanger for humidification.

The ventilator circuit consists of the tubing that is attached to the ventilator and the student's tracheostomy tube and other components such as the humidifier and the exhalation and PEEP valves. The tubing carries the air from the ventilator to the student.
Caution always should be taken not to block or obstruct the exhalation valve with the student's clothing.
Ventilator circuit maintenance: The cleaning of ventilator circuits should be done at home daily or as needed.
Alarms should never be turned off. *All ventilator alarm settings should be written on the emergency card posted on a visible side of the ventilator.*
Each student who travels to school with a ventilator should have a "go bag" containing all of these supplies.

PROCEDURE FOR CHECKING VENTILATOR PARAMETERS

PROCEDURE

Ventilator procedures are prescribed settings for a given student and should be checked several times during the day—every 1–2 hours or more frequently if the student's status changes.

1. Tidal volume

2. Respiratory rate

3. Oxygen percentage

4. Peak inspiratory pressure (PIP)

5. Positive end expiratory pressure (PEEP)

6. Ventilator mode

7. Inspiratory time ("I" Time)

8. High-pressure alarm

9. Low-pressure alarm

10. Power source alarm

11. Temperature alarm

POINTS TO REMEMBER

A safety card, stating the student's ventilator settings, should be mounted on the ventilator and easily visible.

The amount of air in each breath. Determined by the student's size.

Number of breaths delivered in a minute. Determined by student's condition and size.

Percentage is based on the individual student's needs. (Room air is 21%.)

The amount of pressure required to inflate the lungs to the prescribed tidal volume.

The amount of pressure needed to keep the lungs from totally collapsing after exhalation.

The type of respiratory support administered to the student: intermittent mandatory ventilation (IMV), assist-control, or synchronized intermittent mandatory ventilation (SIMV). The prescribed mode will be determined by the student's condition and respiratory ability.

The amount of time in the vent cycle used to deliver a breath.

Reflects an excessive inspiratory pressure. May indicate increased resistance or obstruction.

Indicates a too-low inspiratory pressure. Warns of a leak in the system; may signal that adequate volume is not being delivered.

Indicates a change in power. **Alarms should never be turned off.**

The majority of home care ventilators **do not** *have temperature alarms built into the humidifier unit. The temperature of inspired gas can be checked with an in-line thermometer.*

Respiratory Care

POSSIBLE PROBLEMS WHEN USING A VENTILATOR THAT REQUIRE IMMEDIATE ATTENTION

Observations

Student appears to be in distress:

- Increased shortness of breath
- Agitation
- Blueness or pallor of lips, nailbeds
- Retractions (e.g., pulling in of chest muscles)
- Confusion
- Rapid or pounding pulse

The tracheostomy tube is dislodged

The tracheostomy tube is blocked

The student has increased secretions

The student is wheezing

The student continues to be in distress or becomes unconscious

Distress is relieved by disconnecting from ventilator and using manual resuscitation

The power supply is not functioning

Reason/Action

Immediately check and reassure the student. Call for assistance. **Never leave the student alone.**

The symptoms may be caused by
- *Occlusion of the tracheostomy tube by a plug or secretions*
- *A dislodged tube or other airway problems*
- *Student may be coughing or doing something else to raise pressure transiently*

The symptoms may also be caused by a ventilator malfunction:
- *The exhalation valve may be obstructed.*
- *The student may be disconnected from ventilator.*

Check to see that the power source is functioning and that oxygen supply is adequate.

Disconnect the student from the ventilator and use manual resuscitator bag if needed while attending to the student's needs.

Replace the tube.

Attempt to suction; instill saline if indicated. If unsuccessful, replace tube.

Suction the tracheostomy.

Administer bronchodilators by nebulizer if ordered and suction as necessary.

Continue using manual resuscitator and **activate emergency procedure**.

Check the ventilator while using the manual resuscitator to assist the student's breathing. Check circuit, valves, and tubing for leaks, obstruction, or water condensation in tubing. If unable to locate and correct problem with ventilator, continue using resuscitation bag and call the home care company, family, and other health care providers as specified in student-specific guidelines. **Activate emergency plan.**

Ventilate student with manual resuscitator until back-up power supply is in operation.

An alarm is activated:

- Low-pressure alarm/apnea alarm is a continuous audible alarm and is usually accompanied by a flashing red light on the ventilator front panel.

Always check student first. Remove the student from ventilator and give breaths with resuscitator bag and then check the ventilator.

This alarm may be activated by the following:
- *The student may be disconnected from the ventilator.*
- *The exhalation valve is not working (wet or punctured).*
- *The tracheostomy tube is no longer in place.*
- *The circuit tubing is no longer attached or is loose.*
- *Water is present in pressure or exhalation tubing.*
- *Humidifier is improperly attached or leaking.*
- *Accidental change in ventilator settings.*

Test system after cause of problem is found and fixed. Place student back on ventilator.

- High-pressure alarm is an **intermittent alarm** usually accompanied by a flashing red light.
Note: If the condition that caused this alarm to be triggered is stopped with the next breath, the audible alarm will stop but the visual alarm will need to be reset.

Always check student first, remove the student from ventilator and give breaths with resuscitator ag and then check ventilator.

This alarm may be activated by the following:
- *The student may need to be suctioned for secretions or a mucus plug.*
- *This may indicate increased resistance or obstruction.*
- *The circuit tubing may be blocked by water or pinched off.*
- *The exhalation valve may be obstructed.*
- *The tracheostomy tube may be out of alignment.*
- *The student may be coughing or doing something else to raise pressure transiently (i.e., sneezing, talking, laughing).*
- *Accidental change in ventilator settings*

Test system after cause of problem is found and fixed. Place student back on ventilator.

- Power alarm is **continuous** usually accompanied by a flashing light as well.

*Check to see that power source is functioning (e.g., ac power, internal and external battery). The alarm may sound if power source is interrupted (e.g., power failure, battery change). If all three power sources fail, remove student from ventilator. Give breaths with resuscitator bag and **activate the emergency plan**.*

General Information Sheet

Students Who Use Mechanical Ventilators

Dear (teacher, lunch aide, bus driver):

_____ [Student's name] has a condition that requires a ventilator (i.e., breathing machine). This machine helps a person breathe by pushing air into the lungs. A student who uses a ventilator usually has a tracheostomy tube—a tube that has been surgically placed into the windpipe in the neck. This tube is attached to the ventilator by soft plastic tubing. Ventilators need a battery or other power source to function. The ventilator must be with the student at all times, including during transportation.

A team including the student's family and educational and health personnel will develop a specific health care plan for the school. Classroom issues, such as the accommodation of health care during the day with minimal disruption of the class; feeding issues; and the avoidance of infectious exposures, such as colds, will be addressed in the care plan.

The student will have a caregiver with him or her at all times. This person will be trained to manage the ventilator and care for the student.

The following staff members also have been trained to deal with any problems that might arise:

_____

_____

_____

All staff who have contact with students who use ventilators should be familiar with the emergency plan and how to initiate it in their setting. It is recommended that they participate in cardiopulmonary resuscitation training with specialized training for tracheostomies.

For more information about ventilators, tracheostomies, or the student's needs, consult the school nurse or the family.

Suggested Readings

Bleile, K.M. (Ed.). (1993). *The care of children with long-term tracheostomies.* San Diego: Singular Publishing Group.

Branson, R.D., Campbell, R.S., Chatburn, R.L., & Covington, J. (1992). AARC clinical practice guideline: Patient-ventilator system checks. *Respiratory Care, 37*(8), 882–886.

Buzz-Kelly, L., & Gordin, P. (1993). Teaching CPR to parents of children with tracheostomies. *The American Journal of Maternal/Child Nursing, 18*(3), 158–163.

California Department of Education. (1990). *Guidelines and procedures for meeting specialized physical health care needs of pupils.* Sacramento: Author.

Chatburn, R.L. (1991). A new system for understanding mechanical ventilators. *Respiratory Care, 36*(10), 1123–1155.

Connecticut State Department of Education. (1992). *Serving students with special health care needs.* Hartford: Author.

Dettelbach, M.A., Gross, R.D., Mahlmann, J., & Eibling, D.E. (1995). Effect of the Passey-Muir valve on aspiration in patients with tracheostomy. *Head and Neck, 17*(4), 297–300.

Erl, B., & Robbins, P. (1990). Hand-held nebulization therapy. *Journal of Pediatric Nursing, 5*(6), 408–409.

Fitton, C.M. (1994). Nursing management of the child with a tracheostomy. *Pediatric Clinics of North America, 41*(3), 513–523.

Giganti, A.W. (1995). Lifesaving tubes, lifetime scars? *The American Journal of Maternal/Child Nursing, 20*(4), 192–197.

Jackson, D., & Albamonte, S. (1994). Enhancing communication with the Passey-Muir valve. *Pediatric Nursing, 20*(2), 149–153.

Kacmarek, R.M., & Hess, D. (1991). The interface between patient and aerosol generator. *Respiratory Care, 36*(9), 952–976.

Leder, S.B. (1990a). Importance of verbal communication for the ventilator dependent patient. *Chest, 98*(4), 792–793.

Leder, S.B. (1990b). Verbal communication for the ventilator dependent patient: Voice intensity with the Portex "Talk" tracheostomy tube. *Laryngoscope, 100*(10), 1116–1121.

Leder, S.B. (1994). Perceptual rankings of speech quality produced with one-way tracheostomy speaking valves. *Journal of Speech and Hearing Research, 37*, 1308–1312.

Lewis, D., Barnes, T.A., Beattie, K., Beytas, L.J.R., O'Donohue, W.J., Perlman, N., Ritz, R.H., & Salyer, J. (1992). AARC clinical practice guideline: Oxygen therapy in the home or extended care facility. *Respiratory Care, 37*(8), 918–922.

National Asthma Education Program, National Institutes of Health. (1991). *Managing asthma: A guide for schools.* Bethesda, MD: Author.

National Asthma Education Program, National Institutes of Health. (1992). *Teach your patients about asthma: A clinician's guide.* Bethesda, MD: Author.

Manzano, J.L., Lubillo, S., Henríquez, D., Martin, J.C., Pérez, M.C., & Wilson, D.J. (1993). Verbal communication of ventilator-dependent patients. *Critical Care Medicine, 21*(4), 512–517.

Mathews, P.J., Mathews, L.M., & Mitchell, R.R. (1992). Artificial airways: Resuscitation guidelines you can follow. *Nursing 92, 22*(1), 53–59.

Miller, M.D., Steele, N.F., Nadell, J.M., Tilton, A.H., & Gates, A.J. (1993). Ventilator-assisted youth: Appraisal and nursing care. *Journal of Neuroscience Nursing, 25*(5), 287–295.

O'Donohue, W.J., Giovannoni, R.M., Keens, T.G., & Plummer, A.L. (1986). Long-term mechanical ventilation: Guidelines for management in the home and at alternate community sites. *Chest, 90*(1), 1S–37S.

Runton, N. (1992). Suctioning artificial airways in children: Appropriate technique. *Pediatric Nursing, 18*(2), 115–118.

Scharf, T. (1993). Yes, there is life after ventilation. *Chest, 103*, 1319.

Sherman, L.P., & Rosen, C.D. (1990). Development of a preschool program for tracheostomy dependent children. *Pediatric Nursing, 16*(4), 357–361.

Sly, R.M. (1991). Aerosol therapy in children. *Respiratory Care, 36*(9), 994–1007.

Ventilator Assisted Care Program and Respiratory Care Department, Children's Hospital. (1987). *Getting it started and keeping it going: A guide for respiratory home care of the ventilator assisted individual.* New Orleans, LA: Author.

Wessel, G.L., Prumo, M.O., & Harrison, P. (1989). School placement and the oxygen-dependent child. *Journal of Pediatric Nursing, 4*(6), 435–436.

Respiratory Care

Skills Checklists

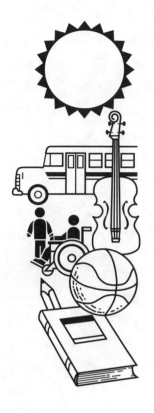

Student's name: _____

Person trained: _____

Position: _____

Instructor: _____

Gastrostomy Feeding Bolus Method
Skills Checklist

Explanation/Return Demonstration	Expl./ Demo. Date	Explanation/Return Demonstration					
		Date	Date	Date	Date	Date	Date
A. States name and purpose of procedure							
B. Preparation:							
1. Identifies student's ability to participate in procedure							
2. Reviews universal precautions							
3. Completes at _____ time(s)							
4. _____ cc (amount) _____ Formula/feeding (type of feeding)							
5. Feeding to be completed in _____ minutes							
6. Position for feeding _____							
7. Identifies possible problems and appropriate actions							
C. Identifies supplies:							
1. Catheter _____ (size) _____ (type) Balloon size _____ cc							
a. Small port plug							
b. Feeding port							
2. Gloves							
3. Formula at room temperature							
4. 60-cc catheter–tipped syringe							
5. Clamp and plug							
6. Small glass of tap water, if prescribed							
7. Rubber bands, safety pins							
D. Procedure:							
1. Washes hands							
2. Gathers equipment							
3. Positions student and explains procedure							
4. Washes hands, puts on gloves							
5. Removes plug from feeding tube							
Student-Specific: (Steps 6–12 need to be individualized for each student.)							
6. Checks for proper placement of tube: Attaches syringe and aspirates stomach contents by pulling plunger back							
7. Measures contents							

(continued)

Format adapted from Children's Hospital Chronic Illness Program, Ventilator Assisted Care Program. (1987). *Getting it started and keeping it going: A guide for respiratory home care of the ventilator assisted individual.* New Orleans, LA: Author; adapted by permission.

Children and Youth Assisted by Medical Technology in Educational Settings (2nd ed.) © 1997 Paul H. Brookes Publishing Co., Baltimore.

Student's name: _____

Explanation/Return Demonstration	Expl./ Demo. Date	Explanation/Return Demonstration					
		Date	Date	Date	Date	Date	Date
8. Returns stomach contents to stomach							
9. If stomach contents are over _____ cc, sub-tract from feeding							
10. If more than _____ cc, hold feeding							
11. Pinches or clamps off tube							
12. Removes syringe							
13. Attaches syringe without plunger to feeding port							
14. Pours formula (room temperature) into syringe (approximately 30cc–40cc)							
15. Releases or unclamps tube and allows feed-ing to go in slowly							
16. Lowers the syringe if feeding is going too fast							
17. When feeding gets to 5-cc marker, adds more formula							
18. Continues this procedure until the feeding has been completed							
19. Takes about 30 minutes to complete feeding (the higher the syringe is held, the faster the feeding will flow)							
20. Makes feeding like mealtime (young children may suck on a pacifier)							
21. Flushes tube with _____ cc of water when feeding is complete							
22. Vents G-tube if ordered							
23. Pinches off tubing, removes syringe, and closes off clamp Reinserts cap or plug into end of G-tube							
24. Applies dressing, if needed, using universal precautions							
25. Removes gloves and washes hands							
26. Makes sure tubing is secured and tucked inside clothing							
27. Refers to student-specific guidelines regard-ing position and activity after feeding							
28. Washes syringe and other reusable equip-ment with soap and warm water; rinses thor-oughly; dries and stores in clean area; stores formula as instructed							
29. Documents feeding/medication, residual amount, and feeding tolerance							
30. Reports any changes to family							

Checklist content approved by:

Parent/Guardian signature _____ Date _____

Children and Youth Assisted by Medical Technology in Educational Settings (2nd ed.) © 1997 Paul H. Brookes Publishing Co., Baltimore.

Gastrostomy Feeding
Slow Drip or Continuous Method
Skills Checklist

Student's name: _____

Person trained: _____

Position: _____

Instructor: _____

Explanation/Return Demonstration	Expl./ Demo. Date	Explanation/Return Demonstration					
		Date	Date	Date	Date	Date	Date
A. States name and purpose of procedure							
B. Preparation:							
1. Identifies student's ability to participate in procedure							
2. Reviews universal precautions							
3. Completes at _____ time(s)							
4. _____ cc (amount) _____ Formula/feeding							
5. Feeding to be completed in _____ minutes							
6. Position for feeding _____							
7. Identifies where procedure is done and student's activity level							
8. Identifies possible problems and appropriate actions							
C. Identifies supplies:							
1. Gastrostomy tube _____ (size) _____ (type) Balloon size _____ cc							
a. Small port plug							
b. Feeding port							
2. Gloves							
3. Feeding solution at room temperature							
4. 60-cc catheter–tipped syringe							
5. Pump and IV stand (if used)							
6. Clamp and plug/cap							
7. Tap water							
8. Feeding container and tubing							
9. Rubber bands, safety pins							
D. Procedure:							
1. Washes hands							
2. Assembles equipment							
3. Positions student and explains the procedure							
4. Washes hands, puts on gloves							
5. Removes plug from feeding tube							
Student-Specific: (Steps 6–11 need to be individualized for each student.)							

_____

(continued)

Format adapted from Children's Hospital Chronic Illness Program, Ventilator Assisted Care Program. (1987). *Getting it started and keeping it going: A guide for respiratory home care of the ventilator assisted individual.* New Orleans, LA: Author; adapted by permission.

Children and Youth Assisted by Medical Technology in Educational Settings (2nd ed.) © 1997 Paul H. Brookes Publishing Co., Baltimore.

Student's name: _____

Explanation/Return Demonstration	Expl./ Demo. Date	Explanation/Return Demonstration					
		Date	Date	Date	Date	Date	Date
6. Checks for proper placement of tube: Attaches syringe and aspirates stomach contents by pulling plunger back							
7. Measures contents							
8. Returns contents to stomach							
9. If volume is more than _____ cc, subtract from feeding							
10. If more than _____ cc, hold feeding							
11. Pinches or clamps off tubing and removes syringe							
12. Pours feeding/fluids into feeding container, runs feeding through tubing to the tip, and clamps tubing							
13. Hangs container on pole at height required to deliver prescribed flow; if pump is used, places tubing into pump and sets flow rate							
14. Opens plug and inserts tubing into the tube							
15. Opens clamp on tubing and adjusts flow to prescribed rate (if pump is used, opens clamp completely)							
16. For a *continuous feeding* with a pump, adds more fluid to container when empty							
17. Checks rate and flow periodically and adjusts if needed							
18. When *single feeding* is completed (bag empty), clamps tubing and G-tube and disconnects from G-tube							
19. Makes feeding like mealtime (young children may suck on pacifier)							
20. Attaches catheter-tipped syringe with plunger removed and flushes G-tube with _____ cc water							
21. After flushing, lowers syringe below stomach level or leaves elevated and open for specified time to vent G-tube							
22. Clamps or caps G-tube							
23. Applies dressing, if needed, using universal precautions							
24. Removes gloves and washes hands							
25. Secures tubing and tucks inside clothing							
26. Refers to student-specific guidelines regarding position and activity after feeding							

(continued)

Children and Youth Assisted by Medical Technology in Educational Settings (2nd ed.) © 1997 Paul H. Brookes Publishing Co., Baltimore.

Student's name: _____

Explanation/Return Demonstration	Expl./ Demo. Date	Explanation/Return Demonstration					
		Date	Date	Date	Date	Date	Date
27. Washes syringe and other reusable equipment; rinses thoroughly; dries and stores in clean area; stores formula as instructed							
28. Documents feeding/medication, residual amount, and feeding tolerance							
29. Reports any changes to family							

Checklist content approved by:

Parent/Guardian signature _____ Date _____

Student's name: _____

Person trained: _____

Position: _____

Skin-Level Gastrostomy Feeding—
Bolus Method
Skills Checklist

Instructor: _____

Explanation/Return Demonstration	Expl./ Demo. Date	Explanation/Return Demonstration					
		Date	Date	Date	Date	Date	Date
A. States name and purpose of procedure							
B. Preparation:							
1. Identifies student's ability to participate in procedure							
2. Reviews universal precautions							
3. Completes at _____ time(s)							
4. _____ cc (amount) _____ Formula/feeding (type of feeding)							
5. Feeding to be completed in _____ minutes							
6. Position for feeding _____							
7. Identifies possible problems and appropriate actions							
C. Identifies supplies:							
1. Size and type of gastrostomy device							
2. Gloves							
3. Formula at room temperature							
4. 60-cc catheter–tipped feeding syringe							
5. Adaptor with tubing and clamp							
6. Tap water (if prescribed)							
D. Procedure:							
1. Washes hands							
2. Gathers equipment							
3. Positions student and explains procedure							
4. Washes hands, puts on gloves							
5. Attaches the adaptor to feeding syringe without plunger							
6. Opens safety plug and attaches the adaptor and tubing with feeding syringe to the skin-level feeding device							
7. Clamps or pinches off tubing Pours feeding into syringe until about one half full							

(continued)

Format adapted from Children's Hospital Chronic Illness Program, Ventilator Assisted Care Program. (1987). *Getting it started and keeping it going: A guide for respiratory home care of the ventilator assisted individual.* New Orleans, LA: Author; adapted by permission.

Children and Youth Assisted by Medical Technology in Educational Settings (2nd ed.) © 1997 Paul H. Brookes Publishing Co., Baltimore.

Student's name: _____

Explanation/Return Demonstration	Expl./ Demo. Date	Explanation/Return Demonstration					
		Date	Date	Date	Date	Date	Date
8. Elevates the feeding above the level of the stomach Opens clamp Allows feeding to go in slowly, 20–30 minutes The higher the syringe is held, the faster the feeding will flow Lowers syringe if the feeding is going too fast							
9. Refills the syringe before it empties to prevent air from entering stomach							
10. Makes feeding like mealtime (young children may suck on a pacifier)							
11. Flushes the feeding device with _____ cc of water when feeding is complete							
12. After flushing, lowers the syringe below the stomach level to facilitate burping							
13. Removes the adaptor with feeding syringe and snaps safety plug in place							
14. Removes gloves, washes hands							
15. Washes syringe and tubing with soap and warm water, rinses and stores in clean area; stores formula as instructed							
16. Refers to student-specific guidelines regarding position and activity after feeding							
17. Documents feeding/medication, residual amount, and feeding tolerance							
18. Reports any changes to family							

Checklist content approved by:

Parent/Guardian signature _____ Date _____

Student's name: _____

Person trained: _____

Position: _____

Skin-Level Gastrostomy Feeding—
Slow Drip or Continuous Method
Skills Checklist

Instructor: _____

Explanation/Return Demonstration	Expl./ Demo. Date	Explanation/Return Demonstration					
		Date	Date	Date	Date	Date	Date
A. States name and purpose of procedure							
B. Preparation:							
1. Identifies student's ability to participate in procedure							
2. Reviews universal precautions							
3. Completes at _____ time(s)							
4. _____ cc (amount) _____ Formula/feeding solution							
5. Feeding to be completed in _____ minutes							
6. Position for feeding _____							
7. Identifies where procedure is done and student's activity level							
8. Identifies possible problems and appropriate actions							
C. Identifies supplies:							
1. Gastrostomy device _____ (size and type)							
2. Gloves							
3. Feeding solution in container (bag) at room temperature							
4. 60-cc catheter–tipped syringe							
5. Pump and IV stand (if used)							
6. Adaptor with tubing and clamp							
7. Tap water							
8. Pole to hold feeding container							
D. Procedure:							
1. Washes hands							
2. Assembles equipment							
3. Positions student and explains the procedure							
4. Washes hands, puts on gloves							
5. Attaches adaptor to tubing							
6. Pours feeding/fluids into feeding container, runs feeding through tubing to the tip, and clamps tubing							
7. Hangs container on pole at height required to deliver prescribed flow (if pump is used, places tubing into pump and sets flow rate)							

(continued)

Format adapted from Children's Hospital Chronic Illness Program, Ventilator Assisted Care Program. (1987). *Getting it started and keeping it going: A guide for respiratory home care of the ventilator assisted individual.* New Orleans, LA: Author; adapted by permission.

Children and Youth Assisted by Medical Technology in Educational Settings (2nd ed.) © 1997 Paul H. Brookes Publishing Co., Baltimore.

Student's name: _____

Explanation/Return Demonstration	Expl./ Demo. Date	Explanation/Return Demonstration					
		Date	Date	Date	Date	Date	Date
8. Opens safety plug and inserts tubing into the button							
9. Opens clamp on tubing and adjusts flow to prescribed rate (If pump is used, opens clamp completely)							
10. For a *continuous feeding* with a pump, adds more fluid to bag when empty							
11. Checks rate and flow periodically and adjusts if needed							
12. When *single feeding* is completed (bag empty), clamps feeding bag tubing and removes							
13. Makes feeding like mealtime: young children may suck on a pacifier							
14. Attaches catheter-tipped syringe and flushes adapter tubing and feeding device							
15. After flushing, lowers syringe below stomach level to facilitate burping							
16. Removes adaptor and tubing from feeding device and snaps safety plug in place							
17. Removes gloves, washes hands							
18. Refers to student-specific guidelines regarding position and activity after feeding							
19. Washes feeding bag and tubing with soap and warm water, rinses and stores in clean area, stores formula as instructed							
20. Documents feeding/medication, residual amount, and feeding tolerance							
21. Reports any changes to family							

Checklist content approved by:

Parent/Guardian signature _____   Date _____

Student's name: _____

Person trained: _____

Position: _____

Instructor: _____

Explanation/Return Demonstration	Expl./ Demo. Date	Explanation/Return Demonstration					
		Date	Date	Date	Date	Date	Date
A. States name and purpose of procedure							
B. Preparation:							
1. Identifies student's ability to participate in procedure							
2. Reviews universal precautions							
3. Completes at _____ time(s)							
4. _____ cc (amount) _____ Formula/feeding solution							
5. Feeding to be completed in ____ minutes							
6. Position for feeding _____							
7. Identifies where procedure is done and student's activity level							
8. Identifies possible problems and appropriate actions							
C. Identifies supplies:							
1. NG-tube _____ (size) _____ (type)							
2. Gloves							
3. Feeding solution at room temperature							
4. 60-cc catheter–tipped syringe							
5. Cap and clamp for tubing							
6. Rubber bands, safety pins							
7. Tap water							
8. Stethoscope							
D. Procedure:							
1. Washes hands							
2. Assembles equipment							
3. Positions student and explains the procedure							
4. Washes hands, puts on gloves							
5. Checks for proper NG-tubing placement:							
a. Connects syringe to NG-tubing after removing cap/plug							
b. Places stethoscope over mid-left abdomen and gently pushes in 5–10 cc of air with syringe							
c. Listens with stethoscope and identifies sounds heard with proper placement							

(continued)

Format adapted from Children's Hospital Chronic Illness Program, Ventilator Assisted Care Program. (1987). *Getting it started and keeping it going: A guide for respiratory home care of the ventilator assisted individual.* New Orleans, LA: Author; adapted by permission.

Children and Youth Assisted by Medical Technology in Educational Settings (2nd ed.) © 1997 Paul H. Brookes Publishing Co., Baltimore.

Nasogastric Tube Feeding—Bolus Method
Skills Checklist

Student's name: _____

Explanation/Return Demonstration	Expl./ Demo. Date	Explanation/Return Demonstration					
		Date	Date	Date	Date	Date	Date
Student-Specific: (Steps 6–11 need to be individualized for each student.)							
6. Aspirates stomach contents by pulling plunger back							
7. Measures stomach contents and returns to stomach							
8. If volume is over _____ cc, subtracts from feeding							
9. If volume is more than _____ cc, holds feeding							
10. Clamps/pinches NG-tubing							
11. Attaches syringe without plunger to NG-tube							
12. Pours 30–40 cc feeding into syringe							
13. Opens clamp on NG-tubing, allows feeding to run in slowly (The higher the syringe is held, the faster the feeding will flow.)							
14. Adds more formula when liquid is at 5-cc mark Continues to add until feeding is completed over prescribed time. (Lowers syringe if flow is too fast)							
15. Makes feeding like mealtime (young children may suck on a pacifier)							
16. Flushes NG-tube with _____ cc water							
17. Pinches or clamps NG-tubing. Disconnects syringe							
18. Clamps and/or caps NG-tube							
19. Makes sure NG-tube is secured							
20. Removes gloves and washes hands							
21. Refers to student-specific guidelines regarding position and activity after feeding							
22. Cleans, rinses, and stores syringe; stores formula as instructed							
23. Documents feeding/medication, residual amount, and feeding tolerance							
24. Reports any changes to family							

Checklist content approved by:

Parent/Guardian signature _____ Date _____

Student's name: _____

Person trained: _____

Position: _____

**Nasogastric Tube Feeding—
Slow Drip or Continuous Feeding**
Skills Checklist

Instructor: _____

Explanation/Return Demonstration	Expl./ Demo. Date	Explanation/Return Demonstration					
		Date	Date	Date	Date	Date	Date
A. States name and purpose of procedure							
B. Preparation:							
1. Identifies student's ability to participate in procedure							
2. Reviews universal precautions							
3. Completes at _____ time(s)							
4. _____ cc (amount) _____ Formula/feeding at room temperature							
5. Feeding to be completed in _____ minutes							
6. Position for feeding _____							
7. Identifies where procedure is done and student's activity level							
8. Identifies possible problems and appropriate actions							
C. Identifies supplies:							
1. NG-tube _____ (size) _____ (type)							
2. Gloves (optional)							
3. Feeding solution in container (bag)							
4. 60-cc catheter–tipped syringe							
5. Pump and IV stand (if used)							
6. Clamp or cap							
7. Rubber bands, safety pins							
8. Tap water							
9. Stethoscope							
D. Procedure:							
1. Washes hands							
2. Assembles equipment							
3. Positions student and explains the procedure							
4. Washes hands, puts on gloves							
5. Checks for proper NG-tubing placement:							
a. Connects syringe to NG-tubing							
b. Places stethoscope over mid-left abdomen and gently pushes in 5–10 cc of air with syringe							

(continued)

Format adapted from Children's Hospital Chronic Illness Program, Ventilator Assisted Care Program. (1987). *Getting it started and keeping it going: A guide for respiratory home care of the ventilator assisted individual.* New Orleans, LA: Author; adapted by permission.

Children and Youth Assisted by Medical Technology in Educational Settings (2nd ed.) © 1997 Paul H. Brookes Publishing Co., Baltimore.

Student's name: _____

Explanation/Return Demonstration	Expl./ Demo. Date	Explanation/Return Demonstration					
		Date	Date	Date	Date	Date	Date
c. Listens with stethoscope and identifies sounds heard with proper placement							
Student-Specific: (Steps 6–11 need to be individualized for each student.)							
6. Aspirates stomach contents by pulling plunger back							
7. Measures volume of contents and returns to stomach							
8. If volume is over _____ cc, subtracts from feeding							
9. If volume is more than _____ cc, holds feeding							
10. Clamps/pinches NG-tubing. Disconnects syringe							
11. Pours feeding into container, running fluid through tubing to tip, and clamps tubing							
12. Hangs container on pole at height required to deliver prescribed flow rate. (If a pump is used, places tubing into pump mechanism and sets to prescribed rate.)							
13. Inserts tip of feeding container tubing into NG-tube and tapes securely, unclamps NG-tube							
14. Opens clamp on feeding bag tubing and adjusts flow to prescribed rate							
15. For a *continuous feeding* with a pump, adds more fluid to bag when empty							
16. Checks rate and flow periodically and adjusts if needed							
17. When *single feeding* is completed (bag empty), clamps feeding bag tubing and pinches or clamps NG-tubing Disconnects feeding container tubing							
18. Makes feeding like mealtime (young children may suck on a pacifier)							
19. Flushes NG-tube with _____ cc water							
20. Clamps and/or caps NG-tube							
21. Makes sure NG-tube is secured							
22. Removes gloves and washes hands							
23. Refers to student-specific guidelines regarding position and activity after feeding							
24. Cleans, rinses, and stores feeding container and tubing; stores formula as instructed							

(continued)

Children and Youth Assisted by Medical Technology in Educational Settings (2nd ed.) © 1997 Paul H. Brookes Publishing Co., Baltimore.

Student's name: _____

Explanation/Return Demonstration	Expl./ Demo. Date	Explanation/Return Demonstration					
		Date	Date	Date	Date	Date	Date
25. Documents feeding/medication, residual amount, and any changes							
26. Reports any changes to family							

Checklist content approved by:

Parent/Guardian signature _____ Date _____

Jejunostomy Feeding—
Continuous Method Feeding by Pump
Skills Checklist

Student's name: _____

Person trained: _____

Position: _____

Instructor: _____

Explanation/Return Demonstration	Expl./ Demo. Date	Explanation/Return Demonstration					
		Date	Date	Date	Date	Date	Date
A. States name and purpose of procedure							
B. Preparation:							
1. Determines student's ability to participate in procedure							
2. Reviews universal precautions							
3. Position for feeding _____							
4. Identifies where procedure is done and student's activity level							
5. Identifies possible problems and appropriate actions							
C. Identifies supplies:							
1. J-tube _____ (size) _____ (type)							
a. Small port plug							
b. Feeding port							
2. Clamp and plug/cap							
3. Gloves (optional)							
4. Feeding solution at room temperature							
5. 10-cc syringe							
6. Feeding container and tubing							
7. Pump							
8. Tap water							
9. Pole to hold feeding container							
D. Procedure:							
1. Washes hands							
2. Assembles equipment							
3. Positions student and explains procedure							
4. Washes hands, puts on gloves							
Student-Specific (Steps 5–10 need to be individualized for each student.)							
5. Checks for proper placement of tube							
6. Pours feeding/fluids into feeding container, runs feeding through tubing to the tip, and clamps tubing							
7. Hangs container on pole at height required to deliver prescribed flow							
8. Vents G-tube or skin-level feeding device if indicated during feeding							

(continued)

Format adapted from Children's Hospital Chronic Illness Program, Ventilator Assisted Care Program. (1987). *Getting it started and keeping it going: A guide for respiratory home care of the ventilator assisted individual.* New Orleans, LA: Author; adapted by permission.

Children and Youth Assisted by Medical Technology in Educational Settings (2nd ed.) © 1997 Paul H. Brookes Publishing Co., Baltimore.

Student's name: _____

Explanation/Return Demonstration	Expl./ Demo. Date	Explanation/Return Demonstration					
		Date	Date	Date	Date	Date	Date
9. Inserts tip of feeding bag tubing into J-tube							
10. Opens clamp on tubing completely and sets rate on pump							
11. For a *continuous feeding* with a pump, adds more fluid to container before completely empty							
12. Checks rate periodically for proper infusion rate							
13. If *single feeding* is completed during school time, clamps tubing and J-tube and disconnects from J-tube							
14. Flushes J-tube with _____ cc water							
15. Clamps or caps J-tube and secures tubing, applies dressing as needed							
16. Cleans and stores feeding container, tubing, and syringe; stores formula as instructed							
17. Washes hands							
18. Documents feeding and observations							
19. Reports any changes to family							

Checklist content approved by:

Parent/Guardian signature _____   Date _____

**Central Venous Catheter
Dressing Change**

Skills Checklist

Explanation/Return Demonstration	Expl./ Demo. Date	Explanation/Return Demonstration					
		Date	Date	Date	Date	Date	Date
A. States name and purpose of procedure							
B. Preparation:							
1. Identifies student's ability to participate in procedure							
2. Reviews universal precautions							
3. Identifies catheter placement and exit site							
4. Identifies CVC catheter type and parts							
5. Identifies where procedure is done (respects privacy)							
6. Identifies possible problems and appropriate actions							
C. Identifies supplies:							
1. Dressing kit:							
a. Sterile gloves							
b. Alcohol swabsticks							
c. Povidone iodine swabsticks or student-specific cleansing supplies							
d. Povidone ointment or student-specific antibacterial ointment							
e. Sterile gauze							
2. Adhesive tape							
3. Mask							
4. Transparent occlusive dressing							
5. Spare clamp							
6. Catheter cap							
7. Spare catheter dressing kit							
8. 3-cc syringe for normal saline							
D. Procedure:							
1. Washes hands							
2. Assembles equipment							
3. Positions student and explains procedure							
4. Puts on mask							
5. Washes hands							
6. Arranges equipment							
7. Removes wet or soiled dressing							
8. Inspects exit site							

(continued)

Format adapted from Children's Hospital Chronic Illness Program, Ventilator Assisted Care Program. (1987). *Getting it started and keeping it going: A guide for respiratory home care of the ventilator assisted individual.* New Orleans, LA: Author; adapted by permission.

Children and Youth Assisted by Medical Technology in Educational Settings (2nd ed.) © 1997 Paul H. Brookes Publishing Co., Baltimore.

Student's name: _____

Explanation/Return Demonstration	Expl./ Demo. Date	Explanation/Return Demonstration					
		Date	Date	Date	Date	Date	Date
9. Puts on sterile gloves							
10. Cleanses skin with alcohol swabs 3 times and allows solution to dry 30 seconds							
11. Cleanses skin with povidone swabs 3 times and allows povidone to dry about 30 seconds							
12. Dries skin with sterile gauze							
13. Applies antibacterial ointment to site							
14. Places sterile gauze over ointment							
15. Covers gauze with sterile dressing							
16. Secures catheter with tape							
17. Disposes of gloves, mask, and supplies appropriately							
18. Washes hands							
19. Documents procedure and observations							
20. Writes date and time of dressing change on dressing							
21. Reports any changes to family							

Checklist content approved by:

Parent/Guardian signature _____ Date _____

Children and Youth Assisted by Medical Technology in Educational Settings (2nd ed.) © 1997 Paul H. Brookes Publishing Co., Baltimore.

Student's name: _____

Person trained: _____

Position: _____

Instructor: _____

Heparin Flush
Skills Checklist

Explanation/Return Demonstration	Expl./ Demo. Date	Explanation/Return Demonstration					
		Date	Date	Date	Date	Date	Date
A. States name and purpose of procedure							
B. Preparation:							
1. Identifies student's ability to participate in procedure							
2. Reviews universal precautions							
3. Completes at _____ time(s)							
4. Identifies where procedure is done							
5. Identifies possible problems and appropriate actions							
C. Identifies supplies:							
1. IV catheter and male adaptor							
2. Heparinized saline of prescribed concentration							
3. 3-ml syringe with a 21- to 23-gauge needle							
4. Two alcohol swabs							
5. Gloves							
6. Adhesive tape							
D. Procedure:							
1. Washes hands							
2. Assembles equipment							
3. Positions student and explains procedure							
4. Washes hands, puts on gloves							
5. Cleanses top of heparinized saline container with alcohol							
6. Draws prescribed dose of heparinized saline into syringe							
7. Cleanses male adaptor hub with alcohol swab							
8. Slowly injects dose of heparinized saline into hub							
9. Removes syringe/needle without dislodging IV catheter							
10. Disposes of syringe and needle in appropriate container							
11. If problems with injection, inspects IV site and removes IV catheter if infiltrated							
12. Reinforces dressing, if needed							
13. Removes gloves and washes hands							

_____

(continued)

Format adapted from Children's Hospital Chronic Illness Program, Ventilator Assisted Care Program. (1987). *Getting it started and keeping it going: A guide for respiratory home care of the ventilator assisted individual.* New Orleans, LA: Author; adapted by permission.

Children and Youth Assisted by Medical Technology in Educational Settings (2nd ed.) © 1997 Paul H. Brookes Publishing Co., Baltimore.

Student's name: _____

Explanation/Return Demonstration	Expl./ Demo. Date	Explanation/Return Demonstration					
		Date	Date	Date	Date	Date	Date
14. Documents procedure and observations							
15. Reports any changes to family							

Checklist content approved by:

Parent/Guardian signature _____ Date _____

Student's name: _____

Person trained: _____

Position: _____

Instructor: _____

**Clean Intermittent
Catheterization—Male**
Skills Checklist

Explanation/Return Demonstration	Expl./ Demo. Date	Explanation/Return Demonstration					
		Date	Date	Date	Date	Date	Date
A. States name and purpose of procedure							
B. Preparation:							
1. Identifies student's ability to participate in procedure							
2. Reviews universal precautions							
3. Completes at _____ time(s) (in emergency complete earlier rather than later)							
4. Completes where _____ (consider privacy and access to bathroom)							
5. Position for catheterization: _____							
6. Identifies body parts:							
a. Scrotum							
b. Foreskin							
c. Meatus							
d. Glans							
7. Identifies possible problems and appropriate actions							
C. Identifies supplies:							
1. Water-soluble lubricant							
2. Type of catheter							
3. Wet wipes or cotton balls							
4. Cleansing supplies							
5. Storage receptacle for catheter							
6. Container for urine							
7. Gloves							
D. Procedure:							
1. Washes hands							
2. Gathers equipment							
3. Arranges equipment for procedure							
4. Positions student and explains procedure							
5. Washes hands, puts on gloves							
6. Lubricates catheter and places on clean surface							
7. Cleans:							
a. Prepares cleaning materials							
b. Retracts foreskin (if needed)							

(continued)

Format adapted from Children's Hospital Chronic Illness Program, Ventilator Assisted Care Program. (1987). *Getting it started and keeping it going: A guide for respiratory home care of the ventilator assisted individual.* New Orleans, LA: Author; adapted by permission.

Children and Youth Assisted by Medical Technology in Educational Settings (2nd ed.) © 1997 Paul H. Brookes Publishing Co., Baltimore.

Student's name: _____

Explanation/Return Demonstration	Expl./ Demo. Date	Explanation/Return Demonstration					
		Date	Date	Date	Date	Date	Date
c. Holds penis at 45-degree–90-degree angle from the abdomen							
d. Pulls penis straight							
e. Cleans meatus and glans							
f. Uses swab only once							
g. Wipes a minimum of three times							
8. Grasps catheter about 4 inches from tip							
9. Inserts well-lubricated catheter into penis with consistent pressure (if muscle spasm occurs, stop momentarily and then again use slow even pressure) **Never force a catheter.**							
10. When urine flow stops, inserts slightly more and withdraws a little							
11. Rotates catheter so all catheter openings reach all bladder areas							
12. Allows urine to flow by gravity into the shallow pan or toilet							
Student-Specific (Steps 13–15 need to be individualized for each student.)							
13. If ordered, gently press bladder to help empty							
14. Pinches catheter and withdraws slowly when urine stops flowing							
15. If not circumcised, pulls foreskin over glans							
16. Removes gloves and washes hands							
17. Assists student in dressing							
18. Puts on gloves, measures and records urine volume, disposes of urine, and cleans equipment and stores in home container							
19. Washes hands							
20. Documents procedure and observations							
21. Reports any changes to family							

Checklist content approved by:

Parent/Guardian signature _____ Date _____

Children and Youth Assisted by Medical Technology in Educational Settings (2nd ed.) © 1997 Paul H. Brookes Publishing Co., Baltimore.

Student's name: _____

Person trained: _____

Position: _____   Instructor: _____

Explanation/Return Demonstration	Expl./ Demo. Date	Explanation/Return Demonstration					
		Date	Date	Date	Date	Date	Date
A. States name and purpose of procedure							
B. Preparation:							
1. Identifies student's ability to participate in procedure							
2. Reviews universal precautions							
3. Completes at _____ time(s) (in emergency, complete earlier rather than later)							
4. Completes where _____ (consider privacy and access to bathroom)							
5. Position for catheterization: _____							
6. Identifies body parts:							
a. Labia majora							
b. Labia minora							
c. Meatus							
d. Urethra							
7. Identifies possible problems and appropriate actions							
C. Identifies supplies:							
1. Lubricant (water soluble)							
2. Type of catheter							
3. Wet wipes or cotton balls							
4. Cleansing supplies							
5. Storage receptacle for catheter							
6. Container for urine							
7. Gloves							
8. Mirror							
D. Procedure:							
1. Washes hands							
2. Gathers equipment							
3. Arranges equipment for procedure							
4. Positions student and explains procedure							
5. Washes hands, puts on gloves							
6. Lubricates catheter and places on clean surface							
7. Cleans:							
a. Prepares cleaning materials							

(continued)

Format adapted from Children's Hospital Chronic Illness Program, Ventilator Assisted Care Program. (1987). *Getting it started and keeping it going: A guide for respiratory home care of the ventilator assisted individual.* New Orleans, LA: Author; adapted by permission.

Children and Youth Assisted by Medical Technology in Educational Settings (2nd ed.) © 1997 Paul H. Brookes Publishing Co., Baltimore.

Student's name: _____

Explanation/Return Demonstration	Expl./ Demo. Date	Explanation/Return Demonstration					
		Date	Date	Date	Date	Date	Date
b. Opens labia minora and majora							
c. Cleans from front of folds to back of meatus							
d. Uses swab only once							
e. Wipes a minimum of three times							
8. Grasps catheter about 3 inches from tip							
9. Inserts into urethra until urine begins to flow							
10. Advances ½ inch more							
11. Rotates catheter so all catheter openings reach all bladder areas							
12. Allows urine to flow by gravity into shallow pan or toilet							
Student-Specific (Steps 13–15 need to be individualized for each student.)							
13. If ordered, gently press bladder to help empty							
14. Pinches catheter and withdraws slowly when urine stops flowing							
15. Stops and waits until all urine has drained if urine begins to flow again during removal							
16. Removes gloves and washes hands							
17. Assists student in dressing							
18. Puts on gloves, measures and records urine volume, disposes of urine, and cleans equipment and stores in home container							
19. Washes hands							
20. Documents procedure and observations							
21. Reports any changes to family							

Checklist content approved by:

Parent/Guardian signature _____ Date _____

Student's name: _____

Person trained: _____

Position: _____

Instructor: _____

Explanation/Return Demonstration	Expl./ Demo. Date	Explanation/Return Demonstration					
		Date	Date	Date	Date	Date	Date
A. States name and purpose of procedure							
B. Preparation:							
1. Identifies student's ability to participate in procedure							
2. Reviews universal precautions							
3. Completes at _____ time(s)							
4. Identifies where procedure is done (consider privacy and access to bathroom)							
5. Position for ostomy care: _____							
6. Identifies possible problems and appropriate actions							
C. Identifies supplies:							
1. Cleanser and water							
2. Skin preparation							
3. Soft cloth or gauze							
4. Clean pouch							
5. Belt, if needed							
6. Measuring guide							
7. Gloves							
8. Tape, if needed							
9. Protective powder and paste							
10. Scissors							
D. Procedure:							
1. Washes hands							
2. Assembles equipment							
3. Positions student and explains procedure							
4. Washes hands, puts on gloves							
5. Empties contents of pouch before removal, if ordered							
6. Removes used pouch and skin barrier							
7. Washes the stoma and skin area and disposes of gauze or cloth							
8. Inspects skin for redness/irritation							
9. Dries stoma and skin; applies protective powder							
10. Places skin barrier around stoma							

(continued)

Format adapted from Children's Hospital Chronic Illness Program, Ventilator Assisted Care Program. (1987). *Getting it started and keeping it going: A guide for respiratory home care of the ventilator assisted individual*. New Orleans, LA: Author; adapted by permission.

Children and Youth Assisted by Medical Technology in Educational Settings (2nd ed.) © 1997 Paul H. Brookes Publishing Co., Baltimore.

Student's name: _____

Explanation/Return Demonstration	Expl./ Demo. Date	Explanation/Return Demonstration					
		Date	Date	Date	Date	Date	Date
11. Applies paste to pouch or removes backing from adhesive							
12. Applies pouch closure							
13. Centers new pouch over stoma							
14. Presses pouch firmly against skin barrier to prevent leaks							
15. Disposes of used pouch in appropriate receptacle							
16. Removes gloves and washes hands							
17. Documents procedure and observations							
18. Reports any changes to family							

Checklist content approved by:

Parent/Guardian signature _____ Date _____

Student's name: _____

Person trained: _____

Position: _____

Ileostomy Pouch Change
Skills Checklist

Instructor: _____

Explanation/Return Demonstration	Expl./ Demo. Date	Explanation/Return Demonstration					
		Date	Date	Date	Date	Date	Date
A. States name and purpose of procedure							
B. Preparation:							
1. Identifies student's ability to participate in procedure							
2. Reviews universal precautions							
3. Completes at _____ time(s)							
4. Identifies where procedure is done (consider privacy and access to bathroom)							
5. Position for ostomy care: _____							
6. Identifies possible problems and appropriate actions							
C. Identifies supplies:							
1. Cleanser and water							
2. Soft cloth or gauze							
3. Clean pouch and belt, if needed							
4. Skin barrier							
5. Scissors and measuring guide							
6. Clean gloves							
7. Tape, if needed							
8. Protective powder and paste							
D. Procedure:							
1. Washes hands							
2. Assembles equipment							
3. Positions student and explains procedure							
4. Washes hands, puts on gloves							
5. Empties contents of pouch into toilet before removal, if ordered							
6. Removes used pouch							
7. Washes the stoma area and places gauze over stoma							
8. Inspects skin for redness/irritation							
9. Dries stoma and skin, applies protective powder							
10. Places skin barrier around stoma							
11. Applies paste to pouch, removes backing from adhesive, removes gauze from stoma and disposes							
12. Applies pouch closure							

(continued)

Format adapted from Children's Hospital Chronic Illness Program, Ventilator Assisted Care Program. (1987). *Getting it started and keeping it going: A guide for respiratory home care of the ventilator assisted individual.* New Orleans, LA: Author; adapted by permission.

Children and Youth Assisted by Medical Technology in Educational Settings (2nd ed.) © 1997 Paul H. Brookes Publishing Co., Baltimore.

Ileostomy Pouch Change
Skills Checklist

Explanation/Return Demonstration	Expl./ Demo. Date	Explanation/Return Demonstration					
		Date	Date	Date	Date	Date	Date
13. Centers new pouch over stoma							
14. Presses pouch firmly against skin barrier to prevent leaks							
15. Disposes of used pouch in appropriate receptacle							
16. Removes gloves and washes hands							
17. Documents procedure and observations							
18. Reports any changes to family							

Checklist content approved by:

Parent/Guardian signature _____ Date _____

Children and Youth Assisted by Medical Technology in Educational Settings (2nd ed.) © 1997 Paul H. Brookes Publishing Co., Baltimore.

Student's name: _____

Person trained: _____

Position: _____

Urostomy Pouch Change

Skills Checklist

Instructor: _____

Explanation/Return Demonstration	Expl./ Demo. Date	Explanation/Return Demonstration					
		Date	Date	Date	Date	Date	Date
A. States name and purpose of procedure							
B. Preparation:							
1. Identifies student's ability to participate in procedure							
2. Reviews universal precautions							
3. Completes at _____ time(s)							
4. Identifies where procedure is done (consider privacy and access to bathroom)							
5. Position for ostomy care: _____							
6. Identifies possible problems and appropriate actions							
C. Identifies supplies:							
1. Cleanser and water							
2. Soft cloth or gauze							
3. Skin preparation							
4. Clean pouch and belt, if needed							
5. Gloves							
6. Scissors and measuring guide							
7. Tape, if needed							
8. Adhesive							
9. Container to store used pouch							
10. Disinfectant solution to clean used pouch							
D. Procedure:							
1. Washes hands							
2. Assembles equipment							
3. Positions student and explains procedure							
4. Washes hands, puts on gloves							
5. Empties contents of pouch into toilet before removal							
6. Removes used pouch							
7. Washes the stoma area and places gauze over stoma							
8. Inspects skin for redness/irritation							
9. Dries stoma and skin							
10. Places skin barrier around stoma							
11. Applies adhesive to pouch or removes backing from adhesive; disposes of gauze							

(continued)

Format adapted from Children's Hospital Chronic Illness Program, Ventilator Assisted Care Program. (1987). *Getting it started and keeping it going: A guide for respiratory home care of the ventilator assisted individual.* New Orleans, LA: Author; adapted by permission.

Children and Youth Assisted by Medical Technology in Educational Settings (2nd ed.) © 1997 Paul H. Brookes Publishing Co., Baltimore.

Student's name: _____

Explanation/Return Demonstration	Expl./ Demo. Date	Explanation/Return Demonstration					
		Date	Date	Date	Date	Date	Date
12. Removes gloves							
13. Centers new pouch over stoma							
14. Presses pouch firmly against skin barrier to prevent leaks							
15. Attaches belt, if used							
16. Disposes of used pouch in appropriate receptacle							
17. Washes hands							
18. Documents procedure and observations							
19. Reports any changes to family							

Checklist content approved by:

Parent/Guardian signature _____ Date _____

Student's name: _____

Person trained: _____

Position: _____

Continent Urostomy/Vesicostomy
Catheterization
Skills Checklist

Instructor: _____

Explanation/Return Demonstration	Expl./ Demo. Date	Explanation/Return Demonstration					
		Date	Date	Date	Date	Date	Date
A. States name and purpose of procedure							
B. Preparation:							
1. Identifies student's ability to participate in procedure							
2. Reviews universal precautions							
3. Completes at _____ time(s) (in emergency, complete earlier rather than later)							
4. Completes where _____ (Consider privacy and access to bathroom)							
5. Position for catheterization: _____							
6. Identifies possible problems and appropriate actions							
C. Identifies supplies:							
1. Cleanser and water or alcohol-free towelettes							
2. Disposable gloves							
3. Type of catheter							
4. Lubricant (water soluble)							
5. Container for urine							
6. Small adhesive bandage or stoma covering							
7. Storage receptacle for catheter							
D. Procedure:							
1. Washes hands							
2. Assembles equipment							
3. Positions student and explains procedure							
4. Washes hands and puts on clean gloves							
5. Lubricates catheter and places on clean surface							
6. Washes stoma using cleansing supplies							
7. Inserts catheter into stoma until urine begins to flow							
8. Advances ½ inch–1 inch further							
9. Allows urine to flow by gravity into shallow pan or toilet							
10. Leaves catheter in until urine flow stops							
11. Pinches catheter and withdraws slowly							
12. Removes gloves and washes hands							

(continued)

Format adapted from Children's Hospital Chronic Illness Program, Ventilator Assisted Care Program. (1987). *Getting it started and keeping it going: A guide for respiratory home care of the ventilator assisted individual.* New Orleans, LA: Author; adapted by permission.

Children and Youth Assisted by Medical Technology in Educational Settings (2nd ed.) © 1997 Paul H. Brookes Publishing Co., Baltimore.

Student's name: _____

Explanation/Return Demonstration	Expl./ Demo. Date	Explanation/Return Demonstration					
		Date	Date	Date	Date	Date	Date
13. Reapplies small adhesive bandage on stoma covering							
14. Assists student in dressing							
15. Puts on gloves, measures and records urine volume; disposes of urine, and cleans equipment and stores in home container							
16. Washes hands							
17. Documents procedure and observations							
18. Reports any changes to family							

Checklist content approved by:

Parent/Guardian signature _____ Date _____

Student's name: _____

Person trained: _____

Position: _____

Oxygen Cylinder
Skills Checklist

Instructor: _____

Explanation/Return Demonstration	Expl./ Demo. Date	Explanation/Return Demonstration					
		Date	Date	Date	Date	Date	Date
A. States name and purpose of procedure							
B. Preparation:							
1. Identifies student's ability to participate in procedure							
2. Reviews universal precautions							
3. Identifies where procedure is done							
4. Identifies possible problems and appropriate actions							
5. States oxygen safety procedures							
C. Identifies supplies:							
1. Oxygen cylinder with key							
2. Oxygen regulator							
3. Flowmeter							
4. Delivery device with oxygen tubing							
5. Humidifier, if needed							
6. Tank stand							
D. Procedure:							
1. Positions student and explains procedure							
2. Washes hands							
3. Prepares tank and regulator							
4. Turns on tank							
5. Checks pressure in tank							
6. Estimates amount of time tank will last							
7. Connects delivery device and humidifier (if needed) to cylinder							
8. Adjusts flow to prescribed LPM; checks delivery device to make sure oxygen is coming out							
9. Provides oxygen to student using prescribed delivery device							
10. Monitors PSI, flow, and time while tank is in use							
11. Monitors student for hypoxia while oxygen is in use							
12. Turns off tank before turning off flowmeter, when tank is no longer needed or must be changed; removes delivery device from student							
13. Stores tank safely							

(continued)

Format adapted from Children's Hospital Chronic Illness Program, Ventilator Assisted Care Program. (1987). *Getting it started and keeping it going: A guide for respiratory home care of the ventilator assisted individual.* New Orleans, LA: Author; adapted by permission.

Children and Youth Assisted by Medical Technology in Educational Settings (2nd ed.) © 1997 Paul H. Brookes Publishing Co., Baltimore.

Student's name: _____

Explanation/Return Demonstration	Expl./ Demo. Date	Explanation/Return Demonstration					
		Date	Date	Date	Date	Date	Date
14. Washes hands							
15. Documents procedure and observations							
16. Reports any changes to family							

Checklist content approved by:

Parent/Guardian signature _____ Date _____

Student's name: _____

Person trained: _____

Position: _____

Oxygen Liquid System
Skills Checklist

Instructor: _____

Explanation/Return Demonstration	Expl./ Demo. Date	Explanation/Return Demonstration					
		Date	Date	Date	Date	Date	Date
A. States name and purpose of procedure							
B. Preparation:							
1. Identifies student's ability to participate in procedure							
2. Reviews universal precautions							
3. Identifies where procedure is done							
4. Identifies possible problems and appropriate actions							
5. States oxygen safety procedures							
C. Identifies supplies:							
1. Liquid oxygen system							
2. Delivery device with oxygen tubing							
3. Humidifier, if needed							
D. Procedure:							
1. Positions student and explains procedure							
2. Washes hands							
3. Prepares unit							
4. Checks level of fluid							
5. Connects delivery device and humidifier to liquid system							
6. Adjusts flow to prescribed LPM							
7. Checks delivery device to make sure oxygen is coming out							
8. Provides oxygen to student using prescribed delivery device							
9. Monitors flow while in use							
10. Monitors student for hypoxia while oxygen is in use							
11. Turns off cylinder before turning off flow-meter, when cylinder is no longer needed; removes delivery device from student							
12. Washes hands							
13. Monitors level of the liquid daily and stores cylinder safely							
14. Documents procedure and observations							
15. Reports any changes to family							

Checklist content approved by:

Parent/Guardian signature _____ Date _____

Format adapted from Children's Hospital Chronic Illness Program, Ventilator Assisted Care Program. (1987). *Getting it started and keeping it going: A guide for respiratory home care of the ventilator assisted individual.* New Orleans, LA: Author; adapted by permission.

Children and Youth Assisted by Medical Technology in Educational Settings (2nd ed.) © 1997 Paul H. Brookes Publishing Co., Baltimore.

Student's name: _____   **Oxygen Concentrator**

Person trained: _____   Skills Checklist

Position: _____   Instructor: _____

	Explanation/Return Demonstration	Expl./ Demo. Date	Explanation/Return Demonstration					
			Date	Date	Date	Date	Date	Date
A.	States name and purpose of procedure							
B.	Preparation:							
	1. Identifies student's ability to participate in procedure							
	2. Reviews universal precautions							
	3. Identifies where procedure is done							
	4. Identifies possible problems and appropriate actions							
	5. States oxygen safety procedures							
C.	Identifies supplies:							
	1. Oxygen concentrator							
	2. Flowmeter							
	3. Delivery device with oxygen tubing							
	4. Humidifier, if needed							
D.	Procedure:							
	1. Positions student and explains procedure							
	2. Washes hands							
	3. Checks filter							
	4. Turns on concentrator							
	5. Tests power-failure alarms							
	6. Connects delivery device to concentrator with oxygen tubing							
	7. Adjusts flow to prescribed LPM; provides oxygen to student using prescribed delivery device							
	8. Checks delivery device to make sure oxygen is coming out							
	9. Monitors flow while in use							
	10. Monitors student for hypoxia while oxygen is in use							
	11. Turns off tank before turning off flowmeter, when tank is no longer needed; removes delivery device from student							
	12. Washes hands							
	13. Documents procedure and observations							
	14. Reports any changes to family							

Checklist content approved by:

Parent/Guardian signature _____ Date _____

Format adapted from Children's Hospital Chronic Illness Program, Ventilator Assisted Care Program. (1987). *Getting it started and keeping it going: A guide for respiratory home care of the ventilator assisted individual.* New Orleans, LA: Author; adapted by permission.

Children and Youth Assisted by Medical Technology in Educational Settings (2nd ed.) © 1997 Paul H. Brookes Publishing Co., Baltimore.

Student's name: _____

Person trained: _____

Position: _____

Go Bag Supplies

Skills Checklist

Instructor: _____

Explanation/Return Demonstration	Expl./ Demo. Date	Explanation/Return Demonstration					
		Date	Date	Date	Date	Date	Date
A. States name and purpose of procedure							
B. Identifies use of each essential supply:							
1. Resuscitator bag							
2. Extra tracheostomy tube with ties and obturator (if indicated)—one the same size (If student has a cuffed tracheostomy tube, have an uncuffed tube of same size available. Second tracheostomy tube should be one size smaller.)							
3. Syringe (3 cc)							
4. Saline vials							
5. Suction catheters							
6. Bulb syringe							
7. Portable suction machine							
8. Blunt scissors							
9. Tissues							
10. Cotton-tipped applicators and pipe cleaners							
11. Hydrogen peroxide							
12. Gloves							
13. Tracheal gauge or sponges							
14. Water-soluble lubricant or saline							
15. Passive condenser							
16. Emergency phone numbers							
17. Go Bag list							
18. Other individualized items							
19. Emergency telephone number list							
C. Demonstrates plan for checking emergency supplies							

Checklist content approved by:

Parent/Guardian signature _____ Date _____

Format adapted from Children's Hospital Chronic Illness Program, Ventilator Assisted Care Program. (1987). *Getting it started and keeping it going: A guide for respiratory home care of the ventilator assisted individual.* New Orleans, LA: Author; adapted by permission.
Children and Youth Assisted by Medical Technology in Educational Settings (2nd ed.) © 1997 Paul H. Brookes Publishing Co., Baltimore.

Student's name: _____

Person trained: _____

Position: _____

Tracheostomy Tube Care

Skills Checklist

Instructor: _____

Explanation/Return Demonstration	Expl./ Demo. Date	Explanation/Return Demonstration					
		Date	Date	Date	Date	Date	Date
A. States name and purpose of procedure							
B. Preparation:							
1. Identifies student's ability to participate in procedure							
2. Reviews universal precautions							
3. Identifies where procedure is done							
4. Identifies possible problems and appropriate actions							
C. Identifies supplies:							
1. Tracheostomy tie or tracheostomy tube holder							
2. One half hydrogen peroxide and one half normal saline or distilled water							
3. Cotton-tipped applicators							
4. Pipe cleaners							
5. Tracheal gauze or sponges							
6. Two clean containers							
7. Gloves							
D. Procedure:							
1. Washes hands							
2. Assembles supplies							
3. Positions student and explains procedure							
4. Washes hands thoroughly and puts on gloves							
5. Removes old gauze or sponges from tracheostomy							
6. Cleans stoma with hydrogen peroxide and cotton swabs							
7. If tracheostomy has inner cannula, removes inner cannula							
8. Replaces old tracheostomy ties or holder with a new one							
a. Holds flange, cuts old ties, and removes ties or holder							
b. Replaces used ties or holder							
c. Ties ends securely with double knot or secure holder							
d. Inserts tracheostomy sponge under the tracheostomy tube phalanges							

(continued)

Format adapted from Children's Hospital Chronic Illness Program, Ventilator Assisted Care Program. (1987). *Getting it started and keeping it going: A guide for respiratory home care of the ventilator assisted individual.* New Orleans, LA: Author; adapted by permission.

Children and Youth Assisted by Medical Technology in Educational Settings (2nd ed.) © 1997 Paul H. Brookes Publishing Co., Baltimore.

Student's name: _____

Explanation/Return Demonstration	Expl./ Demo. Date	Explanation/Return Demonstration					
		Date	Date	Date	Date	Date	Date
9. Cleans removed inner cannula:							
a. Soaks inner cannula in one half hydrogen peroxide and one half normal saline or distilled water and cleans with a small brush, pipe cleaners, or cotton swabs							
b. Rinses with saline							
c. Replaces inner cannula and locks in place							
10. Discards cleaning solution							
11. Removes gloves and washes hands							
12. Documents procedure and observations							
13. Reports any changes to family							

Checklist content approved by:

Parent/Guardian signature _____ Date _____

Student's name: _____

Person trained: _____

Position: _____

Tracheal Suctioning—Sterile Technique
Skills Checklist

Instructor: _____

Explanation/Return Demonstration	Expl./ Demo. Date	Explanation/Return Demonstration					
		Date	Date	Date	Date	Date	Date
A. States name and purpose of procedure							
B. Preparation:							
1. Identifies student's ability to participate in procedure							
2. Reviews universal precautions							
3. Identifies where procedure is done							
4. Identifies possible problems and appropriate actions							
C. Identifies supplies:							
1. Suction machine with tubing							
2. Sterile catheter kit with gloves							
3. Sterile saline							
4. Cup of tap water							
5. Resuscitator bag with tracheostomy adaptor							
6. Gloves (nonsterile)							
D. Procedure:							
1. Washes hands							
2. Assembles supplies							
3. Positions student and explains procedure							
4. Washes hands							
5. Turns on suction machine and checks for function							
6. Opens package and removes kit							
7. Opens kit without touching inside of package, and opens saline and fills container with saline							
8. Removes gloves by holding inside of cuff and pulling gloves over hands that will hold catheter							
9. Picks up catheter and removes catheter							
10. Attaches end of catheter to suction tubing							
11. Uses resuscitator to give three to five breaths, _if ordered_							
12. Inserts catheter into tracheostomy tube without suction							
13. Advances catheter to end of tracheostomy tube or until student coughs							
14. Applies suction by putting thumb on suction catheter adaptor							

(continued)

Format adapted from Children's Hospital Chronic Illness Program, Ventilator Assisted Care Program. (1987). *Getting it started and keeping it going: A guide for respiratory home care of the ventilator assisted individual.* New Orleans, LA: Author; adapted by permission.

Children and Youth Assisted by Medical Technology in Educational Settings (2nd ed.) © 1997 Paul H. Brookes Publishing Co., Baltimore.

Student's name: _____

Explanation/Return Demonstration	Expl./ Demo. Date	Explanation/Return Demonstration					
		Date	Date	Date	Date	Date	Date
15. Twirls catheter between fingers as it is pulled out of tracheostomy tube, leaving in no more than 10 seconds							
16. Gives three to five breaths with resuscitator bag after catheter has been removed from tracheostomy tube							
17. Places drops of saline or prescribed solution in tracheostomy tube (if secretions are thick), follows with extra breaths, then suction							
18. Repeats suctioning in above order (Steps 11–17) until secretions are removed							
19. Suctions nose and mouth with same catheter the same way, if indicated							
20. Completes suctioning, disconnects catheter from suction tubing, wraps catheter around gloved hand, and pulls gloves off inside out; disposes of catheter and gloves appropriately							
21. Rinses suctioning tubing with tap water							
22. Washes hands							
23. Documents procedure and observations							
24. Reports any changes to family							

Checklist content approved by:

Parent/Guardian signature _____ Date _____

Children and Youth Assisted by Medical Technology in Educational Settings (2nd ed.) © 1997 Paul H. Brookes Publishing Co., Baltimore.

**Tracheostomy Suctioning—
Bulb Technique**

Skills Checklist

Instructor: _____

Explanation/Return Demonstration	Expl./ Demo. Date	Explanation/Return Demonstration					
		Date	Date	Date	Date	Date	Date
A. States name and purpose of procedure							
B. Preparation:							
1. Identifies student's ability to participate in procedure							
2. Reviews universal precautions							
3. Identifies where procedure is done							
4. Identifies possible problems and appropriate actions							
C. Identifies supplies:							
1. Go-Bag supplies (see Go Bag Supplies skills checklist on p. 355)							
D. Procedure:							
1. Washes hands							
2. Assembles supplies							
3. Positions student and explains procedure							
4. Washes hands and puts on gloves							
5. Squeezes bulb syringe; places tip in tracheostomy tube and releases							
6. Removes bulb syringe from tracheostomy tube							
7. Squeezes and releases bulb into tissue, expelling secretions							
8. Repeats Steps 5–7 until secretions are removed							
9. Squeezes bulb syringe for **nose/mouth**; places tip in mouth/nose and releases							
10. Removes bulb syringe from nose/mouth							
11. Squeezes and releases bulb into tissue; expelling secretions							
12. Repeats Steps 9–11 until secretions are removed							
13. Cleans bulb syringes and disposes of tissues							
14. Removes gloves, washes hands							
15. Documents procedure and observations							
16. Reports any changes to family							

Checklist content approved by:

Parent/Guardian signature _____ Date _____

Format adapted from Children's Hospital Chronic Illness Program, Ventilator Assisted Care Program. (1987). *Getting it started and keeping it going: A guide for respiratory home care of the ventilator assisted individual.* New Orleans, LA: Author; adapted by permission.

Children and Youth Assisted by Medical Technology in Educational Settings (2nd ed.) © 1997 Paul H. Brookes Publishing Co., Baltimore.

Student's name: _____

Person trained: _____

Position: _____

Instructor: _____

Explanation/Return Demonstration	Expl./ Demo. Date	Explanation/Return Demonstration					
		Date	Date	Date	Date	Date	Date
A. **In a school setting, this procedure should be done only in an emergency situation.** States name and purpose of procedure							
B. Preparation:							
1. Identifies student's ability to participate in procedure							
2. Reviews universal precautions							
3. Identifies where procedure is done							
4. Identifies possible problems and appropriate actions							
C. Identifies supplies:							
1. Type and size of tracheostomy tube							
2. Twill tape or other ties							
3. Obturator, if applicable							
4. Stethoscope							
5. Resuscitation bag							
6. Oxygen, if ordered							
7. Suctioning devices and supplies							
8. Water-soluble lubricant or sterile saline							
9. One size smaller tracheostomy tube							
10. Blanket roll, if needed							
11. Gloves							
12. Syringe, if cuffed tube							
D. Procedure:							
1. Washes hands							
2. Assembles equipment							
3. Explains procedure							
4. Washes hands							
5. Opens package							
6. Puts on gloves							
7. Removes from package; if cuffed tube, tests cuff							
8. Puts obturator into tracheostomy tube							
9. Attaches ties							
10. Lubricates tube							
11. Positions student							

(continued)

Format adapted from Children's Hospital Chronic Illness Program, Ventilator Assisted Care Program. (1987). *Getting it started and keeping it going: A guide for respiratory home care of the ventilator assisted individual.* New Orleans, LA: Author; adapted by permission.

Children and Youth Assisted by Medical Technology in Educational Settings (2nd ed.) © 1997 Paul H. Brookes Publishing Co., Baltimore.

Student's name: _____

Explanation/Return Demonstration	Expl./ Demo. Date	Explanation/Return Demonstration					
		Date	Date	Date	Date	Date	Date
12. Suctions tracheostomy, nose, and mouth, if needed							
13. Gives two to four breaths with resuscitation bag, if needed							
14. Cuts ties							
15. If cuffed tracheostomy tube, removes air from cuff with syringe							
16. With new tube ready, removes old tube							
17. If tube does not have obturator, inserts tube at right angle to stoma; holds in place until secured							
18. If tube has obturator, inserts tube straight into stoma; immediately removes obturator after tube insertion							
19. Inserts inner cannula							
20. Listens and feels for air movement through tube; watches chest rise with breath							
21. If tube has cuff, inflates cuff with prescribed amount of air							
22. Secures tracheostomy tube in place with ties or holder							
23. Listens for breath sounds with stethoscope; watches chest rise and fall with breath from resuscitation bag							
24. Does skin care if needed; reapplies gauze around and under tracheostomy and ties							
25. Gives two to four breaths with resuscitation bag; suctions, if needed							
26. Discards used equipment appropriately							
27. Removes gloves and washes hands							
28. Documents procedure and observations							
29. Reports any changes to family							

Checklist content approved by:

Parent/Guardian signature _____ Date _____

Student's name: _____

Person trained: _____

Position: _____

**Manual Resuscitator Bag
with Tracheostomy**
Skills Checklist

Instructor: _____

Explanation/Return Demonstration	Expl./ Demo. Date	Explanation/Return Demonstration					
		Date	Date	Date	Date	Date	Date
A. States name and purpose of procedure							
B. Preparation:							
1. Identifies student's ability to participate in procedure							
2. Reviews universal precautions							
3. Identifies where procedure is done							
4. Identifies possible problems and appropriate actions							
C. Identifies supplies:							
1. Oxygen source with appropriate tubing if needed							
2. Manual resuscitator							
3. Adaptor for tracheostomy tube							
4. Go-Bag items							
D. Procedure:							
1. Washes hands							
2. Positions student and explains procedure							
3. Checks that manual resuscitator is functioning properly							
4. Attaches resuscitator bag to tracheostomy tube							
5. Coordinates manual breaths with student's own breaths, if student breathes independently							
6. Squeezes manual resuscitator at regular rate to give prescribed breaths per minute, if student unable to breathe independently							
7. Removes resuscitation bag from tracheostomy tube when appropriate							
8. Washes hands							
9. Documents procedure and observations							
10. Reports any changes to family							

Checklist content approved by:

Parent/Guardian signature _____ Date _____

Format adapted from Children's Hospital Chronic Illness Program, Ventilator Assisted Care Program. (1987). *Getting it started and keeping it going: A guide for respiratory home care of the ventilator assisted individual.* New Orleans, LA: Author; adapted by permission.
Children and Youth Assisted by Medical Technology in Educational Settings (2nd ed.) © 1997 Paul H. Brookes Publishing Co., Baltimore.

Student's name: _____

Person trained: _____

Position: _____

Respiratory Emergencies—Accidental Removal of the Tracheostomy Tube

Skills Checklist

Instructor: _____

Explanation/Return Demonstration	Expl./ Demo. Date	Explanation/Return Demonstration					
		Date	Date	Date	Date	Date	Date
A. States name and purpose of procedure							
B. Preparation:							
1. Identifies student's ability to participate in procedure							
2. Reviews universal precautions							
3. Identifies where procedure is done							
4. Identifies possible problems and appropriate actions							
C. Identifies Go-Bag supplies (see p. 355), including:							
1. Emergency phone number list							
2. Spare tracheostomy tube with ties or holder attached and obturator							
3. Water-soluble lubricant—jelly or saline							
4. Blunt scissors							
5. Suction supplies and machine							
6. Gloves							
7. Gauze or sponges							
8. Manual resuscitator bag							
D. Procedure:							
1. Describes recognition of problems:							
a. Respiratory distress							
b. Finding tracheostomy tube out of trachea							
c. Low-pressure alarm (ventilator)							
2. Preparation and prevention:							
a. Has spare tracheostomy tube with student at all times							
b. Posts emergency numbers							
c. Answers alarms promptly							
d. Keeps tracheostomy tube midline and straight							
e. Knows cardiopulmonary resuscitation							
3. Action:							
a. Repositions tube if possible or removes old tracheostomy tube and replaces with spare tube (see p. 266)							
b. Assesses student							
c. Calls for emergency help, if needed							

Checklist content approved by:

Parent/Guardian signature _____ Date _____

Format adapted from Children's Hospital Chronic Illness Program, Ventilator Assisted Care Program. (1987). *Getting it started and keeping it going: A guide for respiratory home care of the ventilator assisted individual.* New Orleans, LA: Author; adapted by permission.

Children and Youth Assisted by Medical Technology in Educational Settings (2nd ed.) © 1997 Paul H. Brookes Publishing Co., Baltimore.

Student's name: _____

Person trained: _____

Position: _____

**Respiratory Emergencies—
Blocked Tracheostomy Tube**
Skills Checklist

Instructor: _____

Explanation/Return Demonstration	Expl./ Demo. Date	Explanation/Return Demonstration					
		Date	Date	Date	Date	Date	Date
A. States name and purpose of procedure							
B. Preparation:							
1. Identifies student's ability to participate in procedure							
2. Reviews universal precautions							
3. Identifies where procedure is done							
4. Identifies possible problems and appropriate actions							
C. Identifies Go-Bag supplies (see p. 355), including:							
1. Emergency phone number list							
2. Spare tracheostomy tube with ties or holder attached and obturator							
3. Water-soluble lubricant or saline							
4. Blunt scissors							
5. Suction supplies and machine							
6. Gloves							
7. Gauze or sponges							
8. Manual resuscitator bag							
D. Procedure:							
1. Describes recognition of problems:							
a. Respiratory distress							
b. Air will not go into lungs with a resuscitator bag							
c. Suction catheter will not pass through tracheostomy tube							
d. High-pressure alarm (ventilator)							
2. Preparation and prevention:							
a. Has spare tracheostomy tube with student at all times							
b. Has emergency supplies with student at all times							
c. Posts emergency numbers							
d. Keeps tracheostomy tube humidified properly							
e. Maintains routine tracheostomy tube changes							
f. Always answers alarms promptly							
g. Knows cardiopulmonary resuscitation							

(continued)

Format adapted from Children's Hospital Chronic Illness Program, Ventilator Assisted Care Program. (1987). *Getting it started and keeping it going: A guide for respiratory home care of the ventilator assisted individual.* New Orleans, LA: Author; adapted by permission.
Children and Youth Assisted by Medical Technology in Educational Settings (2nd ed.) © 1997 Paul H. Brookes Publishing Co., Baltimore.

Student's name: _____

Explanation/Return Demonstration	Expl./ Demo. Date	Explanation/Return Demonstration					
		Date	Date	Date	Date	Date	Date
3. Action:							
a. Puts on gloves							
b. Asks student to cough							
c. Puts several drops of saline in tracheostomy tube and suctions							
d. Changes tracheostomy tube *or* replaces inner cannula with spare and checks air movement							
e. Gives breaths with resuscitator bag							
f. Calls for emergency help and begins CPR, if needed							

Checklist content approved by:

Parent/Guardian signature _____ Date _____

Children and Youth Assisted by Medical Technology in Educational Settings (2nd ed.) © 1997 Paul H. Brookes Publishing Co., Baltimore.

Student's name: _____

Person trained: _____

Position: _____

Instructor: _____

Respiratory Emergencies—Aspiration
Skills Checklist

Explanation/Return Demonstration	Expl./ Demo. Date	Explanation/Return Demonstration					
		Date	Date	Date	Date	Date	Date
A. States name and purpose of procedure							
B. Preparation:							
1. Identifies student's ability to participate in procedure							
2. Reviews universal precautions							
3. Identifies where procedure is done							
4. Identifies possible problems and appropriate actions							
C. Identifies Go-Bag supplies (see p. 355), including:							
1. Suction supplies and machine							
2. Emergency phone number list							
3. Spare tracheostomy tube with ties or holder attached and obturator							
4. Blunt scissors							
5. Gloves							
6. Gauze or sponges							
7. Oxygen, if prescribed							
8. Manual resuscitator bag							
D. Procedure:							
1. Describes recognition of problems:							
a. Seeing student "breathe in" food, liquid, or vomit							
b. Seeing signs of aspiration (e.g., coughing, choking, turning blue)							
2. Preparation and prevention:							
a. Keeps suction catheters and saline with student at all times							
b. Uses caution when feeding and suctions before feeding, if ordered							
c. Turns student's head to side and is sure tracheostomy tube opening is covered if vomiting occurs							
d. Posts emergency numbers							
e. Knows cardiopulmonary resuscitation							
3. Action:							
a. Puts on gloves, suctions immediately— does not give breaths with resuscitation bag							
b. Gives breaths with bag after initial suctioning							

(continued)

Format adapted from Children's Hospital Chronic Illness Program, Ventilator Assisted Care Program. (1987). *Getting it started and keeping it going: A guide for respiratory home care of the ventilator assisted individual.* New Orleans, LA: Author; adapted by permission.

Children and Youth Assisted by Medical Technology in Educational Settings (2nd ed.) © 1997 Paul H. Brookes Publishing Co., Baltimore.

Student's name: _____

Explanation/Return Demonstration	Expl./ Demo. Date	Explanation/Return Demonstration					
		Date	Date	Date	Date	Date	Date
c. Checks air movement							
d. Adds saline and gives breaths with resuscitation bag, repeats suctioning, and repeats Steps c and d until aspirated secretions are clear or gone							
e. If tracheostomy tube remains blocked by foreign material, changes tracheostomy tube							
f. Checks air movement							
g. Gives breaths with resuscitation bag if indicated							
h. Gives oxygen if prescribed							
i. If respiratory distress continues, initiates emergency plan and begins CPR, if needed							

Checklist content approved by:

Parent/Guardian signature _____ Date _____

Student's name: _____

Person trained: _____

Position: _____

Suctioning—Nose and Mouth
Skills Checklist

Instructor: _____

Explanation/Return Demonstration	Expl./ Demo. Date	Explanation/Return Demonstration					
		Date	Date	Date	Date	Date	Date
A. States name and purpose of procedure							
B. Preparation:							
1. Identifies student's ability to participate in procedure							
2. Reviews universal precautions							
3. Identifies where procedure is done							
4. Identifies possible problems and appropriate actions							
C. Identifies supplies:							
1. Suction machine with tubing							
2. Catheter							
3. Cup of tap water or saline							
4. Bulb syringe							
5. Gloves							
6. Plastic bag for disposal							
D. Procedure:							
1. Washes hands							
2. Assembles supplies							
3. Positions student and explains procedure							
4. Washes hands							
5. Turns on suction machine and checks functions							
6. Removes catheter from storage bag being careful not to touch the last 5 inches of catheter, puts on gloves							
7. Attaches catheter to suction tubing							
8. Inserts catheter into nose and advances until student coughs without suction (If resistance occurs, do not proceed with catheter. Nasal area bleeds easily.)							
9. Applies suction when student coughs and withdraws catheter while twirling catheter							
10. Puts a few drops of normal saline into nose to thin secretions (if they are thick)							
11. Repeats suctioning in this order (Steps 8–10) until nose is clear							
12. Suctions mouth by advancing catheter into mouth without suction							
13. Applies suction and withdraws catheter while twirling							

(continued)

Format adapted from Children's Hospital Chronic Illness Program, Ventilator Assisted Care Program. (1987). *Getting it started and keeping it going: A guide for respiratory home care of the ventilator assisted individual*. New Orleans, LA: Author; adapted by permission.

Children and Youth Assisted by Medical Technology in Educational Settings (2nd ed.) © 1997 Paul H. Brookes Publishing Co., Baltimore.

Student's name: _____

Explanation/Return Demonstration	Expl./ Demo. Date	Explanation/Return Demonstration					
		Date	Date	Date	Date	Date	Date
14. Repeats suctioning in above order (Steps 12–13) until mouth is clear							
15. Does not suction nose again after suctioning mouth; disposes of catheter							
16. Rinses tubing with tap water							
17. Removes gloves and washes hands							
18. Documents procedure and observations							
19. Reports any changes to family							

Checklist content approved by:

Parent/Guardian signature _____   Date _____

Student's name: _____

Person trained: _____

Position: _____

Suctioning—Nose and Mouth with Bulb Syringe
Skills Checklist

Instructor: _____

Explanation/Return Demonstration	Expl./ Demo. Date	Explanation/Return Demonstration					
		Date	Date	Date	Date	Date	Date
A. States name and purpose of procedure							
B. Preparation:							
1. Identifies student's ability to participate in procedure							
2. Reviews universal precautions							
3. Identifies where procedure is done							
4. Identifies possible problems and appropriate actions							
C. Identifies supplies:							
1. Bulb syringe							
2. Saline							
3. Tissues							
4. Gloves							
D. Procedure:							
1. Washes hands							
2. Assembles supplies							
3. Positions student and explains procedure							
4. Washes hands and puts on gloves							
5. Squeezes bulb syringe, places tip gently in nose or mouth, and releases (Always suction nose before mouth.)							
6. Remove bulb syringe from nose or mouth							
7. Squeezes and releases bulb into tissue, expelling secretions (repeats Steps 5–7 until secretions are removed)							
8. Cleans bulb syringes, disposes of tissues							
9. Removes gloves and washes hands							
10. Documents procedure and observations							
11. Reports any changes to family							

Checklist content approved by:

Parent/Guardian signature _____ Date _____

Format adapted from Children's Hospital Chronic Illness Program, Ventilator Assisted Care Program. (1987). *Getting it started and keeping it going: A guide for respiratory home care of the ventilator assisted individual.* New Orleans, LA: Author; adapted by permission.

Children and Youth Assisted by Medical Technology in Educational Settings (2nd ed.) © 1997 Paul H. Brookes Publishing Co., Baltimore.

Student's name: _____

Person trained: _____

Position: _____

Nebulizer Treatment

Skills Checklist

Instructor: _____

Explanation/Return Demonstration	Expl./ Demo. Date	Explanation/Return Demonstration					
		Date	Date	Date	Date	Date	Date
A. States name and purpose of procedure							
B. Preparation:							
1. Identifies student's ability to participate in procedure							
2. Reviews universal precautions							
3. Identifies where procedure is to be done							
4. Identifies possible problems and appropriate actions							
C. Identifies supplies:							
1. Compressor (or gas cylinder)							
2. Connecting tubing							
3. Nebulizer unit							
4. Mask or T-adaptor and mouthpiece							
5. Medication							
6. Diluent solution							
7. Syringe							
8. Outlet							
9. Inlet							
10. Power switch							
11. Filter disc/exhalation filter, if indicated							
D. Procedure:							
1. Washes hands							
2. Assembles supplies							
3. Positions student and explains procedure							
4. Attaches end of nebulizer tubing to compressor air outlet							
5. Unscrews top from nebulizer cup							
6. Measures medications accurately, draws up medication in syringe or graduated dropper, and injects medication into nebulizer cup							
7. Adds prescribed amount of diluent to nebulizer cup							
8. Reattaches nebulizer cup							
9. Attaches connecting tubing to nebulizer cup							
10. Assesses student:							
a. Takes pulse before starting treatment							
b. Checks respiratory rate and effort							
11. Turns on power switch							

(continued)

Format adapted from Children's Hospital Chronic Illness Program, Ventilator Assisted Care Program. (1987). *Getting it started and keeping it going: A guide for respiratory home care of the ventilator assisted individual.* New Orleans, LA: Author; adapted by permission.

Children and Youth Assisted by Medical Technology in Educational Settings (2nd ed.) © 1997 Paul H. Brookes Publishing Co., Baltimore.

Student's name: _____

Explanation/Return Demonstration	Expl./ Demo. Date	Explanation/Return Demonstration					
		Date	Date	Date	Date	Date	Date
12. Checks mist production and starts treatment and assesses student after 5 minutes							
13. Places mouthpiece in mouth or mask over face/tracheostomy							
14. Allows medication to aerosolize before ending treatment							
15. Asks student to cough and suctions if needed							
16. At end of treatment turns off power switch							
17. Assesses student's status after treatment							
18. Describes proper cleaning method for equipment and stores properly							
19. States frequency for replacement of equipment and supplies							
20. States steps for replacing filter							
21. Washes hands							
22. Documents treatment							
23. Reports any changes to family							

Checklist content approved by:

Parent/Guardian signature _____ Date _____

Children and Youth Assisted by Medical Technology in Educational Settings (2nd ed.) © 1997 Paul H. Brookes Publishing Co., Baltimore.

Student's name: _____

Person trained: _____

Position: _____

Ventilator Machine and Circuit

Skills Checklist

Instructor: _____

Explanation/Return Demonstration	Expl./ Demo. Date	Explanation/Return Demonstration					
		Date	Date	Date	Date	Date	Date
A. States name and purpose of procedure							
B. Describes machine components and settings: 1. Power source							
a. Internal battery							
b. External battery							
c. Accessible, functioning electrical outlets							
d. Back-up battery							
e. Emergency power supply							
2. Oxygen source (if needed)							
a. Connection to ventilator and spare tubing							
b. Oxygen supply, spare tank, and gauge							
c. Flow (LPM) and percentage of oxygen							
3. Humidification source:							
a. Passive condensor							
4. Volume							
5. Rate							
6. Patient pressure manometer							
7. Peak inspiratory pressure (PIP)							
8. Positive end expiratory pressure (PEEP)							
9. Ventilator mode							
10. Inspiratory time							
11. High-pressure alarm							
12. Low-pressure alarm							
13. Power source alarm							
C. Describes circuit components: 1. Patient pressure tubing							
2. Patient port							
3. Exhalation valve							
4. PEEP valve							
5. Additional adaptors							
D. Go-Bag supplies (see p. 355), including: 1. Manual resuscitation bag with adaptor or mask							

(continued)

Format adapted from Children's Hospital Chronic Illness Program, Ventilator Assisted Care Program. (1987). _Getting it started and keeping it going: A guide for respiratory home care of the ventilator assisted individual._ New Orleans, LA: Author; adapted by permission.

Children and Youth Assisted by Medical Technology in Educational Settings (2nd ed.) © 1997 Paul H. Brookes Publishing Co., Baltimore.

Student's name: _____

Explanation/Return Demonstration	Expl./ Demo. Date	Explanation/Return Demonstration					
		Date	Date	Date	Date	Date	Date
2. Spare tracheostomy tube and supplies							
3. Suctioning supplies							

Checklist content approved by:

Parent/Guardian signature _____ Date _____

Student's name: _____

Person trained: _____

Position: _____

Ventilator Troubleshooting Alarms
Skills Checklist

Instructor: _____

Explanation/Return Demonstration	Expl./ Demo. Date	Explanation/Return Demonstration					
		Date	Date	Date	Date	Date	Date
A. States name and purpose of procedure							
B. Steps:							
1. Identifies which alarm is sounding							
2. Checks student first if *low-pressure* alarm sounds							
3. Removes student from ventilator and gives breaths with resuscitator bag							
4. Checks for leaks, if student is fine:							
a. Student disconnected							
b. Disconnected tubing							
c. Kinked tubing							
d. Punctured tubing							
e. Water in exhalation valve							
f. Hole in exhalation valve							
g. Loose-fitting heater humidification source							
h. Check ventilator settings							
5. Tests system after leak is found (Occlude student end of circuit and wait for high-pressure alarm to sound.)							
6. Places student back on ventilator							
7. Checks student first if a *high-pressure* alarm sounds							
8. Checks activity of student:							
a. Needs suctions							
b. Blocked tracheostomy tube							
c. Coughing							
d. Sneezing							
e. Talking							
f. Laughing							
g. Crying							
h. Hiccups							
i. Body position							
j. Holding breath							
9. Suctions, if needed							
10. Realigns or changes tracheostomy tube, if needed							
11. Removes student from ventilator and gives breaths with resuscitator bag							

(continued)

Format adapted from Children's Hospital Chronic Illness Program, Ventilator Assisted Care Program. (1987). *Getting it started and keeping it going: A guide for respiratory home care of the ventilator assisted individual*. New Orleans, LA: Author; adapted by permission.

Children and Youth Assisted by Medical Technology in Educational Settings (2nd ed.) © 1997 Paul H. Brookes Publishing Co., Baltimore.

Student's name: _____

Ventilator Troubleshooting Alarms
Skills Checklist

Explanation/Return Demonstration	Expl./ Demo. Date	Explanation/Return Demonstration					
		Date	Date	Date	Date	Date	Date
12. Checks ventilator for obstructions, if student is okay:							
a. Kinks in tubing							
b. Water in tubing							
c. Blocked exhalation valve							
d. Accidental change in ventilator settings							
13. Places student back on ventilator once problem is solved after checking high-pressure circuit							
14. Checks the following if *power source* alarm is on:							
a. AC power							
b. Internal battery							
c. External battery							
15. Removes student from ventilator if all three systems fail and *gives breaths with resuscitator bag*							
16. If bagging is required for longer than 15 minutes, adds drops of saline for humidity or puts passive condensor on resuscitation bag and continues to bag; follows emergency plan							

Checklist content approved by:

Parent/Guardian signature _____ Date _____

GLOSSARY

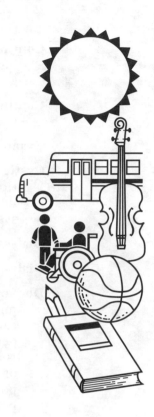

Abdominal distension   The abdomen becomes enlarged or appears stretched out.

Acquired immunodeficiency syndrome (AIDS)   A blood-borne disease representing the final phase of human immunodeficiency virus (HIV) infection.

Americans with Disabilities Act (ADA) of 1990 (PL 101-336)   A law passed in 1990 to supplement civil rights legislation enacted under the Rehabilitation Act of 1973 (PL 93-112), the ADA prohibits discrimination against people with disabilities. This act applies to all employers, including state and local governments, with 25 or more employees after July 26, 1992, and all employers with 15 or more employees after July 26, 1994. This law applies to both adults and children. Places such as hotels, auditoriums, grocery stores, retail stores, public transportation terminals, zoos, museums, parks, schools, and child care centers are just some of the businesses/services covered under the law.

Arteriovenous fistula   An artery and a vein are surgically joined so that arterial blood flows through the vein.

Aspiration   The accidental inhalation of any substance into the windpipe and/or lungs.

Body fluids   Cerebrospinal, synovial, vaginal, semen, pericardial, pleural, peritoneal, or amniotic fluids (e.g., saliva, urine, blood).

Bolus feeding   A specific amount of feeding given at one time (20–30 minutes).

Bronchopulmonary dysplasia   A chronic lung disease often caused by high oxygen concentrations, use of positive pressure ventilation, fluid overload, and prolonged use of these treatments.

Bronchospasm   A spasm of the airways leading into the lungs.

Bruit   Vibration or buzzing sound associated with blood flow.

Case manager/service coordinator   A person who works with a family to plan for services and who communicates with many service providers. A case manager/service coordinator could be a social worker, a nurse, an insurance representative, or a professional from a home care company. A case manager/service coordinator tries to oversee and bring together the many aspects of care needed by the student.

Central venous catheter   A long-term intravenous catheter that is inserted surgically into a deep, large vein in the neck or chest, usually near the heart.

Clean intermittent catheterization A procedure used to empty the bladder using a catheter to drain urine.

Colostomy A surgically created opening in the large intestine.

Confidentiality A limitation on who may see a student's records. Generally, records and information will be shared only with people directly involved in the student's care (i.e., the health care team).

Continuous ambulatory peritoneal dialysis (CAPD) A solution called dialysate is instilled by gravity through a catheter into the abdominal space and drained out by gravity, at regular intervals.

Continuous cycling peritoneal dialysis (CCPD) A machine is set to instill and drain dialysate at timed intervals, usually over a 12-hour period.

Cyanosis Bluish color of mucus membranes and skin.

Cystic fibrosis A hereditary disease resulting from abnormalities in enzyme production in the pancreas, causing an increase in the mucus-producing glands. Cystic fibrosis affects several body systems, most frequently the lungs and gastrointestinal system.

Dialysate Commercially prepared dialysis solution.

Dialysis A therapy that uses a filter to get rid of body waste products and excess fluid.

Do-Not-Resuscitate (DNR) order A written physician order stating that cardiopulmonary resuscitation (CPR) should not be provided to a person in the event of a cardiac/respiratory arrest. A DNR order is written only after consultation with the person involved and/or his or her family or legal guardian. A DNR order may be considered for a person who is terminally ill and is imminently dying, whose illness or injury is irreversible and irreparable, or for whom continuous advanced life support would result in prolonged, unrelieved pain or discomfort with little or no potential for human experience.

Drainage Leakage of food, fluids, or medications that comes into contact with the skin.

Due process procedural safeguards An established complaint mechanism to be used when a student or family disagrees with an individualized education program. It always indicates that there is a way to disagree formally and to work through channels to resolve disagreements.

Dumping syndrome A condition causing too-rapid emptying of the stomach contents into the small intestine. The exact causes are unknown, but it may follow gastric surgery. Symptoms include nausea, sweating, weakness, vomiting, dizziness, and increased heart rate.

Early intervention Any services or programs, for children age 3 and under, created to improve the development of a child who has a disability or is considered at risk. These services are meant to help decrease or eliminate the disabilities or risks as the child grows older.

Education of the Handicapped Act Amendments of 1986 (PL 99-457) Amendments passed by Congress to address the needs of young children with disabilities. PL 99-457 consists of two parts: Title I, Part H, which addresses the child from birth through 2 years, 11 months; and Title II, the extension of special education services to children ages 3–5.

Title I (Part H) of PL 99-457 Section of the law that calls on states to coordinate early intervention services for infants and toddlers and to create a plan for how the services are to be implemented.

Title II of PL 99-457 Extension of the provisions of PL 94-142 to children ages 3–5. This part of the program is run by state departments of education. The educational services may be provided in small integrated groups, in separate programs, or through home-based services. Eligibility requirements for different services vary greatly from state to state.

Elemental formula A formula in which the protein, and sometimes the fats, are broken down into more easily digested parts. Students who have certain food allergies or difficulties with malabsorption may require this type of formula.

Emergency plan Documented plan that details how to intervene in a student health emergency or natural disaster.

Enteral Involves the intestine or digestive system.

Federal Motor Vehicle Safety Standard 213 (FMVSS 213) Applies to child restraint systems designed for children weighing less than 50 pounds.

Federal Motor Vehicle Safety Standard 222 (FMVSS 222) Establishes requirement for school bus seating equipment.

Gastric residual Digested foods or fluids remaining in the stomach.

Gastroesophageal reflux Backup of the stomach contents into the esophagus.

Gastrostomy Surgical opening into the stomach through the surface of the abdomen.

Gastrostomy skin-level indwelling feeding device A T-shape plastic device held in place by a mushroom-shape dome or fluid-filled balloon inside the stomach.

Gastrostomy tube A flexible rubber catheter held in place by a balloon or a widened flat "mushroom" at the tip of the tube inside the stomach.

Hemodialysis The removal of certain waste products by circulating the blood outside of the body through a filter called a dialyzer.

Heparin A medication that prevents blood from clotting.

Heparin lock Intravenous device used for short-term courses of intermittent medication or fluid.

Hepatitis B A virus that is transmitted through blood or body fluids causing a wide range of infections.

Human immunodeficiency virus (HIV) A virus that affects white blood cells (T cells). When enough T cells are destroyed, the body's immune system is unable to fight off infections.

Ileostomy A surgically created opening in the small intestine.

Inclusion A philosophy that reflects the following beliefs: 1) all students can learn; 2) all students have the right to be educated with their peers in age-appropriate, heterogeneous classrooms within their local schools; and 3) it is the responsibility of the school system to meet the diverse educational and psychological needs of all students.

Individualized education program (IEP) A special education service plan for a student's school program that is required for all students receiving special education services. The IEP outlines a student's long-term educational goals, short-term objectives, and any services/assistance the student needs to meet those goals and objectives.

Individualized family service plan (IFSP) A written document that states the details of the early intervention services plan.

Individualized health care plan (IHCP) A document that is based on the health assessment of the student. It outlines the special health care needs, goals, and strategies needed to maintain and/or improve student health and increase student participation in self-care activities.

Individuals with Disabilities Education Act (IDEA) of 1990 (PL 101-476)   A law based on the Education for All Handicapped Children Act of 1975 (PL 94-142). A student must be enrolled in special education in order to receive the services mandated by IDEA. Students with a wide range of disabilities may be eligible for special education and related services. These disabilities include speech impairment, severe vision and hearing problems, learning disabilities, mental retardation, emotional problems, physical disabilities, and other health impairments. There is state-to-state variation in the way in which a child qualifies for special education services, but in general, if a child has a disability that makes it hard for him or her to obtain education without extra services, he or she is eligible for an evaluation to determine what services need to be provided.

Inhaler   A hand-held, metered-dose unit that dispenses inhaled medication when compressed.

Intestinal pseudo-obstruction   Impaired intestinal motility producing episodes of gastrointestinal blockage.

Jejunostomy   A surgical opening into the jejunum.

Jejunostomy tube   A flexible rubber or latex catheter that is held in place on the abdominal wall with tape or is fed through the gastrostomy site through the intestine down to the jejunum and taped to the gastrostomy. The jejunostomy tube may be used to administer food or fluids directly into the jejunum.

Latex allergy   Sensitivity to latex manufactured from the sap from the *Hevea brasiliensis* tree. Some symptoms may include watery eyes, rash, wheezing, hives, and swelling; in severe cases, life-threatening anaphylactic shock may occur.

Least restrictive environment (LRE)   A child with special needs is educated to the extent possible with children who do not have special needs. The school program should still meet all of the student's education needs. Words such as *mainstreaming, integration,* and *inclusion* may be used by teachers, principals, or special education directors when making suggestions for a student's educational program and including a student in the least restrictive environment. It is important to establish what exactly is meant when those terms are used.

Manual resuscitator bag   A self-inflating bag used to deliver breaths manually.

Mechanical nebulizer   A device powered by either oxygen or compressed air that produces a stable aerosol of fluid particles.

Mechanical ventilator   A machine that can be used to provide respiratory support for a person who is unable to breathe independently or may be used to assist someone who is able to breathe but whose respiratory ability is inadequate.

Mediation   A process involving a mediator, a trained neutral person who hears the position of all parties. Mediation provides an opportunity for people to settle differences before a due process hearing begins.

Medicaid (Title XIX)   A joint state–federal health insurance program administered by the states' health department or public welfare department under the Health Care Financing Administration (HCFA). Medicaid makes payments for approved health services that hospitals, health agencies, and private practitioners provide to people who qualify for Medicaid. A person usually qualifies for Medicaid if his or her income is not more than the maximum welfare benefits, he or she has a disability and has limited assets, or he or she spent a certain percentage of his or her income and/or assets on medical expenses.

Medicaid waiver   Allows people who might not otherwise qualify for Medicaid, due to income and asset rules, to receive assistance. These waivers pay for services provided in the home for people who would otherwise need to receive their health care in the hospital or other institutional setting.

Medical services   Services provided by a licensed physician to determine a student's medically related disability that results in that student's need for special education and related services. These services are for diagnostic and evaluative purposes.

Myelodysplasia   The abnormal formation of the spinal cord.

Nasogastric tube   A rubber or plastic tube that passes through a nostril down into the throat and esophagus and into the stomach.

Nebulize   To convert a liquid to a fine spray.

Negative pressure ventilator   A machine that pulls air into the lungs by pulling a person's chest wall outward as the person lies in a vacuum chamber.

Neurogenic bladder   A condition in which the nerves from the spinal cord to the bladder are damaged; it prevents the bladder from emptying completely.

Nurse Practice Act   State regulations passed by the state legislature to address the power and authority for the regulation of nursing practice. The following items are addressed in a Nursing Practice Act: definition and scope of nursing practice, qualifications for advanced nursing specialists, accountability for nursing practice, and accountability for nursing tasks delegated and supervised by nurses.

Occupational Safety and Health Administration (OSHA)   A federal agency dealing with job safety and health programs.

Occupational therapy (OT)   Activities that concentrate on helping a student improve fine motor skills and perceptual abilities (e.g., bathing, feeding, directing a wheelchair, rolling a ball, finger painting) and on making adaptations to equipment.

Parenteral   Descriptive of an act that bypasses the intestine (e.g., fluids, feedings, or medicine given through a vein).

Patency   The state of being open.

Peritoneal dialysis   A procedure in which dialysis occurs using the abdominal lining as a filter for the waste products.

Peritoneal membrane   The lining of the abdomen and pelvic walls.

Personal protective equipment   The equipment used to reduce the risk of contact with blood or other potentially infectious materials, including disposable gloves, protective eyewear, masks, lab coats, cover gowns, and shoe covers.

Physical therapy (PT)   Activities or routines to help a student improve motor skills through exercise, whirlpool, and other methods.

Portable feeding pump   A machine used to deliver feeding at a prescribed rate.

Positive pressure ventilator   A machine that breathes for a person by pushing air or oxygen-rich gas into the lungs.

Raincoat   A portable type of negative pressure ventilator.

Related services   Transportation and such developmental, corrective, and other supportive services as are required to assist a student with a disability to benefit from special education and includes speech pathology and audiology; psychological services; physical and occupational therapy; recreation, including therapeutic recreation; early identification and assessment of disabilities in children; counseling services, including rehabilitation counseling; and medical services for diagnostic or evaluation purposes. The term also includes school health services, social work services in schools, and parent counseling and training.

Renal failure   An inability of a kidney to remove waste materials from the body, produce urine, and conserve important body chemicals.

Retractions   Pulling in of the chest muscles.

School health services   Services provided by a qualified school nurse or other qualified person, not limited to diagnosis or evaluation.

Section 504 of the Rehabilitation Act of 1973 (PL 93-112)   Federal legislation passed to protect the civil rights of people with disabilities. Its definition of handicapped is the basis for later statutes regarding rights and eligibility for services. It also prohibits discrimination against individuals solely on the basis of physical impairment in federally assisted or run programs, including any health or social program supported by federal dollars. The law is aimed also at schools, in an attempt to prevent them from excluding students with health impairments or from restricting an educational program for such students.

Short bowel syndrome   The large loss of small intestine resulting in malabsorption and malnutrition. The large intestine also may be affected.

Slow drip feeding   A feeding given slowly over a number of hours.

Speech therapy   Activities or routines to help a student improve communication skills.

State health department   A department of each state, often called the Department of Public Health, the staff of which educate the public about many health issues. They may have many health-related resources and, in some states, may have case managers/service coordinators available to help families organize a student's care.

Team meeting (educational)   Team members always include people from family and school and may include health care and community service staff. Meetings are held to plan goals, objectives, and services listed in the student's individualized education program.

Title V Programs   The state health department provides students with special health care needs programs.

Total parenteral nutrition   A highly concentrated intravenous nutrition.

Tracheostomy   A surgical opening into the neck into the trachea that allows air to go in and out of the lungs.

Tracheostomy tube   A metal or plastic tube inserted into the opening through a stoma into the trachea.

Ultrasonic nebulizer   A device with fluid in a chamber that is vibrated rapidly, causing the fluid to break down into small particles that are then carried by a flow of compressed air or oxygen to the person.

Universal precautions   Measures intended to prevent transmission of blood-borne and other infections and to decrease the risk of exposure for care providers and others.

Urostomy   A surgically created opening into any part of the urinary tract.

Venting   To open or provide an outlet.

Visiting Nurse Association (VNA)   An organization staffed by community nurses who come into the home for short periods of time. Visiting nurses do assessments and follow-up care and can help do certain nursing procedures. They also may provide home health care services.

Vocational training   Training to help prepare students to work in a particular job or occupation.

Index

Page numbers followed by a "t" indicate tables; those followed by an "f" indicate figures.

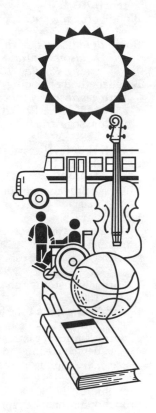

▶ ▶ ▶ ▶ ▶ ▶ ▶ ▶ ▶ *Ordering Information* ◀ ◀ ◀ ◀ ◀ ◀ ◀ ◀ ◀

To order additional copies of **Children and Youth Assisted by Medical Technology,**
photocopy this order form and send it to:

Brookes Publishing Co., Inc.
Department POF
P.O. Box 10624
Baltimore, Maryland 21285-0624

YES! Please send me _____ copy*(ies)* of
Children and Youth Assisted by Medical Technology

Stock #2363 • Price $52.00 each • Maryland orders add 5% sales tax

____ Bill my institution *(purchase order must be attached)*

____ Payment enclosed *(make checks payable to Brookes Publishing Co.)*
FREE shipping and handling on all orders prepaid by check

____ VISA   ____ MasterCard   ____ American Express

Credit card # _____ Expiration date _____

Signature _____

Daytime telephone _____

Name _____

Address _____

_____

City _____ State _____ ZIP _____-_____

Four convenient ways to order:

Mail to **Brookes Publishing Co.** • Post Office Box 10624 • Baltimore, Maryland 21285-0624
Call **1-800-638-3775** • Fax **1-410-337-8539** • E-mail **custserv@pbrookes.com**

Price may be higher outside the United States and are subject to change without notice.